Good Quality Practice (GQP) in Pharmaceutical Manufacturing: A Handbook

Authored By

Jordi Botet

Glez. Tablas 17
Barcelona
Spain

General:

1. Any dispute or claim arising out of or in connection with this License Agreement or the Work (including non-contractual disputes or claims) will be governed by and construed in accordance with the laws of the U.A.E. as applied in the Emirate of Dubai. Each party agrees that the courts of the Emirate of Dubai shall have exclusive jurisdiction to settle any dispute or claim arising out of or in connection with this License Agreement or the Work (including non-contractual disputes or claims).

2. Your rights under this License Agreement will automatically terminate without notice and without the need for a court order if at any point you breach any terms of this License Agreement. In no event will any delay or failure by Bentham Science Publishers in enforcing your compliance with this License Agreement constitute a waiver of any of its rights.

3. You acknowledge that you have read this License Agreement, and agree to be bound by its terms and conditions. To the extent that any other terms and conditions presented on any website of Bentham Science Publishers conflict with, or are inconsistent with, the terms and conditions set out in this License Agreement, you acknowledge that the terms and conditions set out in this License Agreement shall prevail.

Bentham Science Publishers Ltd.
Executive Suite Y - 2
PO Box 7917, Saif Zone
Sharjah, U.A.E.
subscriptions@benthamscience.org

BENTHAM SCIENCE PUBLISHERS LTD.

Dedication

This book is dedicated to the love and support of my parents, who unfortunately will not have the possibility of seeing it,

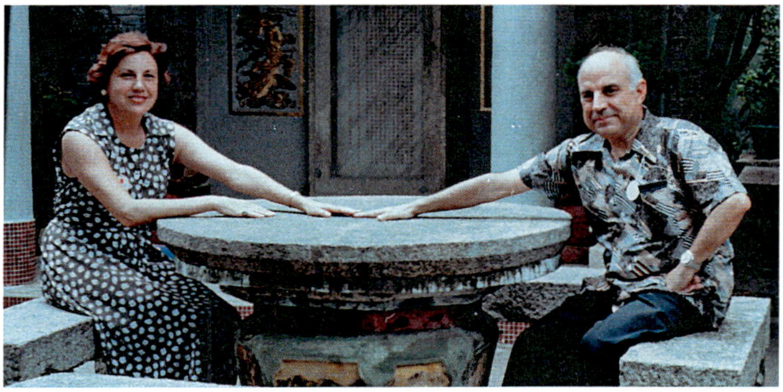

And to Pol on behalf of my whole family.

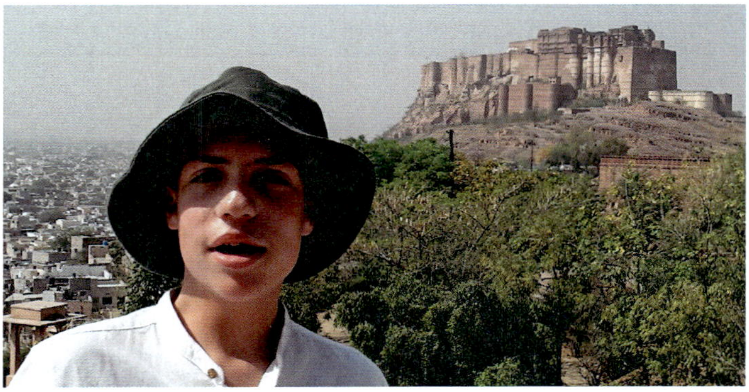

CONTENTS

FOREWORD

As a regulator, scientist, and expert in pharmaceutical quality, I am always searching for the best and most practical tools and reference material available in order to ensure pharmaceutical drug quality. A challenge lies in keeping up with technological advances and frequent updates to the information available. In today's world technical information is so easy to obtain with a few strokes of our fingertips. However, actually understanding and managing the information has become a global challenge. In this age of information overload, it is difficult to determine what of this vast information is actually required and how much understanding on the part of the pharmaceutical personnel is needed to be utilized in practice.

What regulators, consultants, and industry all need is a sensible book that describes GMP topics and international guidance in a simple manner, that both the layman and the expert could understand and put to practical use. Such a book would ultimately benefit the global quality culture.

This handbook responds to the needs previously articulated. It introduces the world of pharmaceuticals in a manner that a layman would understand, but that an expert would also appreciate. It describes GMP topics in a straightforward manner, providing clarity to frequently discussed topics related to pharmaceutical quality and follows international guidance requirements of "knowledge management," and "continual improvement."

I met the author in Estonia, at an International Pharmaceutical Quality Training Conference he was attending, where I was an instructor. From the questions he asked and comments he made it was evident he had extensive world-wide knowledge of Pharmaceutical GMPs. Whereas books in general may not be as popular as they used to be when I was obtaining my education, this handbook will be. It has a world-wide perspective and achieves its goal to provide a clear GMP understanding in Good Quality Practices in Pharmaceutical Manufacturing.

Diana Amador-Toro
Parsippany
New Jersey
USA

PREFACE

Because of my work as a GMP-consultant I often travel and this allows me to meet people from different countries all around the world. As a result I have come to understand how varied human cultures are but also, curiously enough, how the concerns of the technicians from the pharmaceutical industry are shared.

Thanks to modern technologies, the personnel of the pharmaceutical industry can easily obtain all the necessary information. GMP regulations and associated guidance documents are readily accessible and can be freely downloaded. Specialized literature and standards can be purchased on line and often downloaded too. This means that technical information is immediately available in almost anywhere in the world. In fact, getting informed has never been so easy…

Unfortunately there is a huge difference between having documents and being able to apply them in practice. This is why the personnel of the pharmaceutical industry are deeply worried. The amount of information is not only considerable but is also frequently updated. Coping with it is not a straightforward matter. It is complicated for the average technician to develop manufacturing activities and to spare enough time to read and "digest" the necessary documents. It is true that big companies have many resources and can reduce the importance of this problem, but small and medium-size firms are often extremely affected by it. According to my own practical experience, basic doubts are very common and to be able to obtain a global vision and an integrated approach of all the elements composing GMP is far from being widespread.

This book provides an answer to this common worldwide problem. It exposes GMP topics as simply as possible. They are described in an integrated way and as straightforward and as practical as possible. It responds openly to the "frequently asked questions" about hot topics such as the Pharmaceutical Quality System, qualification, process validation, cleaning validation, lifecycle, documentation, training, risk management, *etc.* Many tables and figures help in making the description of these subjects clear and logical.

The global aim is to provide a clear GMP understanding to serve both to face practical everyday manufacturing and to create a steady basis to acquire further knowledge. This follows the GMP requirements of "knowledge management" and of "continual improvement".

Jordi Botet
Barcelona
Spain
E-mail: jbotetfregola@gmail.com

2

CHAPTER 1

Introducing the Particular World of Pharmaceuticals

Abstract: Pharmaceuticals are specialized products because of their characteristics and use and also because of their meticulous regulation. A failure in the quality of a pharmaceutical can put life at risk. Consequently, a specialized manufacturing standard (GMP) is applied with the intention of ensuring quality. Although still different GMP texts exist, there is a steady effort towards their harmonization. GMP is not just practical pharmaceutical common sense, but also a guideline which determines the organization of a pharmaceutical plant. The aim of the pharmaceutical industry is not only manufacturing products with the purported quality, but also delivering them to the patients timely and without any loss of quality. This is why attention should be paid to the whole supply chain of pharmaceuticals and thus complementary standards (GSP, GDPs, and GTDP) have been developed. The globalization of the pharmaceutical market has not only supposed an increase in complexity of the supply chains, but also of contract manufacturing or analysis (outsourcing). Keeping under control such a complex and global market is not easy and this explains why counterfeiting has become a significant matter of concern.

Keywords: API, bulk, counterfeiting, dosage form, excipient, GDPs, GLP, GMP, GSP, GTDP, harmonization, intermediate, key personnel, MAH, outsourcing, packaging, quality assurance, quality control, route of administration, supply chain.

INTRODUCTION TO PHARMACEUTICALS

Since the dawn of civilization, humankind has tried to cure diseases or, at least, to alleviate their consequences by means of "remedies". Initially these were empirically chosen products derived from plants, animals or minerals. Later on, with the development of science, it became possible to know the root causes of illnesses and the composition of those products used to treat them. As substances, which were at the source of the activity of the traditional remedies were tracked down and their mechanisms of action were identified, it was possible to prepare specific products intended to treat diseases and injuries.

Nowadays, "remedies" are specialized products manufactured in purpose-build facilities and are known as "pharmaceutical products", "pharmaceuticals", "medicinal products", "medicines" or "drug products". In this book all these terms are freely used as synonymous.

Jordi Botet

An introduction to pharmaceutical products has to deal with their three basic aspects: what they are in fact (definition), how they are used (routes of administration) and how they look like (dosage forms).

Definition

Currently a pharmaceutical can be defined as *any substance or combination of substances presented for treating or preventing disease in human beings or animals. Any substance or combination of substances which may be administered to human beings or animals with a view to making a medical diagnosis or to restoring, correcting or modifying physiological functions in human beings or in animals is likewise considered a medicinal product* [1].

Or *as a finished dosage form that contains an active drug ingredient generally, but not necessarily, in association with inactive ingredients. The term also includes a finished dosage form that does not contain an active ingredient but is intended to be used as a placebo* [2].

These definitions demonstrate that the scope of contemporary pharmaceuticals is wider than that of the older remedies (Table **1**).

Table 1. From the primitive "remedy" to the modern "pharmaceutical".

Aspect	(Primitive) "Remedy"	(Modern) "Medicine"
Purpose	- Cure - Relieve	- Treat - Relieve - Prevent - Diagnose - Restore, correct or modify physiological functions - Use as a placebo
Composition	Unknown (natural product)	Known (formula/biological entity)
Action principle	Unknown (empirical)	Known (active entity/active principle)
Mode of action	Unknown (empirical)	Known (pharmacology/biology)
Presentation	Variable (empirical)	Dosage form based on pharmacology
Preparation	Artisanal	Technological

Route of Administration

Excepting the particular case of placebos, modern drug products are built on an active substance or, in some cases, several substances, known as APIs ("active pharmaceutical ingredients"), which have to reach quantitatively and timely their point of action in (or on) the body to produce the intended effect. Access into the body is controlled and limited by physical and chemical barriers. The routes of administration, *e.g.* the ways through which medicinal products reach the parts of the body where they have an effect, can fall into three groups:

The first one takes advantage of the existence of natural openings (mouth, nose eyes, ears, urethra, rectum and vagina). Of these, the oral route is the most common. About seventy per cent of the medicinal products use it. Despite the fact that taking a product by mouth is very easy, it is less practical than it might seem, because swallowed substances endure the combined action of the stomach low pH and of the digestive enzymes and are metabolized by the liver. The other routes are, generally speaking, mainly limited to medicines possessing a local action.

The second obvious alternative would be getting absorbed through the skin, but this is a natural barrier, which seriously restricts absorption. This is why it is also chiefly limited to medicines possessing a local action.

The third and last alternative is to overcome all barriers by injecting the product directly into a part of the body. This is a "traumatic" route as it does not use a natural path but pierces teguments. The drug product can reach the point of action without any metabolic transformation, but this route involves a particularly high risk of infection.

Draw a practical classification of the routes of administration is difficult because they are defined by different criteria at the same time, but Table **2** provides a tentative one.

Table 2. Tentative classification of pharmaceutical routes of administration.

Type of route		Designation	Description
(I) Through body openings	mouth	**oral/enteric**	drug is swallowed and reaches the gastrointestinal tract (*e.g.* tablet or syrup)
		sublabial	between cheek and tongue (*e.g.* tablet)
		sublingual	under the tongue (*e.g.* tablet)
		topical	applied on the mouth mucosa (*e.g.* aphtha lotion)
		inhalational	gaseous form reaching the respiratory system (*e.g.* spray)
	nose	**topical**	introduced into the nose cavity (*e.g.* solution, ointment)
	eye	**topical**	applied on the eye or eyelashes (*e.g.* solution, ointment)
	ear	**topical**	applied in the external ear cavity (*e.g.* solution, ointment)

Table 2: contd...

	urethra	**urethral**	given through the urethra (*e.g.* solution)
	rectum	**transmucosal**	introduced into the rectum (*e.g.* suppositories)
	vagina	**transmucosal**	introduced into the vagina (*e.g.* ovules, rings)
(II) Onto/through the skin		**topical**	applied on the skin for a local effect
		transdermal	applied on the skin for a systemic effect
(III) Parenteral*		**intramuscular**	into a muscle
		intradermal	into the skin
		subcutaneous	under the skin
		intravenous	into a vein
		epidural	into the epidural space
*As the product is injected into a given part of the body the number of possibilities is very large (intra-cerebral, intra-arterial, intra-cardiac, intra-articular, *etc.*). The above-mentioned parenteral routes are the commonest.			

Dosage Form

Active substances are administered in a specified dosage form, which provides a defined amount of drug product prepared for a selected route of administration.

The preparation of a dosage form supposes, usually, the addition to the active ingredient or ingredients (when there are several) of other substances devoid of physiological action on the organism and known globally as excipients. Thus, a drug is presented in a definite dosage form which has an exact composition or formula detailing the quantities of substances (APIs and excipients) intervening in it (Fig. **1**).

The dosage form put into an appropriate packaging and labeled is known as the finished pharmaceutical, which can enclose a single dose (monodose) or several, according to the posology. Thus, active principles are:

- Protected from the environmental conditions (temperature, humidity, light) and from contamination;
- Well identified (product, dosage, manufacturing batch and expiring date);
- Provided with the necessary information regarding their use (posology, precautions, dangers, *etc.*);

- Accompanied, as necessary, by the devices required for its delivery (*e.g.* measuring cups, syringes, pipes, *etc.*);

- Easily transported.

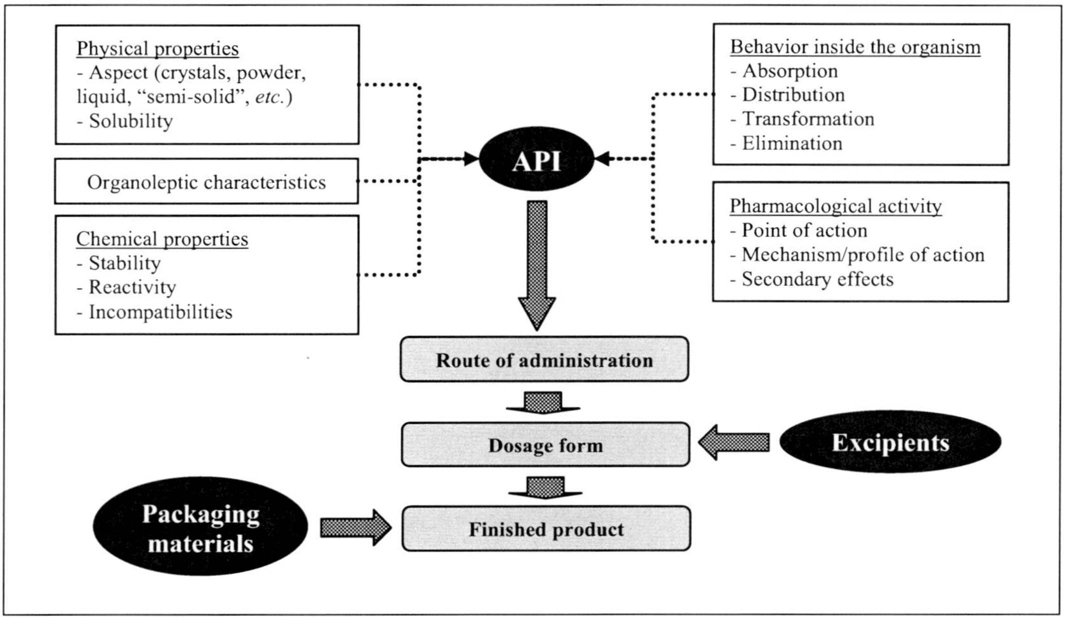

Fig. (1). The characteristics of the API determine the pharmaceutical product.

Dosage forms are quite varied [3]. In practice, however, just a few are commonly used and some are old forms which play limited role nowadays. A quick review of the most common dosage forms would distinguish the following:

- **Tablets:** Solid rounded/elliptical forms obtained by compression of the raw materials. Tablets are a very popular form because of the facility of dosage and preservation and because they are generally administered by the oral route. According to the particular needs there are different types of tablets (coated or enteric, effervescent, chewable).

- **Capsules**: Small containers of gelatin (hard or soft), of starch (amylaceous) or of a similar substance filled with the, usually solid, raw materials. As a dosage form they are considered similar to a tablet, where the solid materials instead of being pressed are packed in. The filling materials can be also coated or enteric.

- **Powders/granulates:** They are easy to prepare (simply a mixture of solid discrete pieces of the materials), but difficult to dose and to preserve, although these difficulties can be overcome by presenting them in single dose sachets. The materials can be also coated or enteric and effervescent. They are mainly used for drug products being administered by the oral route. There are, however, cases of injectable drugs, which API is unstable. Then, they are presented in a sterile container (as powders, granulates or lyophilized products), solved aseptically and immediately injected.

- **Chewable gums/Lozenges**: Solid forms where the API is liberated in the mouth in order to obtain a local action in the mouth or throat.

- **Spheres**: The API is wrapped within tiny polymeric spheres. This denomination comprehends, however, different cases. Microspheres (diameter in the range of micrometers) are often parenterally applied, suspended in liquid. Macroscopic spheres (diameter in the range of millimeters) are used in solid oral forms like tablets or capsules, to obtain specific liberation profiles.

- **Sticks**: The API is dispersed or solved in a base which melts to body temperature. Sticks are rubbed on the skin or mucosa for local absorption.

- **Transdermal devices**: A liquid or semi-solid preparation of the API is disposed in a reservoir externally covered with an impermeable support which is placed on the skin for a sustained release.

- **Solutions/suspensions/emulsions**: These liquid forms can be administered through different routes. In the solutions APIs are solved. In the suspensions, solid non soluble APIs are dispersed in liquids. In the emulsions liquid APIs are dispersed within liquids. Aqueous solutions with a content of at least a 45% w/w of sucrose are known as "syrups" and are taken orally. Solutions, suspensions and emulsions can be presented as "pressurized metered dose aerosols" ("sprays").

- **Ointments/creams/gels/pastes**: Ointments are semi-solid forms where solid or liquid APIs are dispersed on a base. Creams are preparations composed of two phases, lipophilic and hydrophilic. Gels are gelified liquids, either hydrophobic, or hydrophilic. Pastes are preparations where an important concentration of API powder is dispersed in a base.

- **Mousses**: They are dispersions of a gas in a liquid containing the API.
- **Cataplasms/Plaster**: The cataplasms contain a liquid or solid API dispersed in a hydrophilic base and they are applied on the skin. Plasters are constituted by adhesive masses spread on a solid support which contains the API.
- **Suppositories/ovules and slow release rings**: In them the API is dispersed or solved in a base which melts at body temperature. The firsts are administered by rectal route, whereas the seconds use the vaginal route.

Again the classification of dosage forms is not easy. The reasons are the same aforesaid (*i.e.* different intervening criteria at the same time). Table **3** intends to classify in a practical way the above mentioned dosage forms.

Table 3. Simplified table of the commonest dosage forms.

Physical aspect	Route of administration	Dosage forms
Solid forms	oral/enteric	tablet, powder, granulate, capsule, amylaceous capsule, chewable gum, lozenge
	parenteral	powder, micro-spheres, pellets
	topical/transdermal	powder, stick, transdermal device
Liquid forms	oral	solution, suspension, emulsion
	topical/transdermal	solution
	transmucosal	solution
	parenteral	solution, suspension, emulsion
	oral/nose/ear	solution, suspension
	ophthalmic	solution, suspension, emulsion
Semi-solid forms	topical/transdermal	ointment, cream, gel, paste, cataplasm, plaster, mousse
	transmucosal	ointment, cream, gel, paste, cataplasm, plaster, mousse, suppository, ovule, ring
	ophthalmic	ointment

In practical manufacturing terms and taking into account two criteria, physical form and sterility requirements, this array of pharmaceutical dosage forms can be grouped in four types:

- Non sterile solid forms;
- Sterile solid forms;
- Non sterile liquid and semi-solid forms;
- Sterile liquid and semi-solid forms.

QUALITY OF PHARMACEUTICALS

It is evident that any product is expected to possess the intended quality attributes. Every day we face lots of items and we judge them in terms of "quality". If they correspond to our expectations or meet our requirements, we say that they are "good", that they have "good quality" or, simply, that they possess "quality".

This can be applied to drug products as well. Thus, quality can be defined as *the suitability of either a drug substance or drug product for its intended use. This term includes such attributes as identity, strength, and purity* [4]. There is, however, an important practical difference, most of everyday products can be evaluated by their consumers and this creates a pressure on the manufacturer. Even if a producer deems them as possessing the required quality, consumers have the last word and if they don't like the product, they don't buy it. Differently enough and by evident reasons, pharmaceutical products can hardly be judged by their direct consumers. Evaluation is mainly performed by third parts like medical doctors or health authorities.

Hence, medicinal products, as any other product, have to possess the purported quality, but also because they are special products used to cure or relieve health problems if they do not meet the anticipated requirements they might even be harmful. This is why the quality of drug products is a social concern and they are submitted to a three-level control. Firstly, their quality is controlled by an elaborate system of sampling and testing against a background of specifications known as "quality control". Secondly, they have to be manufactured within a "quality assurance" system. And thirdly, they are subjected to a tight "regulatory frame" by competent national authorities.

Quality Control

Quality control (QC) *is the part of GMP concerned with sampling, specifications and testing, and with the organization and documentation which ensure that the necessary and relevant tests are actually carried out and that materials are not released for use, nor products released for sale or supply, until their quality has been judged to be compliant with the requirements. QC is not confined to laboratory operations, but may be involved in many decisions concerning the quality of the product* [5].

Any laboratory must have a QC function possessing an adequate laboratory (although it is possible to outsource some specialized analysis).

QC duties comprise not only sampling, inspecting and testing of materials and products, but also retention of samples and environmental and stability monitoring. All these tasks require a reliable QC laboratory. Ensuring appropriate laboratory performance in connection with its many elements (personnel, organization, documentation, reactives, standards, culture media, equipment, *etc.*) is a complex task. This is why, besides the general pharmaceutical quality guidelines which are described below, a specific standard known as "good laboratory practice" (GLP) has been developed [6]. See chapter 12.

Quality Assurance

Quality assurance (QA) *is a wide-ranging concept covering all matters that individually or collectively influence the quality of a product. It is the totality of arrangements made with the object of ensuring that pharmaceutical products are of the quality required for their intended use* [7]. Unfortunately, it is easier understanding the need of ensuring quality than finding a practical way for doing it. This is why along the way three different approaches have been used.

"Analyzed Quality"

Traditionally, following completion of a batch, samples of the finished product were taken and analyzed. If they met specifications the lot was considered correct and it was liberated for selling. It is true that starting and packaging materials were sampled and analyzed and that in-process controls were performed too, but the decision on the approval of a given lot of product relied, in principle, solely on the analysis of the final product. This approach known as "analyzed quality" has been in use until, roughly speaking, the middle of the 20th century, when its important flaws were acknowledged:

- Analysis is generally destructive. Thus, it is performed on a limited amount of units and the results are then extended to the whole batch. Even if the samples are taken using a statistically sound procedure, their analysis cannot ensure the quality of the batch when just a small part of it is contaminated or degraded.

- Analytical methods are limited in number and scope and thus an unknown contamination or degradation incident might pass undetected. Quality control analyses are basically performed to determine if a substance or product meets established requirements.

- If a finished product batch is out of specification, the possibility of reworking is far from being assured and this represents a severe economical loss.

"Built-in Quality"

As the above-mentioned problems were highlighted a new approach was deemed necessary. If we study a product in detail and we detect all the elements which determine its quality and we monitor them during the process of production, the product should possess the specified quality. Then, the analysis of the finished product would become, beside production monitoring, just one of the elements to be taken into account for the approval of the batch. This approach, used during the second half of the 20th century, was known as "built-in quality".

An important element of this approach was the introduction of "Good Manufacturing Practice for Pharmaceutical Products" (GMP), which is *the part of quality assurance which ensures that products are consistently produced and controlled to the quality standards appropriate to their intended use and as required by the marketing authorization.*

GMP incorporated an important element, "validation" which *is the action of proving, in accordance with the principles of GMP, that any procedure, process, equipment, material, activity or system actually leads to the expected results* [8].

If appropriate procedures regarding all the elements from which quality depends (processes, equipment, utilities and materials) were set-up and then validated, their subsequent reproduction should ensure quality.

Anyway, at the beginning of the 21st century, this second approach was showing some shortcomings too. Let us consider them briefly.

- A process was validated by performing a limited number of batches. The compliance of any posterior batch was based on them. Yes, if everything remained exactly as validated, the process might be considered in "state of validation". A change control system was put in place to handle any change produced after the validation and this involved revalidation if the state of validation was deemed lost, but what about small involuntary and unnoticed changes? The answer to this question was increased monitoring (trend study, quality reviews, *etc.*), but the full effectiveness of the system in place remained dubious.

- Even if the manufacturing process was validated, was it possible to ensure that the process itself was robust? If the parameters from which depends quality are not well known and scientifically sound, how can we rely on its validation? This, again, raised some doubts.

"Quality by Design"

This is why a new approach was devised. It was called "quality by design" and it took into account three elements:

1st quality must be built into the product, yes, but previously has to be designed;

2nd products and processes have to be scientifically based;

and

3rd risk management must be used.

In fact, the three approaches to quality assurance are complementary. Analysis remains a significant quality element. Quality has to be built into the processes, which have to be validated. Quality has to be designed. And all this has to be seen across the glass of science and risk analysis.

Regulation

Competent authorities authorize the drug products and inspect the pharmaceutical units where they are manufactured. The above mentioned GMP is used as the reference and regulatory standard since 1963 when it was introduced in the United States of America.

Although GMP meant basically "codified pharmaceutical common sense", notwithstanding this, it supposed a revolutionary step because it was made compulsory for all the manufacturers and because it was based on the assumption that if work is done carefully and methodically, controlling each step of a process, the probability of contamination, error or accident diminishes drastically. Thus, for instance, GMP states that critical operations have to be supervised by a second person.

In 1969 the World Health Organization (WHO) recommended that GMP be adopted by every country.

When GMP was introduced into pharmaceutical manufacturing it was a quite basic text [9] in comparison with its later development and present-day complexity (GMP is regularly updated to express the pharmaceutical state of the art).

Nowadays GMP is the world-wide pharmaceutical manufacturing standard, both for human and veterinary drug products. Its main principles are completed and enlightened by other documents (guides, guidelines, guidances, standards, handbooks, *etc.*), published by competent authorities or by national and international organizations. From all this information a pharmaceutical practice, accepted by health authorities and by the pharmaceutical industry, has been created. This book follows this practice.

Although in the pharmaceutical world GMP (Good Manufacturing Practice) or GMPs (Good Manufacturing Practices) are frequently used terms, it should be kept in mind that speaking in such a global way is not quite correct. Even if a large amount of harmonization has been reached, a unified and world-wide GMP text does not exist yet. As there are different GMP texts, accepted by a single country or group of countries, an implicit or explicit adjective should be applied to GMP (*e.g.,* WHO GMP, European GMP, *etc.*). Although GMP texts share common objectives and philosophy and rather similar contents, it is important to remember that national competent authorities perform inspections referring back to the nationally-adopted GMP text.

Let us then cast an eye on the present-day GMP panorama.

USA

American GMP is integrated in the code of federal regulations (CFR) which title 21 writes about food and drugs. The text on GMP is basically developed in parts 210 through 226 of this title. From these seventeen parts, two refer particularly to the manufacture of medicinal products,

- Part 210: Current good manufacturing practice in manufacturing, processing, packing, or holding of drugs; general.
- Part 211: Current good manufacturing practice for finished pharmaceuticals.

The regulations set forth in this part and in parts 211 through 226 of this chapter contain the minimum current good manufacturing practice for methods to be used in, and the facilities or controls to be used for, the manufacture, processing, packing, or holding of a drug to assure that such drug meets the requirements of the act as to safety, and has the identity and strength and meets the quality and purity characteristics that it purports or is represented to possess.

The failure to comply with any regulation set forth in this part and in parts 211 through 226 of this chapter in the manufacture, processing, packing, or holding of a drug shall render such drug to be adulterated. and such drug, as well as the person who is responsible for the failure to comply, shall be subject to regulatory action [10].

In the USA instead of GMP it is usually used CGMP, where C stands for "current".

CGMP is published in the United States of America by the Food and Drug Administration (FDA). Besides the CGMP basic principles exposed in CFR Title 21, FDA publishes specialized Guidelines/Guidances, which develop and describe them in detail [11].

In August 2002, the US FDA proclaimed a new initiative called "Pharmaceutical Current Good Manufacturing Practices (CGMPs) for the 21st Century", with the aim of intensifying and updating the regulations pertaining to pharmaceutical manufacturing and product quality. The founding principles of this initiative are:

- *Risk-based orientation;*
- *Science-based policies and standards;*
- *Integrated quality systems orientation;*
- *International cooperation;*
- *Strong public health protection* [12].

This initiative was adopted by the "International Conference on Harmonization of Technical Requirements for the Registration of Pharmaceuticals for Human Use" (ICH) as the "Quality new paradigm" (Brussels, 2003).

WHO

The first WHO text on GMP was drafted in 1967 and accepted in 1969. Since then these "WHO GMP main principles for pharmaceutical products" have been regularly modified and expanded. They have been supplemented with "WHO GMP on starting materials" (APIs and pharmaceutical excipients) and "WHO GMP on specific pharmaceutical products" (sterile pharmaceutical products, biological products, investigational pharmaceutical products for clinical trials, herbal medicines, *etc.*) and on related subjects (water for pharmaceutical use, guidelines on quality risk management, guidelines on good manufacturing practices for heating, ventilation and air-conditioning systems for non-sterile pharmaceutical dosage forms, *etc.*). All these texts on GMP are published as annexes to the "Technical Reports Series" (TRS) [13].

Europe

In 1991, the European Commission approved two Directives establishing the principles and the course of action of good manufacturing practice for medicinal products. The first one was devoted to products for human use (Directive 91/356/EEC substituted later on by Directive 2003/94/EC to include investigational medicinal products), whereas the second dealt with the veterinary medicinal products (Directive 91/412/EEC).

This common European GMP has been regularly revised and expanded. Therefore at the present time it is composed of two general parts plus specialized annexes. Part I develops the basic requirements for the manufacture of medicinal products in nine chapters ("quality management, personnel, premises and equipment, documentation, production, quality control, contract manufacture and analysis, complaints and product recall and self inspection"). Part II establishes the requirements for the manufacture of APIs. Annexes are devoted to specific manufacturing activities (sterile medicinal products; radiopharmaceuticals; herbal medicinal products; liquids, creams and ointments; *etc.*) [14].

Other GMP

Although some other countries have their own GMP texts (*e.g.,* Japan or Brazil) the three above-mentioned GMP texts (USA, WHO and Europe) have world-wide influence and are generally used as a reference. When working in a particular country it is necessary to ascertain which the competent authorities approach to GMP is.

GMP Harmonization

In stark contrast to the above-described GMP diversity there is a world-wide integrated pharmaceutical market, where materials and pharmaceuticals move around almost unrestrictedly. This curious contradiction has to be faced both by national regulatory authorities and by pharmaceutical manufacturers.

The previously mentioned ICH supposes a very important step towards harmonization. It was created by 6 parts representing the regulatory authorities and the pharmaceutical industry with investigational base of the USA, Japan and Europe. Later, other parts without vote have been admitted (*e.g.* WHO, Canada, *etc.*) [15].

ICH issues "harmonized guidelines" on different subjects, from which those of the series Q (from "quality") are directly related to GMP.

Harmonization scored a very important success in 2000 when a guideline on GMP for APIs [16] was accepted by the USA, Japan and Europe as their own GMP text. It became the first true international text on GMP. Since then ICH has released guidelines on pharmaceutical development, risk analysis, pharmaceutical quality system and API development. These guidelines are very important because open new ways in the application and interpretation of GMP. In 2010 it was created the "ICH Quality – Implementation Working Group" (ICH Q-IWG) with the aim of proving guidance on the joint application of quality guidelines in the frame of a new paradigm of pharmaceutical quality, which corresponds to the previously discussed "quality by design" approach.

Another important organization is the "Pharmaceutical Inspection Cooperation Scheme" (PIC/S), which, as its name suggests, fosters the harmonization of the inspectors and of their inspections in the member countries. The PIC/S has many members; among them the same three that constitute the kernel of ICH. They publish many interesting documents which clarify different GMP subjects. It is worth to point out that PIC/S has published a GMP text that is practically the same that European GMP [17].

Pharmaceutical manufacturers react to the described GMP panorama in three ways:

- Firstly, they are obliged to respect faithfully the GMP standard adopted by the national competent authorities.
- Secondly, they can benefit from the already existing harmonized documents published by ICH and PIC/S.
- Thirdly, they can create their own "GMP harmonized standard" composed by a medley of GMP and internal company requirements. It is evident that a given inspector will require compliance on the national GMP standard, but if the company shows an even higher standard (*e.g.,* aligned with the strictest GMP text) there will be no problem. For an international company such a standard can be applied world-wide and facilitates compliance, independently of country.

MANUFACTURE OF PHARMACEUTICALS

Medicinal products, whether they are produced in large quantities in specialized pharmaceutical plants or in restricted amounts in small laboratories of hospitals or pharmacies, follow a similar pattern of preparation [18].

It is worth mentioning here that although often production and manufacture are used as synonymous, this is not quite right. In fact, "production" is the activity of preparing finished pharmaceuticals from starting and packaging materials. Thus, production includes the operations of receipt of materials, their processing and the activities of packaging and labeling. Whereas, "manufacture" is a wider activity which besides production embraces the purchase of starting and packaging materials, the storage and distribution of the drug products and all the related quality control and assurance activities [19].

Manufacturing Steps

A medicinal product has an approved formula for the dosage form, but as it is usually prepared in batches or lots, that is to say, *in a defined quantity of starting material, packaging material or product processed in a single process or series of processes so that it is expected to be homogenous* [20], it is necessary to define how many units (forms) will compose a batch and then calculate the batch formula.

As said before, components either active (APIs) or inactive (excipients) both contribute to the building of the dosage form, but in addition to this there are sometimes components which are added because they are needed in the manufacturing process, but which disappear and are not to be found in the finished dosage form (reagents, solvents, process aids). A typical example of these can be alcohol, which is used in a granulation process, but which evaporates during the drying.

The first operation in the manufacturing process is the purchase of the "starting materials" *(any substance of a defined quality used in the production of a pharmaceutical product, but excluding packaging materials* [21]) or "components" *(any ingredient intended for use in the manufacture of a drug product, including those that may not appear in such drug product)* [22]. These materials or components can be either active or inactive. See Fig. (**2**).

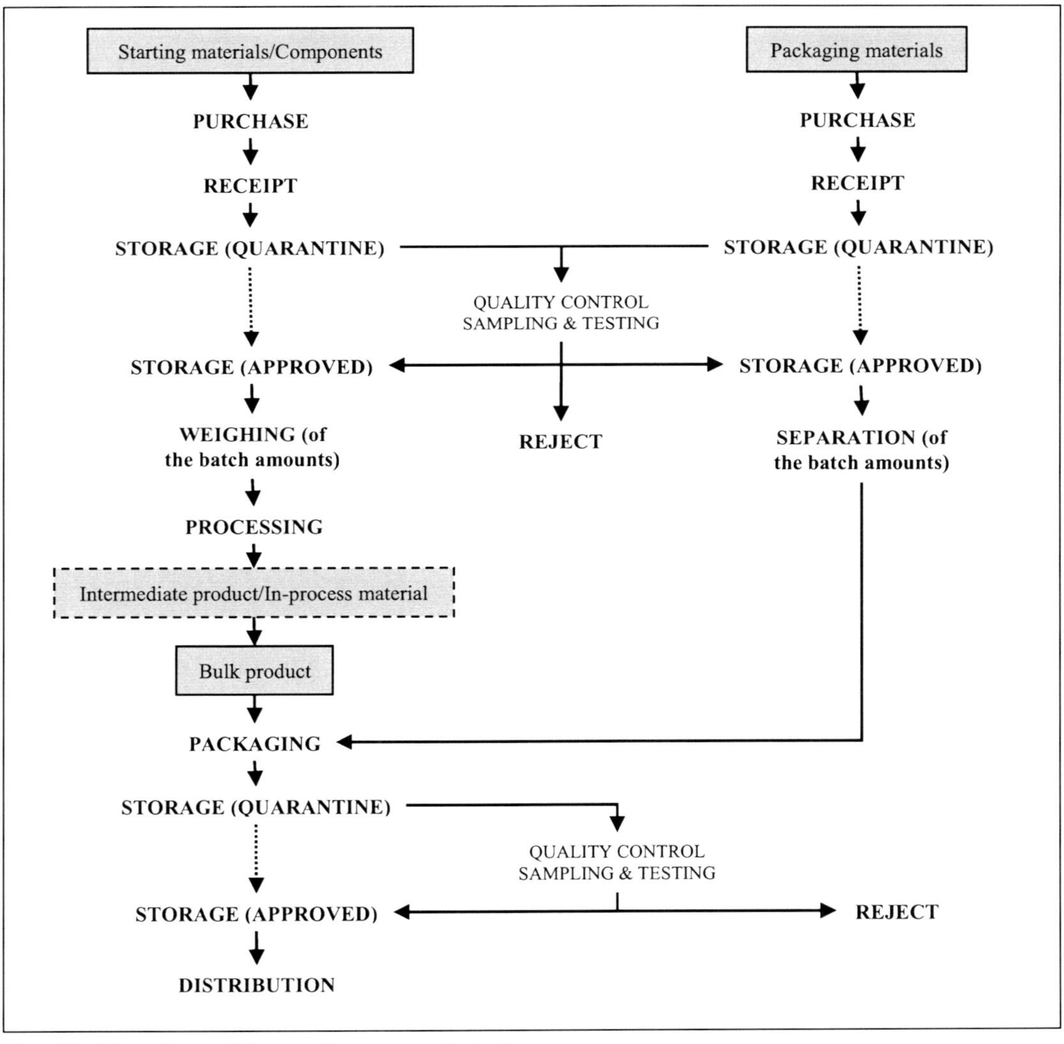

Fig. (2). Flowchart of dosage form manufacturing.

Active ingredient means any component that is intended to furnish pharmacological activity or other direct effect in the diagnosis, cure, mitigation, treatment, or prevention of disease, or to affect the structure or any function of the body of man or other animals. The term includes those components that may undergo chemical change in the manufacture of the drug product and be present in the drug product in a modified form intended to furnish the specified activity or effect. Inactive ingredient means any component other than an active ingredient [23].

Besides starting materials are also purchased packaging materials, which are *any material, including printed material, employed in the packaging of a pharmaceutical, but excluding any outer packaging used for transportation or shipment. Packaging materials are referred to as primary or secondary according to whether or not they are intended to be in direct contact with the product* [24].

Purchased materials are received and examined to confirm that they correspond to the purchase invoice and that they arrive in good state. If they are accepted they are stored in the warehouse in quarantine. Quality control takes samples from them and performs the necessary tests to determine if the materials meet their specifications. If they pass these tests they are released for use in production and are stored out of quarantine, as accepted materials. If they fail they are rejected and transferred to the warehouse area for rejected materials and products pending to be returned to the supplier or to be destroyed in a controlled manner.

When a batch of product has to be prepared the components are weighed and then submitted to the required processes to obtain the "bulk product", that is to say *a product that has completed all processing stages up to, but not including, final packaging* [25]. Sometimes the preparation of the dosage form requires obtaining an "in-process material" defined as *any material fabricated, compounded, blended, or derived by chemical reaction that is produced for, and used in, the preparation of the drug product* [26] or "intermediate product", that is to say, *a partly processed product that must undergo further manufacturing steps before it becomes a bulk product, a product that has completed all processing stages up to, but not including, final packaging* [27]. The existence or not of an intermediate product is dictated by technological or quality reasons (*e.g.*, granulates waiting to be pressed or mixtures being analyzed to confirm that they meet requirements).

All operations, including filling and labeling, that a bulk product has to undergo in order to become a finished product are known collectively as "packaging". Filling of a sterile product under aseptic conditions or a product intended to be terminally sterilized, would not normally be regarded as part of packaging [28].

Only after packaging a medicinal product can be considered a "finished product", that is to say, *a finished dosage form that has undergone all stages of manufacture, including packaging in its final container and labeling* [29].

When a bulk product has to be packaged, the necessary packaging materials are prepared in the warehouse and sent to the packaging area.

Once the packaging of the batch is completed, the finished product is sent to the warehouse, where it is stored under quarantine. Performing a process similar to the one described previously for the starting materials, the finished product is tested by quality control and the batch manufacturing record is studied by quality assurance. Then, the batch is declared either approved or rejected. Exactly as described before, the approved product is stored as such and the rejected product is transferred to the area for rejects.

The approved products can be distributed when receiving requests. Each request starts a consignment (or delivery), defined as *the quantity of a pharmaceutical or pharmaceuticals, made by one manufacturer and supplied at one time in response to a particular request or order. A consignment may comprise one or more packages or containers and may include material belonging to more than one batch* [30].

Distributed pharmaceutical products can be returned, that is to say, *sent back to the manufacturer or distributor of a medicinal product which may or may not present a quality defect* [31]. In this case, returns should be stored in a specific separated area while they are investigated to determine if they present a quality defect and, consequently, their final handling.

Manufacturing Responsibilities

The number of persons in a pharmaceutical manufacturing unit and their organization in departments is very variable and is freely decided by the direction, with the following exceptions established by GMP [32, 33]:

- A "quality unit" should exist performing the tasks of quality control and quality assurance. This quality unit might also be divided into two separated units, "quality control unit" and "quality assurance unit".

- The following "key personnel" should exist: head of production, head of the quality unit (or heads of the quality units) and the authorized person [34].

- The head of production and the head/s of the quality unit/s should be independent of each other. The authorized person may be also responsible for one or for both quality units.

- Key personnel can delegate functions but not responsibilities.

This organization may appear somewhat confusing, but it is a consequence of history. When GMP was introduced in the 1960s the responsibility for the management of pharmaceutical manufacturing was considered divided between two poles: the head of production and the head of QC (quality control). Quality assurance was starting to be seen as an activity but not yet as a self-standing function. The authorized person (in some countries known as "technical director") was to represent the plant before the regulatory authorities and also assumed officially the responsibility of approving batches and liberating them for distribution. Thus, tasks and responsibilities from the GMP point of were to be shared among the aforementioned key personnel. As a matter of fact, as quality assurance became a full-fledged function and its head started to be in practice a member of key personnel, and also, as pharmaceutical plants grew in complexity, some other adjustments were necessary. Taking into account the technical complexity of a pharmaceutical plant, a head of engineering is very important. Considering the significance of environmental and safety issues, a head of HSE (health, safety and environment) came to be indispensable. It is true that in a big pharmaceutical plant we could even add more "key posts", but their intervention would be mainly outside the GMP sphere. See Fig. (**3**).

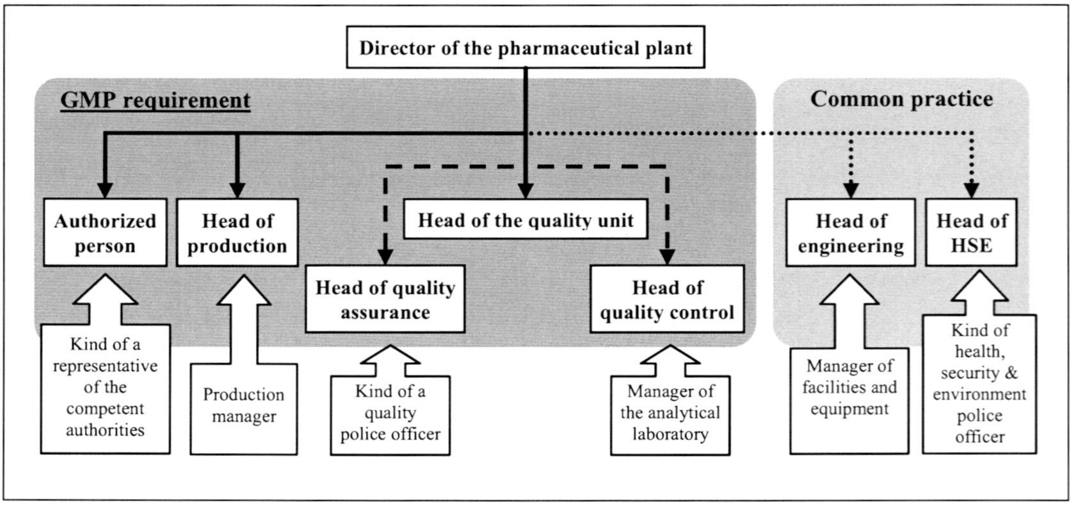

Fig. (3). "Key posts" in a pharmaceutical unit.

GMP responsibilities are distributed among the key posts. Personnel fulfilling these responsibilities can either perform them or just verify/supervise their execution. Usually this depends on the size of the pharmaceutical unit. The annexed figure shows an example of GMP-related key posts in a pharmaceutical plant. It is true that HSE tasks are often outside GMP, but practice has turned its issues so inextricably linked to it that it is better to consider this post too.

(Note: in some countries the following responsibilities may be slightly modified, because of national specific requirements).

Plant Director

The director has the ultimate responsibility in quality and should keep personnel informed about the quality policy of the company. Often the director approves the procedures, not from a GMP point of view, but her/his signature enforces them.

Authorized Person

As a kind of representative of the regulatory authorities, she/he:

- Ensures compliance with the approved requirements for the finished products.
- After checking the batch records certifies and approves the release of the finished product for distribution.
- Informs the authorities in particular situations of critical non-compliance.
- In some cases the authorized person is at the same time the head of the quality unit (if there is a single unit) or of the quality control unit or of the quality assurance unit (when there are two units).

Head of Production

She/he is in charge of the production premises and is responsible for:

- Producing and storing according to the approved procedures;
- Keeping the adequate environmental conditions in the production areas (cleaning, sanitization, monitoring, *etc.*);
- Revising and applying the approved documentation (procedures, instructions, *etc.*) regarding production;

- Revising and applying the approved in-process controls;
- Evaluating the production batch records;
- Validating the production processes;
- Verifying/supervising the implementation of the maintenance plans (premises, facilities and equipment) regarding production;
- Verifying/supervising the implementation of the qualification plan regarding production;
- Verifying/supervising the implementation of the calibration plan regarding production;
- Verifying/supervising the adequate training of production personnel;
- Verifying/supervising and approving the outsourced production.
- Cooperating with the other departments while performing tasks in the production premises (qualification, validation, maintenance, calibration, sampling, *etc.*).

Head of QC (Quality Control)

She/he is in charge of the laboratory of quality control and is responsible for:

- Sampling and monitoring the manufacturing environment;
- Sampling and monitoring the utilities;
- Keeping the adequate environmental conditions in the laboratory areas (cleaning, sanitization, monitoring, *etc.*);
- Sampling, testing and approval/rejection of starting and packaging materials;
- Sampling, testing and approval/rejection of intermediate, bulk and finished products;
- Evaluating the quality control batch records;

- Performing all necessary testing.
- Revising and applying the approved documentation (procedures, instructions, specifications, *etc.*) regarding quality control;
- Performing the analytical validations;
- Verifying/supervising the implementation of the maintenance plans (premises, facilities and equipment) regarding the laboratory;
- Verifying/supervising the implementation of the qualification regarding the laboratory;
- Verifying/supervising the implementation of the calibration plan regarding the laboratory;
- Verifying/supervising the adequate training of quality control personnel;
- Verifying/supervising and approving the outsourced analysis;
- Keeping retention samples of starting materials and of finished products (these latter in their final pack, except when it is exceptionally large);
- Evaluating, maintaining and storing reference standards for substances;
- Ensuring the correct labeling of containers of materials and products;
- Monitoring the stability of the APIs and products;
- Cooperating with the other departments while performing tasks in the laboratory premises (qualification, validation, maintenance, calibration, *etc.*).

Head of QA (Quality Assurance)

She/he is responsible for:

- Establishing, implementing and maintaining the quality system;

- Revising the documentation (procedures, instructions, specifications, *etc.*) to ensure its compliance with GMP and the quality system;
- Verifying/supervising GMP compliance in the plant;
- Performing internal audits or self-inspections;
- Performing external (vendor) audits;
- Approving and monitoring suppliers of materials;
- Defining the validation policy and preparing the Qualification and Validation Master Plans;
- Supervising the qualifications and validations;
- Supervising the results of environmental and utility sampling (air, personnel, water, *etc.*);
- Supervising and monitoring of processes to detect compliance and trends (*e.g.*, quality reviews, change control, CAPA, *etc.*);
- Verifying/supervising the adequate training of QA personnel
- Ensuring the retention of records;
- Preparing (in agreement with other departments) the training program and verifying its implementations;
- Evaluating and approving the complete batch records (production, packaging, quality control) before handling them to the authorized person;
- Cooperating with the other departments regarding quality issues.

Head of Engineering

She/he is responsible for:

- Defining and implementing the engineering policy of the plant;
- Revising and implementing the engineering documentation;

- Stating and implementing the maintenance program;
- Stating and implementing the calibration program;
- Verifying/supervising the adequate training of engineering personnel;
- Verifying/supervising and approving the outsourced engineering services;
- Performing the qualification of facilities and equipment;
- Cooperating with the other departments regarding engineering issues.

Head of HSE

She/he is in charge of the hygiene, safety and environmental policy of the plant (*e.g.,* personnel protection measures, control of insects and pests, fire protection, earthquakes, floods, safe electrical supply, accident handling, effluent and waste disposal, *etc.*) and is responsible for:

- Defining and implementing the HSE policy of the plant;
- Revising and implementing HSE documentation;
- Verifying/supervising and approving the outsourced HSE services;
- Ensuring the adequate training of personnel in HSE matters;
- Cooperating with the other departments regarding HSE issues.

SUPPLY CHAIN

Traditionally regulation and regulators focused on pharmaceutical products and on their manufacturing processes and production units. But, this meant forgetting the real objective of pharmaceutical manufacturing: provide the patients with sure and reliable drug products when they need them. In the 21st century, with the focus shifted towards patients, pharmaceutical industry should be seen like a supply chain (Fig. **4**).

This change of approach, however, not only corresponds to a different attitude but also to a radical modification of the pharmaceutical market. Not longtime ago and generally speaking, the manufacture of pharmaceutical ingredients and of dosage forms was geographically restricted. The actors and steps of the supply chain were just a few and, often, not very far off one from the other. This has changed; actors are often multiple and distributed anywhere on the earth. Thus, supply chains are very complex and difficult to manage. In fact, the supply chain represented in the annexed figure is simplified because it doesn't take in consideration, for instance, that normally before and after any stage there is transportation and storage, and that there are generally several manufacturers of starting materials, ingredients and packaging materials. Although it is preferable to buy any item to the manufacturer (if this is not the case it is very difficult to perform a follow up in order to ensure the quality of the item), this is not always possible for logistic reasons and this is why the corresponding cells have been drawn with discontinuous line.

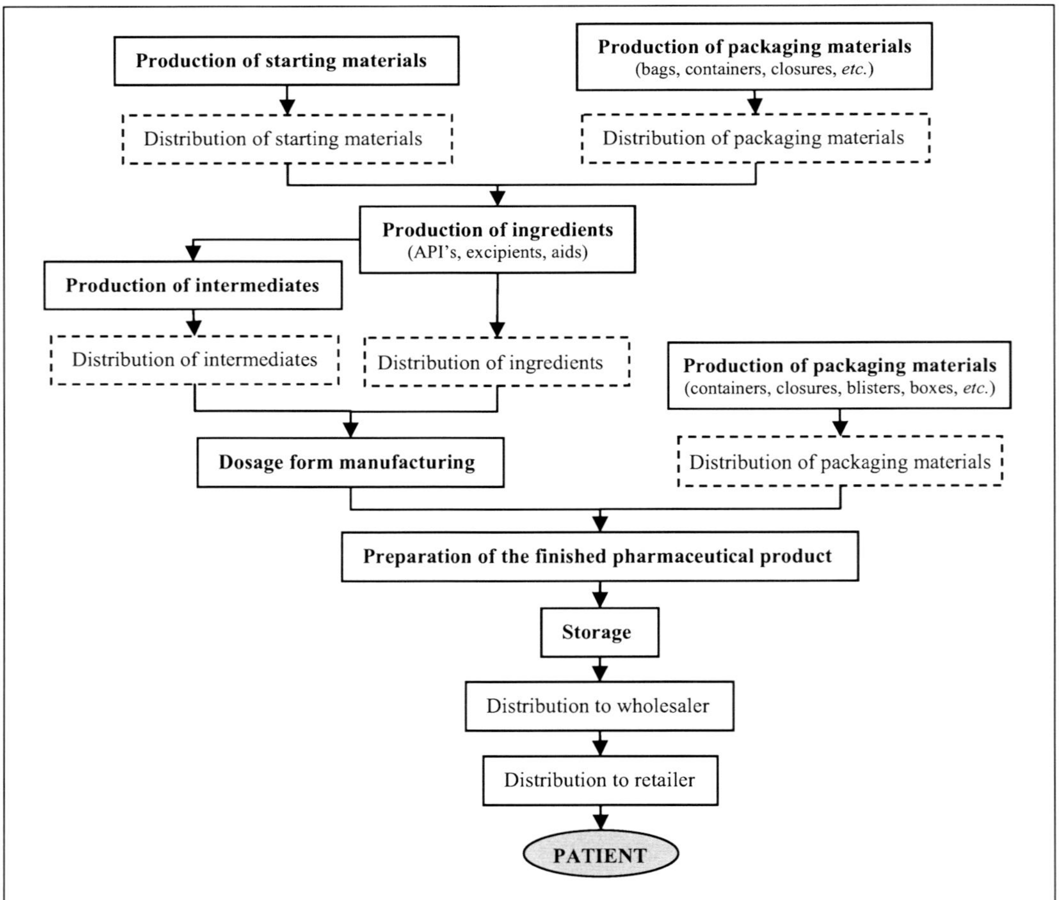

Fig. (4). Approximate outline of a supply chain.

The consequences of possessing a complex supply-chain are very important. Let us consider them from the responsibility, logistics and regulation points of view.

Responsibility

With so many actors in the same play, who is the responsible for the quality of the product and how this responsibility can be exerted?

The ultimate responsibility for the performance of an authorized medicinal product over its lifetime; its safety, quality and efficacy lies with the marketing authorization holder (MAH) [35].

Thus, the MAH has to be able to control any step of the chain, be close or be far off. Although this is easier to say than to put into practice, the following elements should help:

- Contracts among the MAH and the other parts should describe in detail the respective responsibilities and the quality issues.
- All intervening parts should possess a GMP-certificate concerning their respective activities, but not always a nationally-issued certificate will be recognized by other countries. This is why countries are signing "mutual recognition agreements". A manufacturer can be certified by the competent authorities of the country where the products are intended to be sent, but not all the countries, far from that, have the possibility of sending inspectors to other countries. FDA, for instance, is opening offices in some key countries to be able to certify the manufacturers sending products to the US and thus, possess a better control of the supply-chain.
- A manufacturer has to audit its suppliers of starting materials, but often this is difficult and expensive when they are numerous and scattered far away. A way of solving the problem is performing "grouped audits" of the same supplier by different manufacturers (which buy to this supplier). In theory, another possibility could be asking the supplier to fill a question form on quality issues, but, for evident reasons, this cannot be more than an informative element in the whole dossier and cannot replace a quality audit.

Logistics

Even supposing that the different actors in the chain fulfill their duties, if they are not adequately coordinated, there might be dysfunctions leading to a temporary indisponibility of a drug product. The MAH is again the responsible and it may be accused of not supplying the market with the necessary drug products even if the failure has taken place in some supplier. Thus, manufacturers of dosage forms try not to rely on a single supplier for their starting and packaging materials. Disponibility of a substance does not mean disponibility in the production unit. Transportation and customs procedures can also act as bottlenecks.

Regulation

GMP is the quality standard for the manufacture of medicinal products, but the supply chain is much more than manufacturing. Thus, what counts is not only if a drug product has been appropriately manufactured but if the patients get it timely and in good condition.

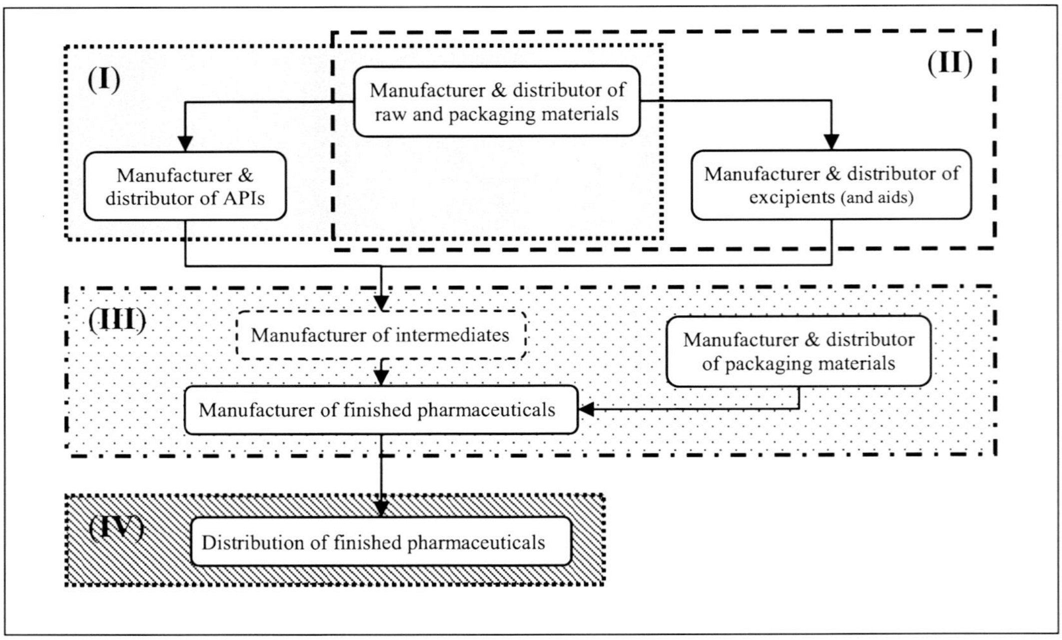

Fig. (5). Regulation of the supply chain.

As shown in Fig. (**5**), from the regulation point of view the supply chain can be divided in four stages.

(I) Preparation and distribution of APIs: The manufacturer of the API, whether prepared by chemical synthesis, by purification of a natural substance or by biotechnology, purchases the necessary raw materials, culture media, reactives and packaging materials. APIs are regulated by a specific GMP [36]. The manufacturer of dosage forms has to ensure that its suppliers meet these GMP.

(II) Preparation and distribution of excipients: The manufacturer of the excipient, normally prepared by chemical synthesis or by purification of a natural substance, purchases the necessary starting materials, reactives and packaging materials, but GMP compliance is not required. Although usually excipients are quantitatively predominant in a dosage form GMP does not include them, firstly, because (at least in principle) they do not possess pharmacological activity and, secondly, because as they are inactive, it can be supposed that their impurities will be inactive too. From a realistic point of view, it is necessary to bear in mind that many excipients (*e.g.,* sugar) are overwhelmingly used by non pharmaceutical industries, which do not require meeting GMP standards. Notwithstanding that, excipients used for the pharmaceutical industry have to be fit for the intended use in terms of purity and of physico-chemical specifications. Excipients should:

- Possess stable composition,
- Be free of cross-contamination
- Be accompanied of appropriate quality control documentation.

In order to help manufacturers simplified GMP guidelines for excipients have been prepared [37-39].

(III) Preparation of medicinal products: The manufacturer of intermediates, of dosage forms and of finished pharmaceutical products (either a single company or several) purchases the necessary APIs, excipients and aids to the above mentioned manufacturers, (I) and (II). Regarding packaging materials, there is again a curious situation, because manufacturers are outside GMP, but their products have to be adequate for the intended use. This state of affairs is solved by agreement between supplier and manufacturers taking into account a reference standard [40]. Although, as is has been mentioned before, the MAH is the global responsible for the quality of the product, even if it is different from the manufacturer of the finished pharmaceutical, it is evident that is this manufacturer who will normally carry the heavy burden of ensuring the GMP compliance of all the three stages (I), (II) and (III).

Once the finished pharmaceutical products are ready they are stored in the warehouse, where they have to be kept in adequate conditions within the defined temperature range for the product (Table **4**). This storage period is considered a part of production and thus, it is under GMP. Notwithstanding that, specific "Good storage practices" (GSP) have been issued [41]. They can be defined as *that part of quality assurance that ensures that the quality of pharmaceutical products is maintained by means of adequate control throughout the storage thereof* [42].

There are three typical storage temperature ranges for finished drug products:

- Room: +15 to +25ºC
- Refrigerator: +2 to +8ºC
- Freezer: -10 to -20ºC

Table 4. Meaning of the labels indicating storage conditions.

Written in the label	Meaning
Do not store above 30°C	Store from +2°C to +30°C
Do not store above 25°C	Store from +2°C to +25°C
Do not store above 15°C	Store from +2°C to +15°C
Do not store above 8°C	Store from +2°C to +8°C
Do not store below 8°C	Store from +8°C to +25°C
Store in freezer	Store from -20°C to -10°C
Store in refrigerator	Store from +2°C to +8°C
Store in cold place	Store below +8°C
Store in cool place	Store between +8°C and +15°C
Store at room temperature	Store between +15°C and +30°C
Heat	From 30°C to 40°C
Excessive heat	More than 40°C

(IV) Distribution of medicinal products: Once the finished pharmaceuticals are formally liberated as required by GMP, they can be sent to the patient. This is normally done indirectly, across distributors. In fact, it is necessary to speak in plural, because distribution is such a complicate task that usually there are at least a wholesaler and a retailer (with the exception of products used in hospitals).

The distribution stage is particularly dangerous for two main reasons. Firstly, because the drug product is finished and will not be subject to further control by the manufacturer or by distributors. And secondly, because the product can go through several stages of transportation and storage which are performed by different actors. It is evident that always that pharmaceutical products are stored they have to meet GMP and GSP requirements.

Complementing these requirements "good distribution practices" (GDPs) [43, 44] and "good trade and distribution practices" (GTDPs) [45] have been issued.

GDPs are described in chapter 12. *GTDPs are that part of quality assurance that ensures that the quality of pharmaceutical products is maintained by means of adequate control throughout the numerous activities which occur during the trade and the distribution process* [46].

Counterfeiting

Even if the supply chain is well managed patients or consumers can receive inappropriate pharmaceuticals because of counterfeiting, that is to say:

- Substitution of a drug product for another counterfeited.
- Uplabeling of a drug product (the labels of the medicament are changed by other ones corresponding to a product of higher value).
- Dilution (the drug product is diluted to obtain more units).
- Repackaging (the product is packaged as a product of higher value).

As it can be seen, these changes (in fact they can be infinite, depending on the imagination of counterfeiters) suppose that the patient is receiving in the best of cases a diluted product.

It is evident that although counterfeiting probably appeared at the same time than the manufacturing of pharmaceuticals, its importance has been growing in the last years, as a consequence of the globalization of the market and of the complexity of the supply chains.

The strict application of GMP, GDPs and GTDPs turns counterfeiting more difficult. Besides that, new measures for preventing counterfeiting are being introduced: codification of all the units to ensure thorough traceability and introduction of new packaging specially designed to detect tampering.

OUTSOURCING

Outsourcing is the contracting of an activity covered by GMP, usually production and/or analysis, by a company to another one. This word became popular in the early 21st century, competing with older terms like "contract or analysis manufacturing".

Sometimes outsourcing is only used when both parts of the contract belong to the same country, and then, offshoring designates contracts with foreign third-parts (at times referred to as "offshore outsourcing"). Insourcing can be used for designing the opposite process, that is to say, performing at the site a process that was realized in other places.

The advantages of outsourcing are evident:

- From the economical point of view: A company can start a process and neither has to invest on facilities and equipment, nor in manpower or training. In any case, it is very useful to see how a process works before investing heavily on it. It is also possible to take advantage of lower costs in other countries and to benefit of economies of scale.

- From the technical point of view: It is not the same starting a production from scratch than benefiting from the experience, skills, contacts, *etc.* of a contract accepter. It is often better concentrating on some well-mastered processes, than trying to assume new unknown ones.

Outsourcing, however, has noticeable inconveniences too:

- Loss of control: It is evident that it is not the same keeping confidential information (formula, technology, know-how, *etc.*) at home than revealing it to a third part. This can be especially important where the protection of intellectual property might be more theoretical than practical. This loss of control can also be extended to logistic aspects (*e.g.,* capacity constraints, responsiveness/flexibility to changes).

- Interaction problems: Sometimes differences in language, culture and quality approaches can be difficult to overcome.

Contract production, analysis and any other activity covered by GMP must be correctly defined, agreed and controlled in order to avoid misunderstandings that could result in a product, or work or analysis, of unsatisfactory quality [47].

From the GMP point of view an outsourcing contract (Table **5**) is a key element for establishing in a clear way the respective responsibilities of the contract giver and the contract acceptor. Although it is evident that a contract will contain many non-GMP terms (amounts, prices, time-limits, *etc.*), GMP terms should be drawn up by competent persons on the aspects covered by the contract and on GMP.

There must be a written contract between the contract giver and the contract acceptor which clearly establishes the responsibilities of each party, covering the outsourced activities, the products or operations to which they are related, communication processes relating to the outsourced activities and any technical arrangements made in connection with it [48].

Table 5. GMP contents of the outsourcing contract.

Feature	Remarks
Batch release/certificate of analysis.	The contract should describe how the authorized person will release each batch of product for sale or emit the certificate of analysis in order to ensure that a batch has been manufactured and examined according to the marketing authorization.
Marketing authorization.	Contract giver and contract acceptor should ensure that both production and analysis of the products are performed in accordance with the marketing authorization.
Responsibilities	In the contract should be clearly stated which persons are responsible for the different activities covered by the contract, such as technology transfer, knowledge management, supply chain and testing and releasing of materials. It should define the responsible persons regarding production, in-process control and quality control. It should also describe who is responsible for sampling and analysis. If the contract refers to analysis, it should define who will take the samples at the premises of the manufacturer, either the contract giver or the contact acceptor.
Records and reference samples	Records regarding the manufacture, analysis and distribution of the products should be at the contract giver's disposal. This includes any record of the contract acceptor concerning the assessment of the quality of products suspected of being defective, fraudulent or falsified. It should be described who is responsible for archiving these records.
Handling of rejects	The contract should describe the handling of rejected starting materials and of rejected intermediate, bulk and finished products. It should also describe how to proceed if the contract analysis shows that the tested product must be rejected. The contract analysis should define how the tested product will be handled if according to the test results it has to be rejected.

Control from Outsourced Activities

Responsibilities of the Contract Giver

- The contract giver's quality system should specify that outsourced activities will be subjected to control and revision.
- The records and results of the outsourced activities should be reviewed and appraised by the contract giver.
- The contract giver should guarantee that the materials and products supplied by the contract acceptor have been prepared in compliance with GMP and with the marketing authorization.
- The contract giver should ensure that the materials and products meet their specifications and that the authorized person has released them in compliance with GMP and with the marketing authorization.
- The level of performance of the contract acceptor should be monitored and assessed. And this should comprise the implementation and the evaluation of the efficacy of any measure of improvement.
- The contract giver should ensure that the contract acceptor will agree to any inspection performed by the competent authorities.

Responsibilities of the Contract Acceptor

- The contract acceptor should only perform changes authorized in the contract.
- The contract acceptor should avoid any action likely to have a negative effect on the manufacture and/or analysis of the products of the contract giver.

Capacity for Performing the Outsourced Activity

Responsibilities of the Contract Giver

- The contract giver should ensure that the contract acceptor is duly authorized by the competent authorities.
- The contract giver should evaluate the contract acceptor in order to ensure that it is appropriate and competent. The contract acceptor should comply with GMP and apply risk management.

Responsibilities of the Contract Acceptor

- The contract acceptor should ensure that her/his premises and equipment are adequate for performing the operations requested by the contract giver.

- The contract acceptor should possess appropriate experience, knowledge and trained personnel for carrying out satisfactorily the operations entrusted by the contract giver. The contract acceptor should own a valid manufacturing authorization and fulfill all the necessary legal requirements.

Information

Responsibilities of the Contract Giver

- The contract giver should supply the contract acceptor with all the documentation necessary to perform adequately the operations described in the contract.

- The contract giver should inform the contract acceptor about any hazard related to the product or to the production or testing operations. She/he should ensure that the contract acceptor understands the associated risks.

Further Outsourcing by the Contract Acceptor

Responsibilities of the Contract Acceptor

- The contract acceptor should not outsource any operation comprised in the contract without the adequate evaluation and agreement by the contract giver.

- Any arrangement made by the contract acceptor and a third part should follow the same above mentioned principles of the contract between contract giver and contract acceptor.

CONCLUDING REMARKS

Pharmaceuticals are "different products" because they can put health at risk and because users cannot judge on their quality. They are subjected to GMP, a basic specific regulation, which is complemented with other specialized standards such as GSP, GDPs and GTDPs.

Medicinal products reach the patient after following an often long and complex supply chain where the marketing authorization holder (MAH) bears the responsibility of ensuring the quality of the product.

CONFLICT OF INTEREST

The author confirms that this chapter contents have no conflict of interest.

ACKNOWLEDGEMENT

Declared None.

REFERENCES

[1] European Commission. Good manufacturing practices. Medicinal products for human and veterinary use. The rules governing medicinal products in the European Union. Volume 4. Brussels.

[2] US National Archives & Records Administration. Federal Register. Code of Federal Regulations (CFR). Title 21 (Food & drugs). 21 CFR 210.3.

[3] Le Hir A, Chaumeil JC, Brossard D. Pharmacie galénique. Bonnes pratiques de fabrication des médicaments. 9th Edition. Elsevier Masson, Issy-les-Moulineaux, France 2009.

[4] ICH (International Conference on Harmonisation of Technical Requirements for registration of Pharmaceuticals for Human Use). Pharmaceutical development. Harmonised Tripartite Guideline. Q8(R2). ICH, Geneva, Switzerland 2009.

[5] WHO (World Health Organization). WHO Good manufacturing practices for pharmaceutical products: main principles. In: WHO Expert Committee on Specifications for Pharmaceutical Preparations. Forty-eighth report (WHO Technical Report Series, No. 986). WHO, Geneva, Switzerland 2014. Annex 2. 17.1.

[6] UNDP (United Nations Development Program)/World Bank/WHO (World Health Organisation). Handbook: Good Laboratory Practice (GLP). Quality practices for regulated non-clinical research and development. Special Programme for Research and Training in Tropical Diseases. TDR/WHO, Geneva, Switzerland 2000.

[7] WHO (World Health Organization). WHO Good manufacturing practices for pharmaceutical products: main principles. In: WHO Expert Committee on Specifications for Pharmaceutical Preparations. Forty-eighth report (WHO Technical Report Series, No. 986). WHO, Geneva, Switzerland 2014. Annex 2. 17.1.

[8] Ibid. 3.

[9] WHO (World Health Organisation). Good practices in the manufacture and quality control of drugs. In: WHO Expert Committee on Specifications for Pharmaceutical Preparations. Twenty-second report (WHO Technical Report Series, No. 418). WHO, Geneva, Switzerland 1969. Annex 2.

[10] US National Archives & Records Administration. Federal Register. Code of Federal Regulations (CFR). Title 21 (Food & drugs). Part 210.1.

[11] http://www.fda.gov

[12] Department of Health and Human Services. U.S Food and Drug Administration. Pharmaceutical cGMPs for the 21st Century: A Risk-Based Approach. Final Report. FDA, Rockville, MD, USA 2004.

[13] http://www.who.int.

[14] http://ec.europa.eu/health/documents/eudralex/vol-4/index_en.htm.

[15] http://www.ich.org.

[16] ICH (International Conference on Harmonisation of Technical Requirements for registration of Pharmaceuticals for Human Use). Active Pharmaceutical Ingredients. Harmonised Tripartite Guideline Q7. ICH, Geneva, Switzerland 2000.

[17] PIC/S (Pharmaceutical Inspection Convention. Pharmaceutical Inspection Co-Operation Scheme). Good Manufacturing Practice for Medicinal Products. Guide PE 009-11. PIC/S, Geneva, Switzerland 2014.
[18] Rosetto Y (editor). φ41. Pharmacotechnie industrielle. I.M.T. Editions, Tours, France 1998.
[19] WHO (World Health Organization). WHO Good manufacturing practices for pharmaceutical products: main principles. In: WHO Expert Committee on Specifications for Pharmaceutical Preparations. Forty-eighth report (WHO Technical Report Series, No. 986). WHO, Geneva, Switzerland 2014. Annex 2. Glossary.
[20] Ibid.
[21] Ibid.
[22] US National Archives & Records Administration. Federal Register. Code of Federal Regulations (CFR). Title 21 (Food & drugs). Part 210.3
[23] Ibid.
[24] WHO (World Health Organization). WHO Good manufacturing practices for pharmaceutical products: main principles. In: WHO Expert Committee on Specifications for Pharmaceutical Preparations. Forty-eighth report (WHO Technical Report Series, No. 986). WHO, Geneva, Switzerland 2014. Annex 2. Glossary.
[25] Ibid.
[26] US National Archives & Records Administration. Federal Register. Code of Federal Regulations (CFR). Title 21 (Food & drugs). 21 CFR 210.3.
[27] WHO (World Health Organization). WHO Good manufacturing practices for pharmaceutical products: main principles. In: WHO Expert Committee on Specifications for Pharmaceutical Preparations. Forty-eighth report (WHO Technical Report Series, No. 986). WHO, Geneva, Switzerland 2014. Annex 2. Glossary.
[28] Ibid.
[29] Ibid.
[30] Ibid.
[31] Ibid.
[32] WHO (World Health Organization). WHO Good manufacturing practices for pharmaceutical products: main principles. In: WHO Expert Committee on Specifications for Pharmaceutical Preparations. Forty-eighth report (WHO Technical Report Series, No. 986). WHO, Geneva, Switzerland 2014. Annex 2.
[33] European Commission. Good manufacturing practices. Medicinal products for human and veterinary use. The rules governing medicinal products in the European Union. Volume 4. Brussels.
[34] WHO (World Health Organisation). Good Manufacturing Practices: Authorized person – role, functions and training. In: WHO Expert Committee on Specifications for Pharmaceutical Preparations. Thirty-fifth report (WHO Technical Report Series, No. 885). WHO, Geneva, Switzerland 1999. Annex 4.
[35] European Commission. Enterprise and Industry Directorate-General. Certification by a Qualified Person and Batch Release. In: EudraLex. The Rules Governing Medicinal Products in the European Union. Volume 4. EU Guidelines to Good Manufacturing Practice. Medicinal Products for Human and Veterinary Use. European Commission, Brussels, Belgium 2013. Annex 16.
[36] ICH (International Conference on Harmonisation of Technical Requirements for registration of Pharmaceuticals for Human Use). Active Pharmaceutical Ingredients. Harmonised Tripartite Guideline Q7. ICH, Geneva, Switzerland 2000.
[37] IPEC (The International Pharmaceutical Excipients Council). PQG (Pharmaceutical Quality Group). The Joint IPEC – PQG Good Manufacturing Practices Guide for Pharmaceutical Excipients. IPEQ, PQG, Arlington, VA, USA 2006.
[38] WHO (World Health Organisation). Good Manufacturing Practices: Supplementary guidelines for the manufacture of Pharmaceutical Excipients. In: WHO Expert Committee on Specifications for Pharmaceutical Preparations. Thirty-fifth report (WHO Technical Report Series, No. 885). WHO, Geneva, Switzerland 1999. Annex 5.
[39] WHO (World Health Organisation). Quality requirements for pharmaceutical aids. In: WHO Expert Committee on Specifications for Pharmaceutical Preparations. Twenty-ninth report (WHO Technical Report Series, No. 704). WHO, Geneva, Switzerland 1984. Annex 2.

[40] ISO (International Organization for Standardization). Primary packaging materials for medicinal products. Particular requirements for the application of ISO 9001:2005 with reference to GMP. International standard ISO 15378:2006(en). ISO, Geneva, Switzerland 2006.
[41] WHO (World Health Organisation). WHO guide to good storage practices for pharmaceuticals. In: WHO Expert Committee on Specifications for Pharmaceutical Preparations. Thirty-seventh report (WHO Technical Report Series, No. 908). WHO, Geneva, Switzerland 2003, Annex 9.
[42] WHO (World Health Organisation). WHO good distribution practices for pharmaceutical products. In: WHO Expert Committee on Specifications for Pharmaceutical Preparations. Forty-fourth report (WHO Technical Report Series, No. 957). WHO, Geneva, Switzerland 2010. Annex 5. Glossary.
[43] European Commission. Guidelines of 5 November 2013 on Good Distribution Practice of medicinal products for human use. Information from European Union Institutions, Bodies, Offices and Agencies. Official Journal of the European Union, C 343/1, 23.11.2013.
[44] PIC/S (Pharmaceutical Inspection Convention. Pharmaceutical Inspection Co-Operation Scheme). Good Distribution Practice for medicinal Products. Guide PE 011-1. PIC/S, Geneva, Switzerland 2014.
[45] WHO (World Health Organisation). Good trade and distribution practices for pharmaceutical starting materials. In: WHO Expert Committee on Specifications for Pharmaceutical Preparations. Thirty-eighth report (WHO Technical Report Series, No. 917). WHO, Geneva, Switzerland 2003. Annex 2.
[46] Ibid.
[47] WHO (World Health Organization). WHO Good manufacturing practices for pharmaceutical products: main principles. In: WHO Expert Committee on Specifications for Pharmaceutical Preparations. Forty-eighth report (WHO Technical Report Series, No. 986). WHO, Geneva, Switzerland 2014. Annex 2. 7.1
[48] Ibid. 7.13.

CHAPTER 2

The Lifecycle Model

Abstract: The performance of any process is both the consequence of its previous development studies and of the adequate transfer of these experimental concepts into practical operation. This is the lifecycle model which reminds us that quality has to be designed, transferred to real routine operation and then maintained within controlled conditions. There is no other way, at least nowadays, to ensure that quality by design will become produced quality too. In a pharmaceutical unit the lifecycle model can be usefully applied both to pharmaceutical products and pharmaceutical projects (premises, facilities, or equipment) and to processes like documentation and personnel. The different lifecycle stages are united like the links of a chain. Therefore, in order to achieve quality, control has to be exerted in a global way. The significance and management of the lifecycle stages of a project (URS, commissioning, admittance, qualification, maintenance and calibration) are analyzed. The practical organization of a qualification program is described in detail, starting with the redaction of a QMP, following with the writing and executing of qualification protocols and finishing with the qualification reports.

Keywords: Admittance, calibration, commissioning, discontinuation, DQ, IQ, maintenance, OQ, PQ, project design, QMP, qualification, qualification protocol, qualification report, qualification testing, requalification, supplier, traceability, URS, verification (checking).

WHAT A LIFECYCLE IS

Pharmaceutical products can be considered a sort of living being. They are initially "conceived" and, after their "birth", they spend a life, which is more or less long, with variable incidences and changes, until the moment their production comes to an end. Thus, *all the phases in the life of a product from the initial development through marketing until the product's discontinuation* [1] are collectively known as "lifecycle".

All lifecycle phases are closely related. Each one is influenced by whatever happened before and, in turn, has an influence on whatever will happen afterwards. Improvement and scientifically sound control are only possible if knowledge and experience gained during one stage are transferred to the next one. This is why the lifecycle model is important.

This model can be usefully applied not only to the products but also to the facilities where they are manufactured and even to the manpower and

Jordi Botet

documentation used for this manufacture. In fact, any process can be considered in terms of a lifecycle.

A lifecycle is typically composed of four stages.

(1) Development/conception: The process is conceived, invented, and its outlook is decided. It consists in gathering, evaluating, comparing and selecting information. And then, on this base, something new is created.

(2) Transfer/realization: What has been created is practically built, adapted or moved to be used for its routine function.

(3) Manufacturing/operation: The process operates routinely during its lifetime.

(4) Discontinuation: The process is no more necessary or useful (*e.g.* it is superseded by a better one or it is unprofitable).

THE PHARMACEUTICAL PRODUCT LIFECYCLE MODEL

As represented in the annexed Fig. (**1**), lifecycles appear intersecting the supply chain, which was considered in chapter 1.

Only two lifecycles are shown in the figure (the first corresponding to the manufacturing of ingredients/intermediates and the second dealing with pharmaceutical products). Practically speaking, these two processes exercise the highest effect on the quality of the pharmaceutical product, as they concern the starting materials and the preparation and packaging of the dosage form. Other processes, however, can have their influence on the pharmaceutical product too (*e.g.* synthesis, extraction, or fermentation of the raw materials used to obtain the pharmaceutical ingredients; manufacturing of the packaging materials employed in the finished product).

In any case, the driving idea is always the same, without a proper study and a scientific design a product will not be adequately understood and consequently the production process will never be enough sure and robust. Also, if the transfer from the development center to the production plant is not adequately performed the quality of the product is doubtful (in research laboratory conditions the product which was obtained met specifications, but what will happen in different conditions).

The last stage, discontinuation, is considered not by taking into account the product itself but the social consequences of its withdrawal. The aim is keeping patients protected (*e.g.* information on the product will continue to be available, there will always exist an alternative product, *etc.*). Pharmaceutical products are not just another commodity, but health assets.

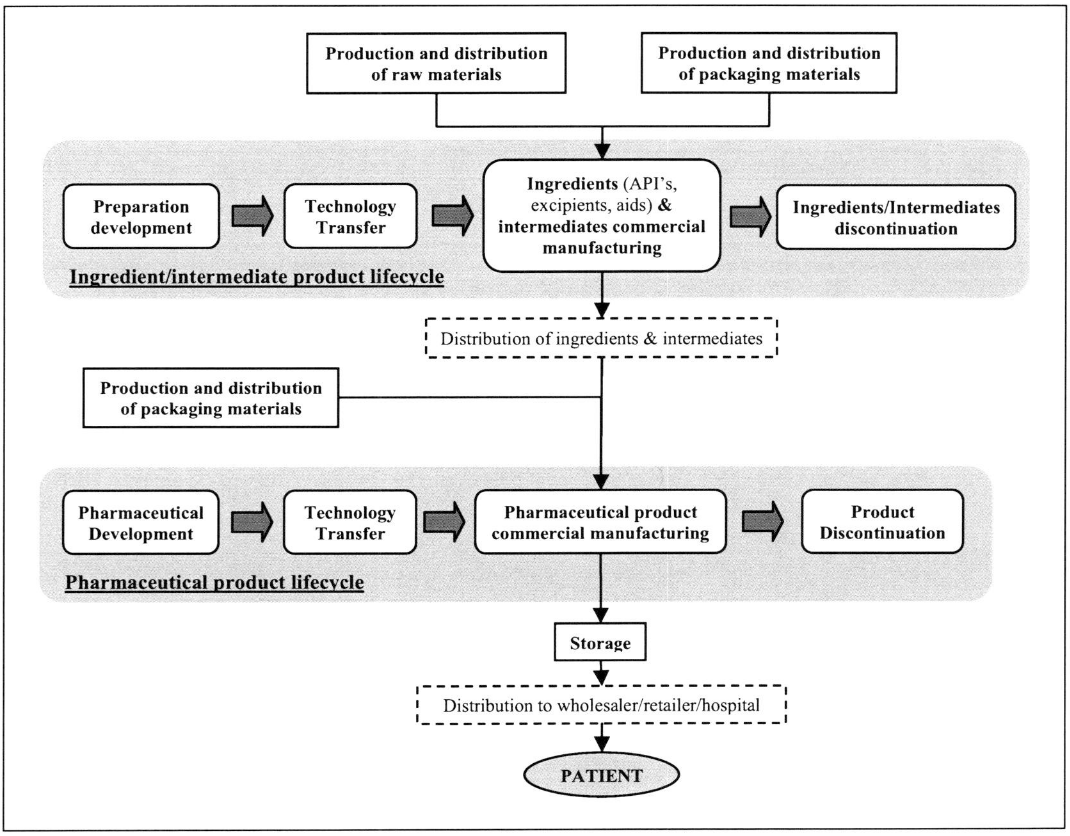

Fig. (1) Intersection of supply chain and lifecycles.

The pharmaceutical product life-cycle is discussed in detail in chapter 11.

THE PREMISES, FACILITIES AND EQUIPMENT LIFECYCLE MODEL

The lifecycle model is usefully applied to a whole plant (with its premises, facilities and equipment), to a definite part of it, or even just to a single system or equipment.

In this case the first stage of development/conception is usually known as "project" and the third one of manufacturing/operation as "service-life". The other two stages can be denominated by the usual general names. See Fig. (**2**).

To simplify matters, in the following paragraphs it is considered a plant project (meaning by this a project comprising premises, facilities and equipment).

1st Stage: Project (Development/Conception)

Following a proposal for a new pharmaceutical plant, different points (technical, financial, strategic, *etc.*) are studied and considered. Each organization has its own procedures, but in the end what counts is determining the viability and opportunity of the proposal and, finally, making a decision about going ahead or not.

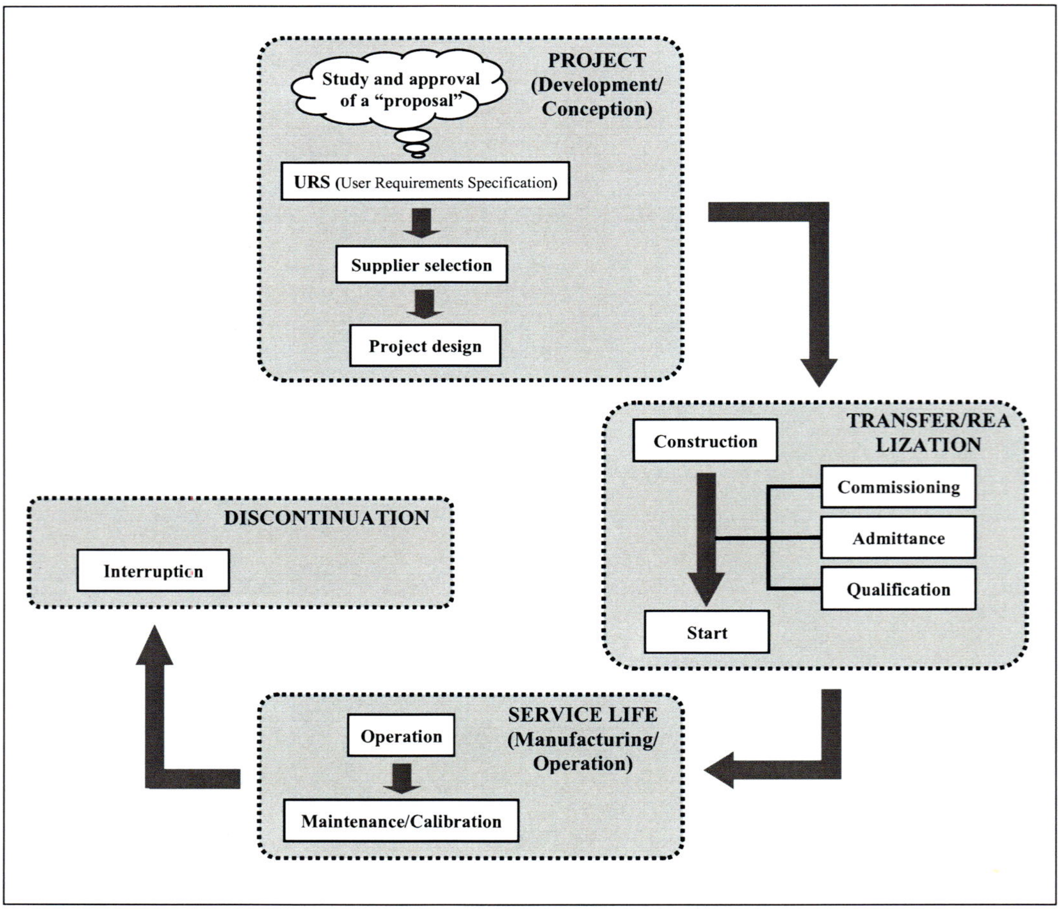

Fig. (2) Pharmaceutical premises, facilities and equipment lifecycle.

URS

Once the viability of the project has been shown and the organization has decided pursuing it, its parameters are set in the "User Requirements Specification"

(URS). In this document the organization establishes which conditions should meet the plant (objective, production capacity, regulations, particular stipulations, *etc.*). This data is used as a base to prepare the tender for the selection of suppliers. In fact, it can truly be said that a project begins only when the URS have been laid down ("zero hour").

Although usually in a complex project several organizations are involved, these are normally hired or coordinated either by the purchaser's task force group or, more often, by the selected supplier. Thus, in a project there are typically just two main characters: purchaser and supplier (vendor). In any case, a clear definition of objectives, conditions and responsibilities on both sides is the key to success, and here documentation plays a fundamental role.

The URS document is the base to which all other documents of the project refer.

Something very important to bear in mind is that the URS should express what is needed and required, but not how to satisfy or perform it, because this is the supplier's task. Although its contents vary according to the particular characteristics of each project, the following points are usually specified in a URS document:

- Objectives: Purpose of the project, including the desired characteristics of the final product/s.

- Framework: Legal and regulatory requirements which should be met by the project. This evidently means GMP and good engineering practice (GEP) [2], but also any other appropriate requirements (standards, internal procedures of the organization, guidelines, *etc.*).

- Project definition: Description of what is needed and expected (functional and non-functional requirements). Integration of the new project into existing systems (computerized control systems, equipment, premises, *etc.*).

- Documentation: It is necessary to keep in mind that the user needs documentation not only for qualification/validation purposes but also for starting and servicing. Although it is evident that the supplier will always prepare documentation to develop the project, this does not entirely cover what the user needs. Therefore it is advisable to indicate in detail which documents the user desires to receive and when.

- Terms and restrictions: Other practical conditions to be fulfilled.

Supplier (Vendor) Selection

The selection of supplier/s is a very important stage in a project (Fig. **3**). Although it is evident that economic and logistic questions play an important role, technical aspects in general and pharmaceutical aspects in particular, should not be overlooked. Suppliers and manufacturers of premises, equipment and utilities should be examined and approved just like any other supplier of materials.

Suppliers should be selected because of the quality and cost of their equipment, but also because of their understanding of GMP and their adherence to a quality system. Their capacity of producing robust quality products should be assessed.

A reliable supplier means adequate and timely documentation as well as simplified and shortened qualification/validation. The advantages of competitive prices could easily turn into disadvantages if, during the commissioning, validation and starting documentation is not appropriate and the URS have not been correctly taken into account.

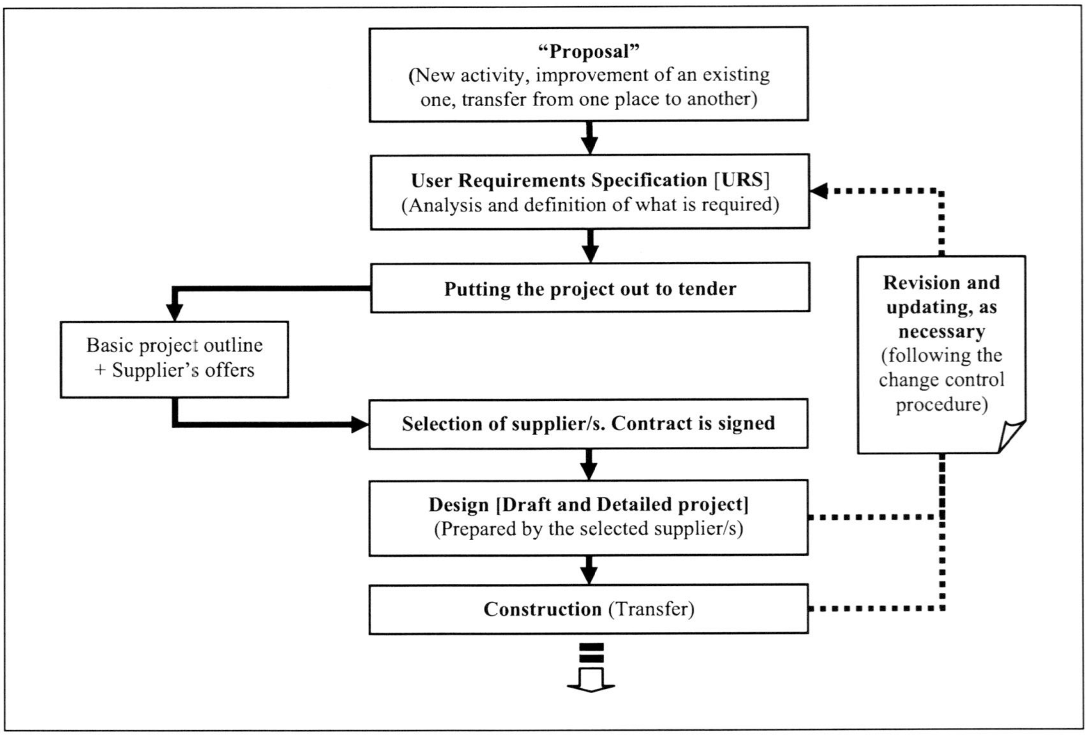

Fig. (3) Project: Supplier selection.

A project team, composed of persons belonging to both user and supplier, lead by the person responsible for the project, is appointed in order to ensure a thorough follow-up.

Project Design

The selected plant supplier, taking into account the requirements set down in the URS, initially prepares a "draft project" (which describes the principles of design and operation of the project – design and functional specifications) and afterwards a "detailed project" (which describes in depth how this project should be constructed). In fact, sometimes, the draft project coincides with the basic project outline which was presented when the supplier tendered for the contract.

The plant functional specifications can be defined *as specifications that document functions, standards and permitted tolerances of systems (plant) or system components (equipment) and which define the operating capabilities of the equipment* [3]. Table **1** summarizes the documents that compose a project.

Table 1. Project documentation.

Prepared by	***Document***		***Comments***
USER	✓ User Requirements Specification (URS)		Base on which the supplier develops the project
SUPPLIER	✓ Design Specifications ✓ Functional Specifications ✓ Project diagrams ✓ List of parts with tags		They constitute the project properly speaking
	✓ "As built" diagrams		They show the actual installation (they are the "final updated" project diagrams).
	✓ Certificates of materials of construction for parts of equipment coming into contact with the products		Also from other parts, as appropriate, to show compliance with specific quality user requirements
	✓ Technical specifications of instrumentation and equipment		They are essential for the change management system
	✓ Spare parts list		
	✓ Commissioning	FAT ("Factory Acceptance Test") reports	Tests performed on the supplier premises
		SAT ("Site Acceptance Test") reports	Tests performed on the user premises

Table 1: contd...

	✓ Operation handbook	Often these are gathered in one document
	✓ Maintenance directions	
	✓ List of critical instrumentation with certificates of calibration for those deemed critical	The "criticality" of instrumentation might be agreed by user and supplier
	✓ Welding documentation (Certificates of equipment and personnel, log-book, P&I welding diagram, welding tests, cleaning and passivation report, *etc.*)	For stainless steel orbital welded parts
	✓ Parameterization of computerized systems ✓ Copy of software	The information which is required depends on the characteristics of the systems

2nd Stage: Transfer/Realization

Construction and Start

Once the detailed project is completed and approved, it can be constructed. What is described on paper becomes a reality. During construction and start, the project is commissioned, admitted and qualified, before being put into routine operation.

Commissioning

Each supplier has its own procedures to check that the project, which has been constructed, conforms to its specifications. These verifications, completed before the formal handing over of the unit to the purchaser, are known as "commissioning", *an engineering term that covers all aspects of bringing a system or sub-system to a position where it is regarded as being ready for use in pharmaceutical manufacture. Commissioning involves all the basis requirements of Installation Qualification (IQ) and Operational Qualification (OQ)* [4].

As commissioning and qualification are close concepts, it is well-worth analyzing which are their differences. While the supplier performs commissioning testing, the customer develops its own verifications (qualification). For the sake of clarity, besides commissioning and qualification admittance is added. See Table **2**.

Both "commissioning" and "qualification" possess the same and unique finality: to demonstrate that the project as designed, installed and started, functions as purported and yields as expected. Thus, it is convenient that supplier and customer act in a coordinated way, limiting the repetition of verifications and taking advantage when performing tests of the knowledge on equipment that the supplier has [5].

Table 2. Commissioning, admittance and qualification.

	Commissioning	Admittance	Qualification
Contents	FAT (factory acceptance tests) and SAT (site acceptance tests)	Equipment/System technical form and Equipment/System file	DQ, IQ, OQ, PQ
Performed by	The supplier/s	The User (Engineering/QA)	The User (Engineering/QA)
Scope	Any element	Any element	"Critical" elements (those which may influence product quality)
Purpose	Showing that the project meets supplier specifications and URS.	Characterize and integrate any new item into the current organization of the plant	Showing that the project meets URS, GMPs and supplier specifications

It is up to the company (or to an external consultant designated by the company) to perform the qualification, whereas commissioning is carried out by the supplier (or suppliers).

Besides, qualification has long been a GMP regulated requirement, whereas commissioning is often agreed by user and supplier. However, because of the quality system requirements of the supplier a more or less complete commissioning is always performed. As it has been mentioned, qualification focuses on critical aspects, whereas commissioning possesses a more general character.

Admittance

By admittance we understand the set of actions performed in order to integrate a new item into the current organization of the plant (*e.g.* codification, tagging, maintenance and calibration programs, opening of a log-book, *etc.*).

This is usually done by the engineering department under the responsibility of its head with the collaboration of the affected departments (production, QC and QA).

This is not a GMP requirement, although it is a very practical method for keeping the plant under control. Every company has the organization that better suits its needs and normally derives from practical experience.

Once that new premises, facilities, or equipment are delivered to the plant and put in place it is necessary to confirm that the received item corresponds to the agreed one. After this formality, it is necessary to complete the equipment/system technical form (Table **3**) and archive the accompanying documentation (Fig. **4**).

Table 3. Simplified example of equipment/system technical form.

EQUIPMENT/SYSTEM TECHNICAL FORM (Associated to the procedure SOP-nnn)		
Equipment/system:		
Code #:		**Log-book reference:**
(1) **DESCRIPTION**	- Manufacturer - Make - Serial number - Manufacturing year - Supplier - Technical service	Photograph
(2) **DIMENSIONS**	- Weight - Height/length/width	
(3) **INSTALLATION**	- Date: - Place:	
(4) **BUILDING MATERIALS** (in contact with products)	- Description: - **Accepted?: Yes** □/No □:	
(5) CALIBRATION	Calibration required? Yes □/No □. Included in the calibration plan? Yes □/No □.	
(6) QUALIFICATION	Qualification required? Yes □/No □. Included in the qualification plan? Yes □/No □. Periodic requalification required? Yes □/No □. Included in the requalification plan? Yes □/No □.	
(7) UTILITIES (connection, supply, consumption)	- Electricity - Compressed air - Steam	
(8) **MAIN OPERATIONAL CHARACTERISTICS**	- Control and safety systems: - Amount of personnel necessary: - Theoretical/Practical yield	
(9) **INSPECTION/AUTHORISATION**		
(10) **SPARE PARTS**		
(11) MAINTENANCE	Maintenance required? Yes □/No □. Included in the maintenance plan? Yes □/No □	
(12) OTHER		

Written by:	**Engineering Head review**	**QC Head review**	**QA Head review**
Date:			
Signature:			

CHANGE CONTROL				
#	**Description**	**Date**	**Written by**	**Reviewed**

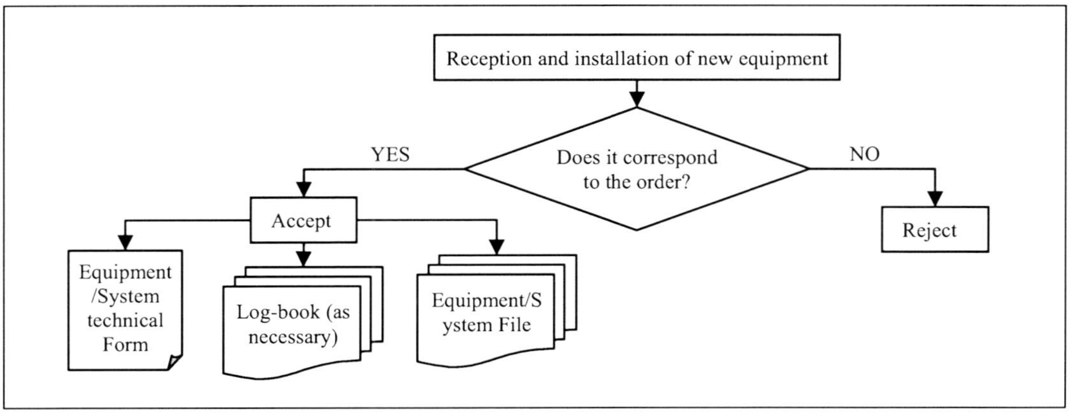

Fig. (4). Admittance.

Qualification

Premises, equipment, and utilities are qualified by the user to ensure that they have been constructed, installed and perform as purported. Qualification, which is *the action of proving that any premises, systems and items of equipment work correctly and actually lead to the expected results* [6], is composed of four elements: DQ, IQ, OQ and PQ. They are defined as follows:

- DQ (Design qualification): *The documented verification that the proposed design of the facilities, systems and equipment is suitable for the intended purpose.*

- IQ (Installation qualification): *The documented verification that the facilities, systems and equipment, as installed or modified, comply with the approved design and the manufacturer's recommendations.*

- OQ (Operational qualification): *The documented verification that the facilities, systems and equipment, as installed or modified, perform as intended throughout the anticipated operating ranges.*

- PQ (performance qualification): *The documented verification that the facilities, systems and equipment, as connected together, can perform effectively and reproducibly, based on the approved process method and product specification* [7].

The V-diagram of qualification shown in Fig. (**5**) explains very well why GMP prescribes these four elements and which their functions are.

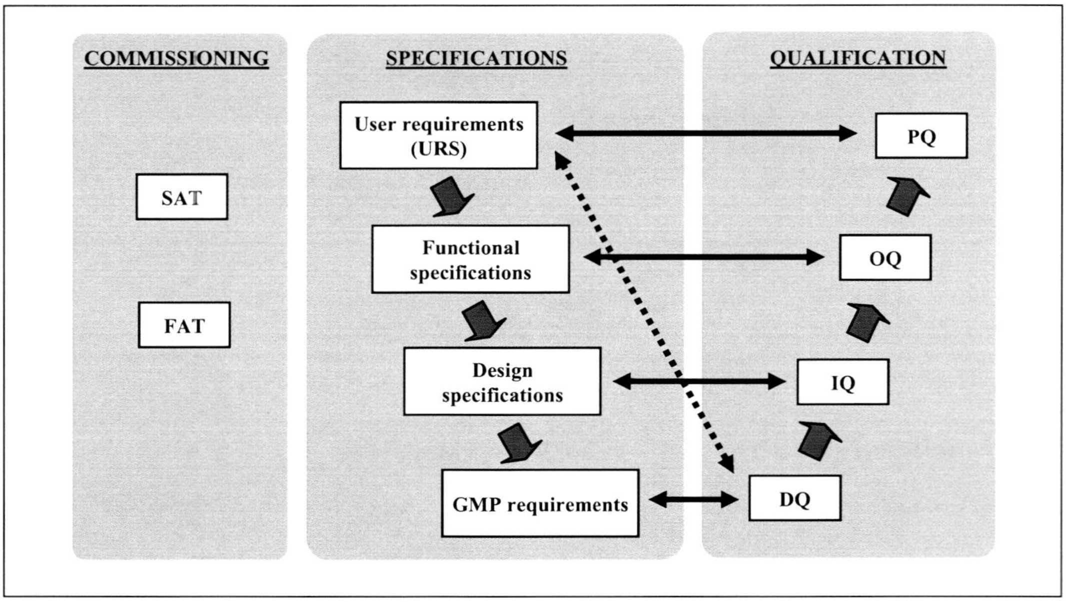

Fig. (5). The "V-diagram" of qualification.

The qualification elements are realized in the given order (DQ>IQ>OQ>PQ) and in principle it is necessary to complete one element before passing to the next one (sometimes it is possible to leave one element unfinished if the deficiency is minor and a delayed finishing does not change much things; *e.g.* a document is missing or a component has not its identification tag).

The purpose of the DQ is verifying that a given project meets GMP requirements and the URS. Logically it is performed, at least ideally, before starting the implementation of the project, in order to have the possibility of modifying it in case of non compliance. DQ is important in purpose-built projects, because there might be important deviations from the URS and even from GMP, but in case of commercially-built equipment DQ is less significant, and if equipment belong to a well known company and the model has been chosen on the base of the URS (in this case very limited, because requirements have to adapt to fit the choice of models), then DQ can be skipped and qualification starts with the IQ.

The objective of the IQ is verifying that what has been installed meets the supplier installation requirements (static trials). In other words, what has been constructed by the supplier is what he stated in the project (piping, equipment, ducts, *etc.*).

The aim of the OQ is verifying that what has been installed meets the supplier operational requirements (dynamic trials), that is to say, the installation performs as expected. Once that the OQ is finished it is possible to say that the installation works adequately. Consequently it can be already used in routine manufacturing.

The OQ tests are performed without the real product, whereas PQ, the last element of qualification, consists in dynamic tests with product. As this distinction is often non realistic (*e.g.* how to qualify the operation of a dosage machine without the intended liquid?) in practice either the OQ includes PQ tests or OQ and PQ are performed at the same time.

The objective of the performance qualification is to verify that the constructed project is capable, under functional routine conditions, of performing as indicated in the URS. Sometimes there is no difference between assay conditions and routine working conditions (*e.g.* for an installation producing compressed air). In these cases PQ is not necessary. However, in a packaging line PQ shows that it yields the intended product as expected, whereas OQ is limited to machine functional tests.

Sometimes PQ is used to show the performance of a system in the long run (*e.g.* in the qualification of pharmaceutical water systems it demonstrates that seasonal variation in feed water do not affect the quality of the produced water).

Note: We have been using the word "qualification" because we were talking about a plant and its premises, facilities and equipment, but "validation" is a closely related term which might also be used. Then which is the difference between qualification and validation?

- Both words have essentially the same meaning, that is: verifying that something is and performs as anticipated. Qualification is typically used for premises, facilities, systems and equipment (this "something" is a machine or installation), whereas validation is usually used for procedures (this "something" is a process).

- Validation, however, is also used with a broader meaning which includes qualification. Then, the validation of a plant starts with the qualification of its premises, facilities and equipment and follows with the validation of the processes to be realized in this plant. Thus, qualification and validation are two links of the same chain. In this book we follow this pattern.

Anyway, these two words are not always used very carefully and sometimes they are synonymous.

It is interesting to underline that although validation is a GMP requirement it represents a quite different approach to quality. Whereas GMP contains general quality principles, validation is case-specific, because it studies each case and performs case-adapted testing in order to ensure the quality of this particular case.

3rd Stage: Service life (Manufacturing/Operation)

Operation

All the previous stages in the lifecycle aim at this one. The target is possessing premises, facilities, or equipment meeting URS and GMP and capable of preparing quality products in the terms specified there.

Moreover, equipment and systems should be kept in an adequate state of control and performance (as qualified), by adequate maintenance and calibration.

Maintenance

According to GMP in order to prevent equipment breakdown it is necessary to implement a preventive maintenance program and also evaluate the data recorded during its implementation. This regular maintenance has to be performed and documented according to established procedures. Maintenance means keeping the plant in good condition, but different approaches can be used.

<u>Preventive maintenance (PM)</u>: The objective is preventing equipment breakdown and keeping it in adequate operational state by performing operations which detect or correct incipient defects. Thanks to preventive maintenance equipment operates normally without having breakdowns and prolonging their service-life.

During the maintenance revisions worn-out parts and service liquids are substituted. The intention is acting before having a breakdown.

PM can be:

- Planned or programmed, when it is scheduled according to calendar time, to real operating time or to performances.

- Condition based maintenance (CBM), when it is scheduled according to the real data obtained by special instrumentation.

Predictive maintenance (PdM): The state of equipment can be evaluated by using different methods in order to determine which type of maintenance is needed. In other words, maintenance is realized when it is necessary and this necessity is scientifically established. This is an important difference in relation to the traditional preventive maintenance, which is realized according to theoretically appraised schedules.

Predictive maintenance supposes determining periodically or continuously the state of the equipment (without affecting their operational readiness) in order to carry out the necessary maintenance tasks before equipment could start having operational problems.

PdM uses on-line non destructive techniques (*e.g.* vibration analysis, acoustic analysis, infrared monitoring, lubricant analysis, *etc.*).

Corrective maintenance (CM): This is what we habitually call repair and it is carried out when the piece of equipment has had a breakdown in order to put it again in good operational state. This is certainly the worst of cases, because of the waste of time and the risk of degradation of equipment.

Summarizing: CBM and PdM are the best choices, but they require either specialized instrumentation or instrument-furnished equipment. PM, either planned or programmed, is the simplest practical choice (and often the only real one), but it is less efficient and reliable.

From the GMP point of view, it is necessary to have a procedure describing the measures to undertake in order to prevent product contamination as a result of any intervention (adjustment, change of format, reparation, or maintenance) on equipment. Equipment should only be restarted for production after approval by a responsible person.

Calibration/Verification

Measuring is an essential working element in the pharmaceutical industry. This is why it is necessary to preserve the metrological quality of the measure instruments. This is achieved by means of calibration and, in a lesser degree, by verification (checking).

Calibration is defined *as the set of operations that establish, under specified conditions, the relationship between values indicated by an instrument or system for measuring (especially weighing), recording, and controlling, or the values represented by a material measure, and the corresponding known values of a reference standard. Limits for acceptance of the results of measuring should be established* [8]. Verification (checking) of an instrument means establishing its capacity for meeting predetermined measure requirements.

4th Stage: Discontinuation

Although discontinuation is not, properly speaking, a lifecycle stage, it has to be taken into account. Discontinuation supposes that the process finishes. From the point of view of the premises, facilities, or equipment, discontinuation supposes mainly a logistic problem (they are either taken to pieces or modified and adapted for other products).

THE PHARMACEUTICAL DOCUMENTATION LIFECYCLE MODEL

Documents are an important element in a pharmaceutical plant. They convey information on how to perform a process or operation (*e.g.* procedure or instruction) or simply data (*e.g.* specification or register) and this is why GMP focuses on them.

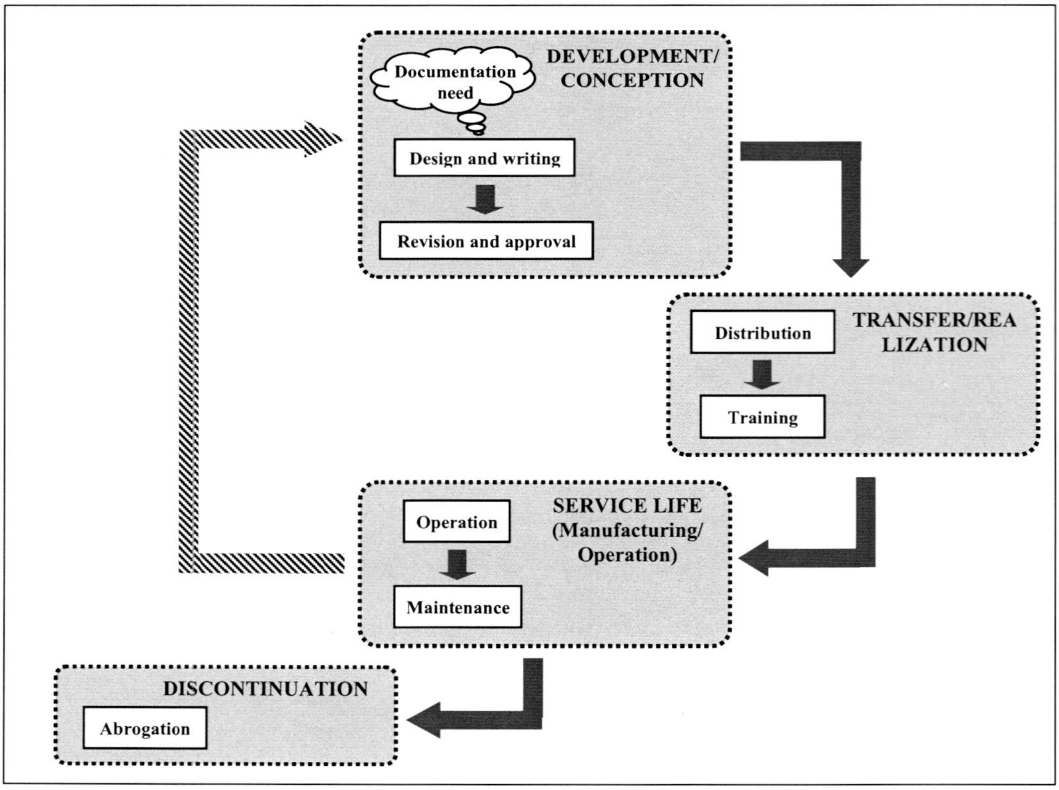

Fig. (6). Pharmaceutical documentation lifecycle.

Thus, documents accompany processes along their life-cycle and they-themselves have a lifecycle, with the typical four stages (Fig. **6**). See chapter 6.

- Development/Conception: When need appears a document is written, reviewed and approved.

- Transfer/Realization: Users get a copy of the document and are given training.

- Service life: The document is used for manufacturing. In order to keep it updated new versions, as necessary, are released. Any new version follows the same cycle.

- Discontinuation: A document can be abrogated because it is no longer necessary or because it is superseded by another one (*e.g.* broader contents, restructuration of operations, *etc.*).

As in any lifecycle "maintenance" is a key element. It is necessary to keep documents in state of validity, namely, reflecting the real situation.

THE PHARMACEUTICAL PERSONNEL LIFECYCLE MODEL

It is not necessary to insist on the importance of manpower in a pharmaceutical plant. As GMP points out, inadequate experience and training can result in critical quality problems. Thus, personnel should also follow the lifecycle model (Fig. **7**), with the typical four stages (see chapter 7):

- Development/Conception: When there are vacant posts or new posts are created, it is necessary to select new personnel meeting the established requirements for these posts.

- Transfer/Realization: Personnel considered suitable for the post receive adequate training and are eventually appointed to the post.

- Manufacturing/Operation: Personnel perform their jobs and receive continual training.

- Discontinuation: A person can leave her/his post because retirement, resignation, or transfer to another position in the plant. In the latter case the cycle starts again for the new post.

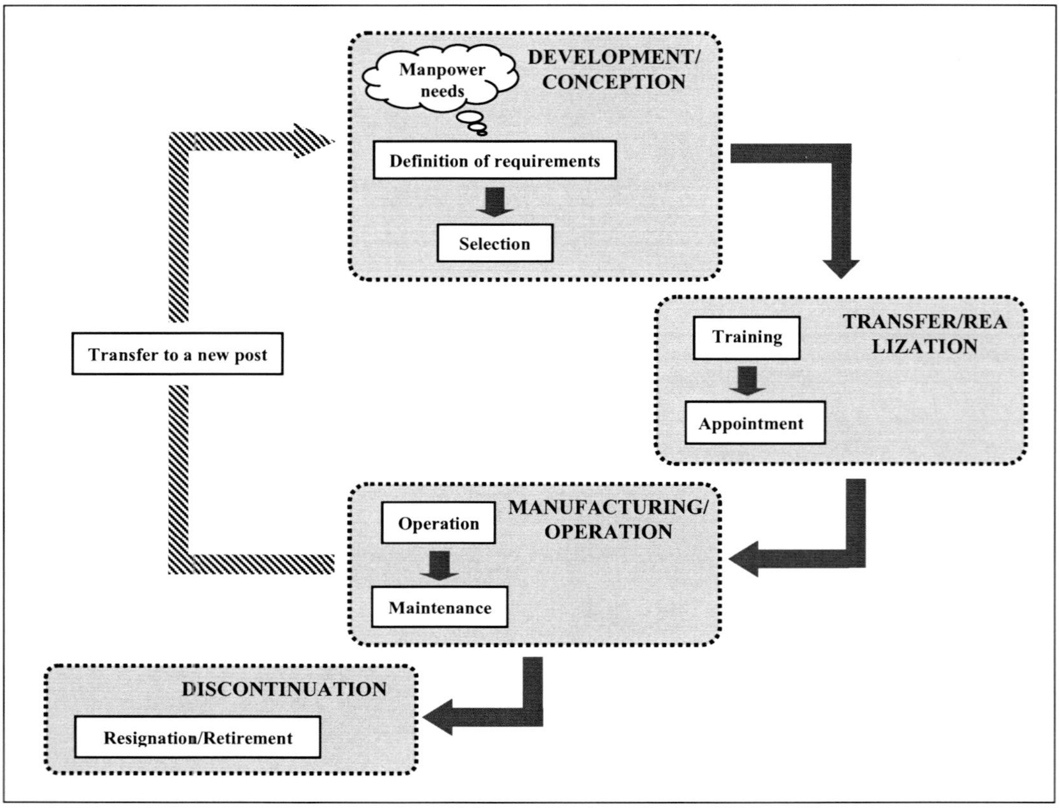

Fig. (7). Personnel lifecycle.

PRACTICAL ORGANIZATION OF A QUALIFICATION PROGRAM

According to GMP the key elements of a qualification and validation program of a company should be clearly defined and documented in a VMP (validation master plan) [9]. However, qualification and validation are different matters involving differentiated approaches and, besides, both subjects require such an amount of attention that in practice it is better to handle them separately. Thus, we propose to have a QMP (qualification master plan) and a VMP (validation master plan); in this case validation is not used as a general word but refers only to the validation of processes.

In this chapter we are going to describe qualification. Validation is dealt with in chapter 11.

Notes: We have mentioned just two separated master plans (QMP and VMP), as generally this suffices largely, but this is not always the case. For example in big plants with differentiated areas or in case of a defined extension project for an existing plant it might be advisable to have several master plans (*e.g.* QMP of oral solids, QMP of injectable drugs, VMP of oral liquids, VMP of biologicals, *etc.*). The number of master plans is not important in itself. What matters is a good control and organization of the qualification and validation tasks. For a better coordination, it is advisable to have a general document describing the qualification/validation approach and how many plans exist and why. See chapter 5.

Preparation of a QMP

QMP is a general document describing how a company will deal with qualification. The contents of a QMP vary according to the particular circumstances, but we could propose these general ones:

1. Objective: This QMP has the following objectives:

- Define how qualification will be organized and performed.
- Ensure the adequate planning of the qualification activities and the allocation of the necessary resources.
- Ensure that the qualification activities will be appropriately documented.
- Provide easy-access information on qualification.

2. Scope: Identification and situation of the plant or unit to be qualified.

3. Responsibilities: There will be a qualification team usually headed by a technician belonging to the QA department and composed by a technician of the engineering department and a technician of the production department.

Table 4. Example of responsibilities regarding qualification documentation.

Task	Personnel			
	Plant Director	QA Head	Qualification Team Head	Qualification technician
QMP	Approves	Reviews	Writes	---
Qualification protocols	---	Approves	Reviews	Writes
Qualification tests	---	---	Reviews	Realizes
Qualification reports	---	Approves	Reviews	Writes

This is, evidently, just a guiding proposal (Table **4**), because the composition of the qualification team will depend on the type and amount of testing to be performed. In any case, the members of the qualification team will always have at their disposal other technicians of the plant for specific tasks, as necessary.

4. Definitions: Introduce the GMP definitions for the main terms (*e.g.* qualification, protocol, report, DQ, IQ, OQ, PQ, *etc.*) and for other words or expressions, as necessary.

5. Summary of premises, facilities and equipment to be qualified: Brief description of the plant. The following is a practical system to describe the different elements of the plant (Fig. **8**).

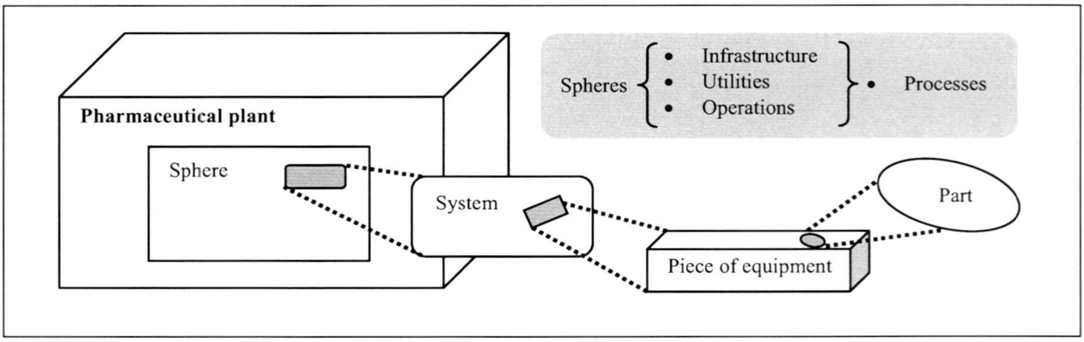

Fig. (8). Practical subdivision of a pharmaceutical plant.

In a systematic way a pharmaceutical plant can be subdivided in "spheres" (groups of systems with similar functions). The systems are constituted by groups of equipment operating in a coordinated way. Equipment transforms inputs in outputs and it can be subdivided into parts, more or less individualized.

Production is performed in the plant premises, within defined rooms (clean or not). These rooms can be grouped in different systems (*e.g.* warehousing, weighing, blending, *etc.*). In this sphere a room can be considered "a piece of equipment", whereas a door would be "a part".

Utilities are systems of equipment which produce or transform and distribute the fluids or energies which are necessary for the manufacturing operations. Well-known systems are HVAC, compressed air or waters for pharmaceutical use, *etc.*

The production operations are performed by equipment systems which transform starting materials into pharmaceutical products.

And lastly these three spheres operating conjointly perform the production processes which are described in chapter 11.

6. Organizational structure of qualification activities: This QMP identifies and lists all items to be qualified, indicating for each of them the elements composing their qualification (DQ, IQ, OQ, and PQ). See Fig. (**9**).

Then, the corresponding qualification protocols will be written and submitted to review and approval. A written protocol should be established that specifies how qualification and validation will be conducted. The protocol should be reviewed and approved. The protocol should specify critical steps and acceptance criteria [10].

Acceptance criteria can be defined as measurable terms under which a test result will be considered acceptable [11]; *or as the criteria assigned, before undertaking testing, to allow evaluation of test results to demonstrate compliance with a test phase of delivery requirement* [12].

The approved protocols will be realized by the qualification team. When completed, the corresponding reports will be written. A report that cross-references the qualification and/or validation protocol should be prepared, summarizing the results obtained, commenting on any deviations observed, and drawing the necessary conclusions, including recommending changes necessary to correct deficiencies. Any changes to the plan as defined in the protocol should be documented with appropriate justification [13].

The approval of a report amounts to the liberation of the item as successfully qualified.

After completion of a satisfactory qualification, a formal release for the next step in qualification and validation should be made as a written authorization [14].

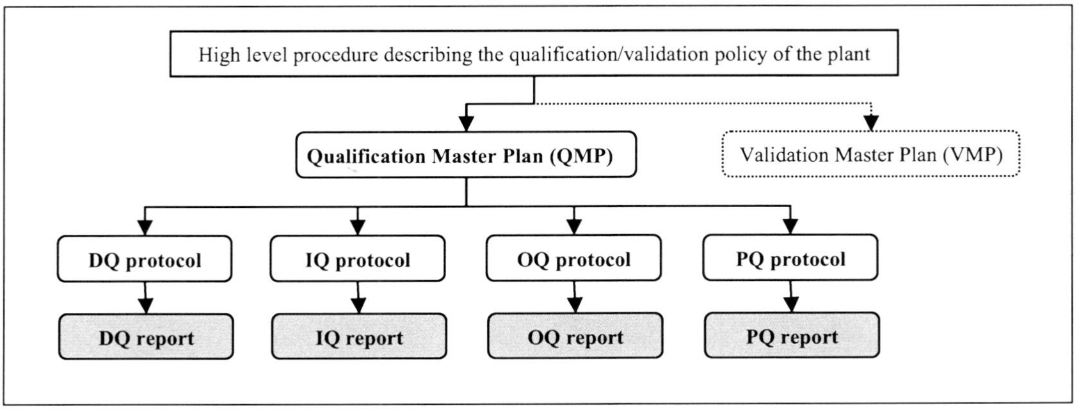

Fig. (9). Qualification documentation.

As we have previously described DQ is usually not necessary for standard models of equipment. IQ and OQ are obviously realized in all cases. PQ is often indispensable but this should be analyzed taking into account the following four different situations:

1st When the item operates independently from any production (*e.g.* compressed air) PQ is not necessary.

2nd When the item is used in production it is necessary to verify that its operational functions are correct (OQ), but also that when operating with the product in real conditions its performance meets requirements; consequently, PQ has to be realized.

3rd Sometimes the item operates independently from any production, but it is necessary to verify its reliability in the long run (*e.g.* pharmaceutical water). PQ is realized as a long period of follow-up.

4th Sometimes there is an intermediate situation. The item in fact works independently from production, but it is necessary to show that it meets requirements in activity and in the long run (*e.g.* HVAC systems). In this case PQ is also performed.

<u>7. Documentation format</u>: Each protocol has a front page identifying the document and providing the adequate spaces for approval, review and writing signatures (name, post, signature and date). See chapter 6.

Then, the protocol describes briefly its object and scope and details the tests to perform.

Every test is composed of the following parts:

- Test # and description.
- Objective of the test;
- Testing procedure;
- Acceptance criteria;
- Test verifications (data matrix);
- Test result: Pass/fail;

- Remarks;
- Signatures (name, date and signature): Performed by/Verified by.

Whereas reports are written and then dated and signed by the writer, the reviewer and the approver (name, post, signature and date). Their contents are summarized as follows:

- Object and scope (reference to the qualification protocol);
- Tests performed and results obtained;
- Comments on deviations and non conformities;
- Recommendations;
- Conclusions.

It is advisable to finish the report with a formal declaration such as:

The installation qualification (IQ) of the system .... of the production unit 1 of the .... plant, has been satisfactorily completed. Consequently it can be released for the realization of the operational qualification (OQ).

8. Codification of the qualification documentation: The above mentioned documents will be identified by a code composed of three letters (identifying the type of document) and three numbers (for successive numbering). See Table **5**.

Table 5. Example of codification of the qualification documents.

Type of document		Identification
Qualification Master Plan		QMP
Qualification protocol	DQ	DQP
	IQ	IQP
	OQ	OQP
	PQ	PQP
Qualification report	DQ	DQR
	IQ	IQR
	OQ	OQR
	PQ	PQR
Note: Requalification protocols/reports keep the initial code, but changing the version number.		

9. Planning: The documents comprising the qualification program are listed (Table **6**).

Table 6. Example of planning of qualification tasks.

Sphere	System/Equipment	Protocols/Reports				
		#	DQ	IQ	OQ	PQ
(I) Premises	Clean rooms	001	DQP-001/DQR-001	IQP-001/IQR-001	N. a.	N. a.
(II) Utilities	HVAC systems	002	DQP-002/DQR-002	IQP-002/IQR-002	OQP-002/OQR-002	PQP-002/PQR-002
	Compressed air	003	DQP-003/DQR-003	IQP-003/IQR-003	OQP-002/OQR-002	N. a.
	Dust extraction	004	DQP-004/DQR-004	IQP-004/IQR-004	OQP-004/OQR-004	PQP-004/PQR-004
	Purified water	005	DQP-005/DQR-005	IQP-005/IQR-005	OQP-005/OQR-005	PQP-005/PQR-005
(III) Operations	Blender	006	DQP-006/DQR-006	IQP-006/IQR-006	OQP-006/OQR-006	PQP-006/PQR-006
	Sifter	007	DQP-007/DQR-007	IQP-007/IQR-007	OQP-007/OQR-007	PQP-007/PQR-007
	Granulator	008	DQP-008/DQR-008	IQP-008/IQR-008	OQP-008/OQR-008	PQP-008/PQR-008
	Compressor	009	DQP-009/DQR-009	IQP-009/IQR-009	OQP-009/OQR-009	PQP-009/PQR-009

10. Scheduling:

Table 7. Qualification chronogram.

Qualification	Period (year: ....)					
	January-February	March-April	May-June	July-August	September-October	November-December
Item #1						
Item #2						
Item #3						
Item #4						
Item #5						

GMP requires that a QMP contains a chronogram detailing how the qualification will be realized (Table **7**). Experience shows that keeping this schedule is often difficult, but, if necessary, new updated versions of the document will be released.

11. Change control: Any change will be handled following the approved procedure (SOP-nnn).

12. Filing: The qualification documentation will be archived by the QA department.

13. Training: All personnel taking part in qualification tasks will be provided with the adequate training.

14. Calibration: All instruments used in qualification should be in state of calibration.

15. Requalification: As shown in Fig. (**10**), the need for requalification will be based on science and risk analysis. Requalification is necessary when equipment possess automated functions, which require verification that they perform as intended.

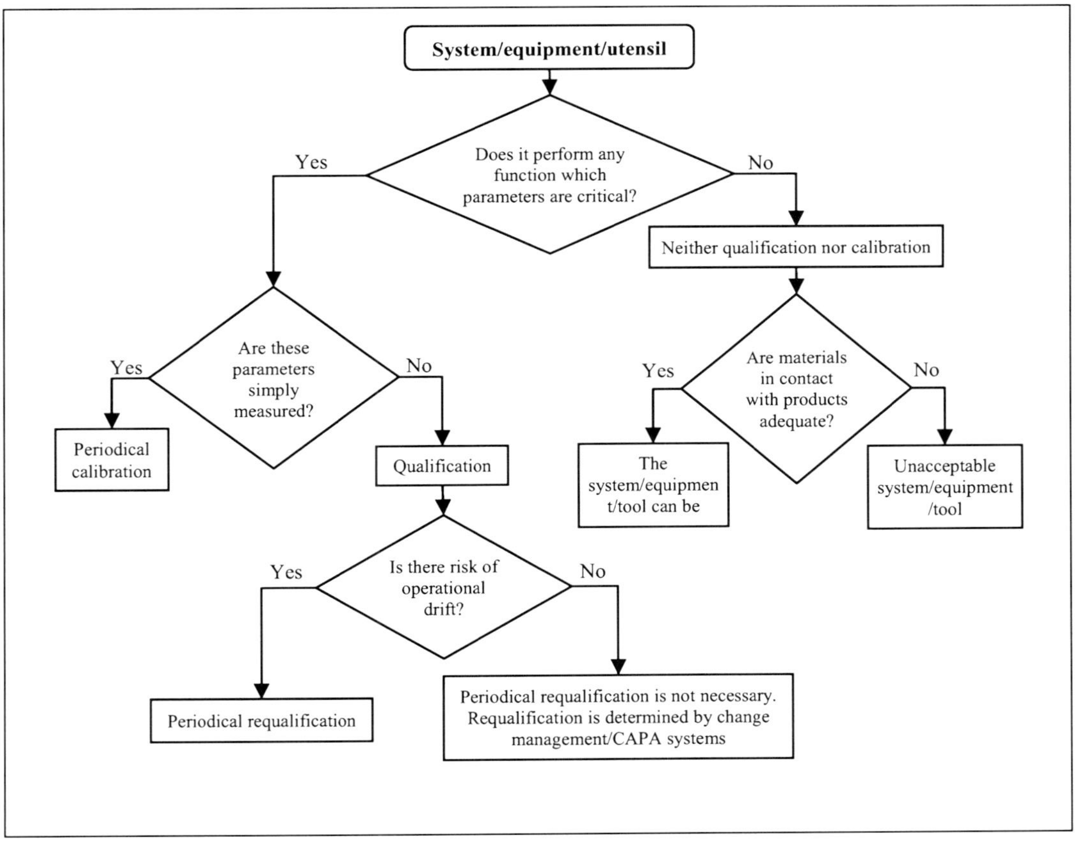

Fig. (10). Approach used to establish the need of requalification.

Once equipment is qualified continual monitoring is necessary in order to ensure that small changes do not lead to operational drift and to the loss of the state of qualification. This is completely unacceptable in case of equipment performing very critical operations which might be affected by tiny unremarked changes (*e.g.* sterilizators). Then, periodical requalification is required. In all the other cases the need of requalification is dictated by continual monitoring, change management and CAPA systems.

Qualification Testing

Tests which compose the qualification elements vary according the characteristics of the item being qualified. In following chapters it is provided more information regarding particular cases (*e.g.* water, HVAC, *etc.*). Here are described the tests which usually compose the qualification of a piece of equipment. However, particular cases might require slight modifications, depending on the characteristics of equipment [15].

DQ

The objective of DQ is verifying that the system/equipment, as proposed/projected, meets GMP/GEP and URS requirements. In practice, this means checking the following matters:

- Design (material/product flows, protection from contamination, cleanability, isolation of service fluids, separation of processing from mechanical parts, *etc.*);

- Construction (materials and surface finish);

- Capacity and performances (meeting requirements).

It is usually very practical performing these verifications by means of a table. See Table **8**.

Table 8. DQ verifications.

#	URS/GMP requirement	Checking	Reference
1	Rooms of differing cleanliness levels should be communicated by airlocks in order to control the airflow.	□ Pass/□ Fail	WHO. TRS 986. Annex 2. Glossary
2	The parts of the production equipment likely of contacting the products which are processed should not affect their quality by having any significant type of reaction, addition or absorption.	□ Pass/□ Fail	WHO. TRS 986. Annex 2. 13.9.

IQ

The objective of IQ is verifying that the system/equipment, as put into position and made it ready to operate, meets the supplier specifications. Thus, usually the following tests are carried out:

- Collect and exam of the supplier documentation (operation and maintenance directions, as-built drawings, instrumentation list - with special mention of those instruments considered critical).
- Verification that installed items correspond to the projected ones and that they are adequately identified with tags fixed onto them (Admittance).
- Verification that items have been installed according to specifications (position, slope, connection of utilities, coupling to drain, *etc.*) and as shown on the as-built plans (P&I diagrams).
- Verification that critical instruments are calibrated (there are calibration certificates and items are provided with calibration labels).
- Verification of materials of construction (there are material certificates).

OQ

The objective of OQ is verifying that the system/piece of equipment functions according to the supplier specifications. Tests are mainly composed of operational verifications which derive from the operational specifications provided by the supplier. Besides routine operation testing it is often necessary worst-case testing.

Worst Case is defined as a condition or *set of conditions encompassing upper and lower processing limits and circumstances, within standard operating procedures, which pose the greatest chance of product or process failure when compared to ideal conditions. Such conditions do not necessarily induce product or process failure* [16].

Thus, usually the following tests are carried out:

- Verification of procedures regarding operation (assembly, verification, use, cleaning, maintenance).

- Verification of operator training.

- Verification of performance (start, stop, breakdown and alarm messages, realization of foreseen functions, working parameters, security mechanisms, *etc.*).

- Verification of computerized systems (access protection, traceability, accessibility and security of data, report printing, *etc.*).

PQ

Although PQ is described as a separate activity, it may in some cases be appropriate to perform it in conjunction with OQ [17].

The objective of the performance qualification is to verify that the system/equipment, under functional routine conditions, performs as required in the URS. Thus, usually the following tests are carried out:

- Verification of the performance in real production conditions (this includes connection with other pieces of equipment). For example:

    - When the item operates with materials (*e.g.* blender, filling machine, *etc.*) functional tests are carried out in actual working conditions using either real production materials or adequate substitutes;

    - When the item operates without materials (*e.g.* HVAC, dust extraction, *etc.*) functional tests are carried out in order to verify that the appropriate working conditions are obtained (*e.g.* temperature, RH, airflows, differential pressure).

- Verification of the behavior of the item in the long run (sustained performance).

Requalification Testing

In order to keep updated the QMP, a qualification program is prepared every year including equipment/systems submitted to periodical requalification and new pieces of equipment/systems.

For requalification it is not necessary to repeat the whole testing realized in the initial qualification, but only those tests which ensure the continued state of qualification of the equipment. If there have not been changes, it is not necessary to repeat IQ testing, whereas all significant OQ testing is usually repeated.

PRACTICAL ORGANIZATION OF A MAINTENANCE PROGRAM

Whenever possible, equipment should be installed so as to enable maintenance and repair in a technical zone (outside from the manufacturing areas). Procedures should describe precautions to be taken to avoid product contamination when an intervention is unavoidable (change of format, adjustment, emergency stops, etc).

Following the life-cycle model, when during admittance the system/equipment technical form is filled, it is necessary to establish if it requires maintenance and, if the answer is yes, which type of maintenance.

Equipment and utensils shall be maintained at appropriate intervals to prevent malfunctions or contamination that would alter the safety, identity, strength, quality, or purity of the drug product beyond the official or other established requirements [18].

Although any approach is acceptable provided it ensures the appropriate maintenance, it involves usually the following steps:

1st Establish the maintenance requirements (usually proposed by the supplier, although experience can help in adapting them to particular situations) indicating tasks and schedules.

2nd Prepare procedures/instructions describing how and when the maintenance tasks of systems/equipment will be realized.

3rd Introduce the above mentioned tasks in the maintenance plan (this plan shows the systems/equipment submitted to maintenance and the temporal distribution of tasks) and approve it.

4th Follow-up of the maintenance plan (execution and detection of deviations or anomalies). If necessary, modify it, but it must be kept up to date and fulfilled as approved.

The maintenance plan can be a spread sheet of paper and followed manually, but in big plants (with many items to follow and with frequent changes) this might be unpractical. This is why there are special items of software specially conceived for maintenance. They are very easy to update, they allow for an easy follow-up and they send a message when, according to the schedule, an intervention on a piece of equipment is due [19].

PRACTICAL ORGANIZATION OF A CALIBRATION/VERIFICATION PROGRAM

As a measurement is usually obtained by comparison to a reference value (a standard), it is evident that it never has an absolute value. This standard is, in turn, measured in relation to another standard of higher level. And this chain, connecting standards, goes up until reaching a universal reference standard (Fig. **11**). This allows for the traceability of the measurement [20].

In a pharmaceutical unit it is often possible to distinguish between primary standards (first level standards), *e.g.* standards of the highest metrological qualities, which are used as a reference and secondary standards (second level standards), whose value is established by comparison with the primary standards.

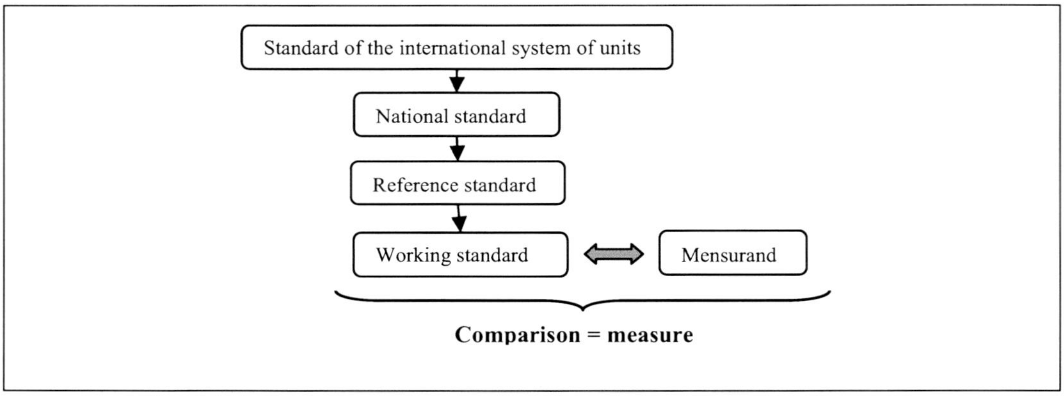

Fig. (11). Principle of calibration.

The accuracy of the standards used for calibration should be higher than the accuracy required for the instrument which is being calibrated and there should be traceability of the calibration certificate to a national or international standard (provided that there is such a standard).

Calibration and verification are close concepts, which are sometimes assimilated. However, they usually have a basic difference. Whereas calibration is the establishment of the relationship existing between measured values and the known values of a mensurand (known standard), verification is checking the capacity of an instrument of meeting its requirements. An instrument is deemed calibrated, when it has the capability to measure a variable to a required accuracy over a determined range of values.

Instruments of measure are classified as "critical" or "non-critical", according to their capacity of having an effect on the quality of the products. Critical instruments should be periodically calibrated, whereas non-critical instruments simply need to be checked (verified).

Thus, with regard to calibration instruments may be classified as:

- Instruments subject to periodic calibration;
- Instruments subject to non-periodic calibration (they are calibrated according to the number of functioning hours, the results of verifications, *etc.*);
- Instruments not subject to calibration.

For the instruments that are periodically calibrated, it is necessary to establish the frequency of this calibration. There is no pre-established calibration frequency. The frequency has to be determined for each case; always taking into account that calibration frequency is a compromise between two opposing factors. On the one hand, it is advantageous to limit the frequency of calibration (because it has a direct cost and also an indirect one, an instrument not being available while being calibrated). On the other hand, a lengthy period of time between calibrations means an increased risk of losing the metrological qualities of the instrument.

The points to be taken into account when establishing the frequency of calibration are the following:

- Characteristics of the instrument;
- Recommendations of the instrument supplier;
- Experience with other similar instruments;
- Frequency and conditions of use of the instrument;
- Maintenance of the instrument;

- Criticality of the measures;
- Required exactitude;
- Regulatory requirements/standard recommendations, as appropriate;
- Experience with this instrument.

Taking into account all these factors it is evident that the frequency of calibration cannot be established in a general way. In practice, however, most instruments are calibrated on an annual or biannual basis. Still, the frequency of calibration has to be "followed" and consequently, it may be appropriate to modify it.

After calibration, adjustment or repair, if it appears that the instrument did not meet its metrological requirements and consequently, the exactitude of the measures might have been jeopardized, there should be a procedure detailing how to study the possible consequences and the corrective actions to be undertaken.

In fact, instruments need neither be calibrated nor be checked over their full range unless they are in fact used over all this range. It is sufficient to ensure that their calibration/verification covers the real process range.

When a group of instruments are connected together to measure a variable, this is known as an instrument loop. These loops should be tested and calibrated together in order to establish their overall performance.

Realization of Calibrations

When an instrument is handed over to be calibrated, it should be accompanied by a written form containing the following information:

- Identification of the instrument submitted for calibration (make, model, serial number/tag number)
- Information on calibration procedures or special instructions, as appropriate
- Statement of the calibration range
- Definition of the required calibration accuracy and failure limits

A calibrated instrument receives a "calibration certificate" containing the following information:

a) Identification of the calibration laboratory

- Name;
- Address;
- Metrological accreditation.

b) Identification of the certificate

- Number of certificate;
- Number of pages of the certificate;
- User (customer) identification;
- Date of the certificate.

c) Identification of the instrument which has been calibrated

- Information on the instrument (make, model, serial number);
- Required calibration accuracy and failure limits;
- Status following calibration (pass or fail).

d) Identification of the standard/test instruments used for the calibration

- Information on the instrument (make, model, serial number);
- Certificate of calibration traceable to recognized standards;
- Certified standards.

e) Information on the calibration

- Date of calibration;
- Environmental conditions during the calibration;

- Calibration range;
- Calibration procedure;
- Calibration results;
- Determination of uncertainty, indicating that the expanded uncertainty of the measure was obtained multiplying the typical uncertainty of the measure by the covering factor k=2 to obtain a level of confidence close to 95% for a normal distribution;
- Observations;
- Adjusting of the instrument (if it was needed and after customer approval);
- Signature of the responsible person.

After calibration, a label is fixed on the instrument, usually a green one, to show conformity. At least the date of calibration should appear on the label if the size of the equipment allows for it (it is also possible to stick the label on the case of the instrument). See Fig. (**12**).

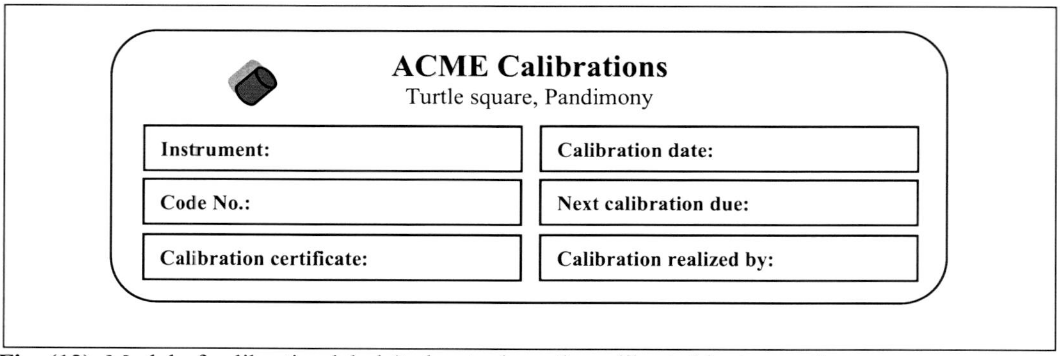

Fig. (12). Model of calibration label (to be stuck on the calibrated instrument).

Metrological Vigilance

Even if critical instruments are periodically calibrated, how is it possible to ensure that an instrument maintains its state of calibration during the length of time going from one calibration to the next one? Different approaches exist for doing this:

- Metrological redundancy: Comparison of critical measures obtained by two different instruments. When there is no coincidence this shows evidence of failure.

- Control of result coherence: Comparison of typical values (*e.g.* standard deviation) allows for the unveiling of anomalies.

- Vigilance standards: Periodical measures using reference standards allows for the detection of deviations. Thus, critical instruments, if possible, are regularly checked (verified) to ensure that they maintain their metrological qualities. Scales are typically checked with calibrated weights to verify that the registered weight falls within the expected range.

Metrological Management

The responsible person in charge of the metrological management should ensure:

- That instruments are adequately chosen to be apt for the appointed use,

- That instruments are controlled (identified, documented, stored, transported and personnel is trained, *etc.*),

- That they perform as required and that they are well maintained,

- That they are periodically calibrated or checked, as appropriate.

- Following a lifecycle model the following steps should be considered:

(1) <u>Analysis and definition of requirements</u>

The analysis of measuring requirements gives the definition of the instruments that should be acquired. In this case, the document of URS (User Requirements Specification) is usually very simple, just a template defining the variable to be measured, the principle of measure chosen, the type of instrument and its technical characteristics (measuring range, exactitude, accuracy, hysteresis, precision, resolution, effect of environmental conditions, data treatment, calibration, maintenance, servicing, *etc.*), and product contact parts (as appropriate).

(2) Instrument selection

Instrument manufacturers supply hand quotes according to the user's requirements. An instrument is chosen according to previous experience, external advice and price.

(3) Reception and first use of the instrument

As previously indicated, when receiving any new piece of equipment/instrument it should be submitted to admittance. In the particular case of measuring instruments the person responsible for metrology should ensure the following:

- confirmation of the supplied instrument (the instrument received corresponds to the order);
- assignment of a code, according to an unambiguous coding system;
- physical tagging by means of an indelible sticker;
- designation of the "the person technically responsible for the instrument";
- inscription of the instrument in the inventory of measuring instruments;
- drafting internal operating, cleaning/decontamination and maintenance instructions including calibration frequency and service measuring range;
- training the users of the instrument;
- keeping an instrument master file or master history record, containing all the documents related to it (URS, approved offer, order, delivery, certificate of calibration, operating and maintenance instructions, personnel training certificates, *etc.*);
- start of the log-book of the instrument.

There are several more or less computerized approaches and all are appropriate. There exist specific programs for metrological management too. These can be useful for big units or for companies with several units, wanting unified metrological management.

Experience shows that it is very useful to appoint a person to be technically responsible for each instrument. She/he cares for it and keeps its related documentation.

Instrument management can be computerized (by using special software or just self-made "Excel" or "Word" spreadsheets). However a classical file, containing all paper documentation, is usually still necessary. An instrument sheet containing all information concerning the instrument can be computerized too.

There should be a procedure in place ensuring that all instruments which do not satisfy requirements are taken out of service, duly labeled (an out of calibration label is attached) and that before being re-used, they are repaired, adjusted or calibrated, as necessary. A non-conformance documented investigation should be carried out, to determine the causes and to assess the consequences on the reliability of the processes and on the quality of the products.

(4) Maintenance

A distinction should be made between preventative maintenance and repairs. Routine preventative maintenance does not usually require calibration, whereas repairs usually do.

Metrological Documentation

Related to instrumentation/equipment, in general

- Coding procedure (premises, equipment and instruments)
- Instrument master files (master history records)
- Inventory of unit instruments
- Personnel education and training records
- Non-conformance procedure
- Log-book handling

Related to calibration, in particular

- Calibration methods and frequencies
- Annual calibration program
- Personnel education and training records

CONCLUDING REMARKS

In order to keep full control over processes the lifecycle model is very practical. It ensures that useful information will be preserved and that decisions will be based on knowledge. URS (user requirements specification) is a key document, which lays the foundations of any pharmaceutical project comprising premises, facilities and equipment. Then qualification is the tool that allows verifying that they work as anticipated and that the specified results are obtained. Qualification is essential for getting to know new pieces of equipment or systems. Afterwards it is necessary to keep the "state of qualification" by a regular program of maintenance, calibration and, when necessary, requalification. Equipment follow-up is very important for ensuring continued satisfactory performance.

CONFLICT OF INTEREST

The author confirms that this chapter contents have no conflict of interest.

ACKNOWLEDGEMENT

Declared None.

REFERENCES

[1] ICH (International Conference on Harmonisation of Technical Requirements for registration of Pharmaceuticals for Human Use). Quality Risk Management. Q9. ICH, Geneva, Switzerland 2005. 7.

[2] ISPE (International Society of Pharmaceutical Engineering). Good Engineering Practice. ISPE Good Practice Guide. ISPE, Tampa, Florida, USA 2008.

[3] PIC/S (Pharmaceutical Inspection Convention/Pharmaceutical Inspection Co-Operation Scheme). Validation Master Plan, Installation and Operational Qualification, Non-sterile Process Validation, Cleaning Validation. Recommendations PI 006-3. PIC/S, Geneva, Switzerland 2007.

[4] Ibid.

[5] ISPE (International Society of Pharmaceutical Engineering). Commissioning and qualification. ISPE Baseline Pharmaceutical Engineering Guides. ISPE, Tampa, Florida, USA 2001.

[6] WHO (World Health Organization). WHO Good manufacturing practices for pharmaceutical products: main principles. In: WHO Expert Committee on Specifications for Pharmaceutical Preparations. Forty-eighth report (WHO Technical Report Series, No. 986). WHO, Geneva, Switzerland 2014. Annex 2. Glossary.

[7] PIC/S (Pharmaceutical Inspection Convention. Pharmaceutical Inspection Co-Operation Scheme). Qualification and validation. In: Good Manufacturing Practice for Medicinal Products. Guide PE 009-11. PIC/S, Geneva, Switzerland 2014. Annex 15. Glossary.
[8] WHO (World Health Organization). WHO Good manufacturing practices for pharmaceutical products: main principles. In: WHO Expert Committee on Specifications for Pharmaceutical Preparations. Forty-eighth report (WHO Technical Report Series, No. 986). WHO, Geneva, Switzerland 2014. Annex 2. Glossary.
[9] Ibid. 4.2.
[10] PIC/S (Pharmaceutical Inspection Convention. Pharmaceutical Inspection Co-Operation Scheme). Qualification and validation. In: Good Manufacturing Practice for Medicinal Products. Guide PE 009-11. PIC/S, Geneva, Switzerland 2014. Annex 15. 6.
[11] WHO (World Health Organisation). Supplementary guidelines on good manufacturing practices for heating, ventilation and air-conditioning systems for non-sterile pharmaceutical dosage forms. In: WHO Expert Committee on Specifications for Pharmaceutical Preparations. Fortieth report (WHO Technical Report Series, No. 937). WHO, Geneva, Switzerland 2006. Annex 2. 3. Glossary.
[12] PIC/S (Pharmaceutical Inspection Convention/Pharmaceutical Inspection Co-Operation Scheme). Validation Master Plan, Installation and Operational Qualification, Non-sterile Process Validation, Cleaning Validation. Recommendations PI 006-3. PIC/S, Geneva, Switzerland 2007. 8. Glossary.
[13] PIC/S (Pharmaceutical Inspection Convention. Pharmaceutical Inspection Co-Operation Scheme). Qualification and validation. In: Good Manufacturing Practice for Medicinal Products. Guide PE 009-11. PIC/S, Geneva, Switzerland 2014. Annex 15. 7.
[14] Ibid. 8.
[15] WHO (World Health Organisation). Supplementary guidelines on good manufacturing practices: validation. In: WHO Expert Committee on Specifications for Pharmaceutical Preparations. Fortieth report (WHO Technical Report Series, No. 937). WHO, Geneva, Switzerland 2006. Annex 4 (Appendix 6: Qualification of systems and equipment).
[16] Ibid. Glossary.
[17] Ibid. 18.
[18] US National Archives & Records Administration – Federal Register: Code of Federal Regulations (CFR) – Title 21 (Food & drugs): 21 CFR 211.67.a.
[19] ISPE (International Society of Pharmaceutical Engineering). Maintenance. Good practice guide. ISPE, Tampa, Florida, USA 2009.
[20] ISPE (International Society of Pharmaceutical Engineering). A risk-based approach to calibration management. GAMP guidance document. Second edition. ISPE, Tampa, Florida, USA 2010.

Chapter 3: Risk Management

CHAPTER 3

Risk Management

Abstract: The quality of pharmaceutical products is permanently threatened by hazards that are potential sources of harm. And hazards have an associated risk, defined as the combination of the probability of occurrence and of the severity of that harm. Therefore, it is necessary to keep these hazards under control by diminishing as much as possible the related risks. This approach to quality assurance is known as risk management. Different tools allow for the assessment of risk. Then, risk can be routinely monitored. Yet, there are no magic tools. Risk assessment requires a good amount of knowledge on the matter submitted to study. This does not exclude, however, that by skillfully using the existing tools it is possible to appraise adequately the level of risk and decide on its acceptance. A high residual risk is, in principle, inacceptable and requires the implementation of measures for its reduction (changes in the process or system or in the way it is monitored), whereas a low residual risk can be accepted. And this allows for the introduction of continual improvement, understood as the progressive diminution of the residual risk level. The whole process of risk management is explained step by step and the most useful tools used in risk assessment are described providing practical examples.

Keywords: Cpk, Fishbone diagram, FMECA, FTA, HACCP, Hazard, HAZOP, histogram, Pareto chart, PHA, process capability, risk, risk assessment, risk communication, risk control, risk monitoring, risk review, RRF, specific tools, unspecific tools.

INTRODUCTION TO RISK MANAGEMENT

Risk management designates an approach to the organization and monitoring of items (premises, facilities, processes, *etc.*) that analyzes the risks which might put in danger their reliability with the aim of applying corrective and preventive measures for ensuring that reliability will be maintained.

An anecdote can help us to understand why risk management is advantageous: Many years ago, we were in the Pyrenees and we wanted to visit a small and secluded glacier lake high up in the mountains. The dirt track leading there was steep and in bad condition. Consequently, we decided to rent a powerful Land Rover adapted to the harsh conditions of our excursion. To our great surprise when we reached the lake we saw a small city car parked beside it. Our Land Rover driver could not refrain from complimenting the proprietary of the car for being so bold as to drive there with such a kind of car. I have always remembered the answer he gave. "You know. This is not a question of boldness, but of sheer ignorance".

Jordi Botet

This story reminds us of an approach that we had in the past, pharmaceutical industry included, which ignored formal risk management.

Pharmaceutical products have to be safe and meet approved requirements or, said in other words, they have to posses the purported quality. This was and is out of discussion. Notwithstanding that, different types of "hazards" (contamination, degradation and error or mix-up) loom during their manufacturing and distribution processes and put quality at stake. Thus, if we have to manufacture quality products, we are bound to know and understand these "hazards" in order to take measures to keep them under control. This approach has been fully incorporated into GMP by the WHO [1] and by the ICH [2], which means adoption by the USA, Japan, and Europe (incorporated as Annex 20 to European GMP) [3].

A "hazard" is *a potential source of harm* and "harm" can be defined as *damage to health, including the damage that can occur from loss of product quality or availability*. Then, "risk" is *the combination of the probability of occurrence of harm and the severity of that harm* [4]. See Fig. (**1**).

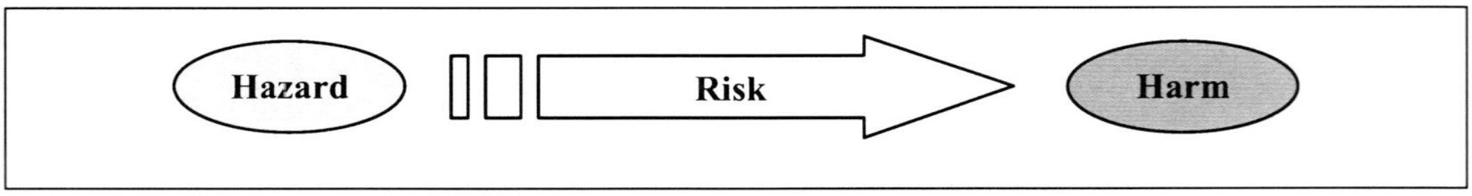

Fig. (1). Relations between hazard and harm.

In our everyday's life we often talk about "risk" and, unconsciously, we apply this definition. Thus, we say that a given activity is risky because we estimate that there is a significant possibility of being seriously injured. Or we do not want to go on board of a very old and rusty aircraft, whereas we might happily seat in a brand-new airplane. The reason is clear: although the severity of an accident might be about the same, its probability seems to be much higher in the first case!

Medicinal products supplied to patients have to correspond exactly to the marketing authorization and possess the purported quality, but as we are bound to accept that the quality of products and processes is always at risk (because hazards are ordinarily there, independently from our wishes), it is evident that we have to manage that risk. Risk management is *the systematic application of quality management policies, procedures, and practices to the tasks of assessing, controlling, communicating and reviewing risk* [5].

Therefore, risk management is a methodical and cyclical process (Fig. **2**) that starts by identifying the hazards and assessing their risk. Then, once the risk is known, it is necessary to decide if it is acceptable or not. If the answer is negative that means that either we modify things in order to reduce the risk or we have to stop what we are doing. If the answer is positive, than we have to put into practice measures for keeping it under control. The accepted risk can be communicated to third parts (*e.g.* inspectors, clients) and submitted to periodic revision to see if it can be further reduced by applying improved procedures.

Risk management can be applied both to production and to supporting processes.

Let us then see risk management in detail.

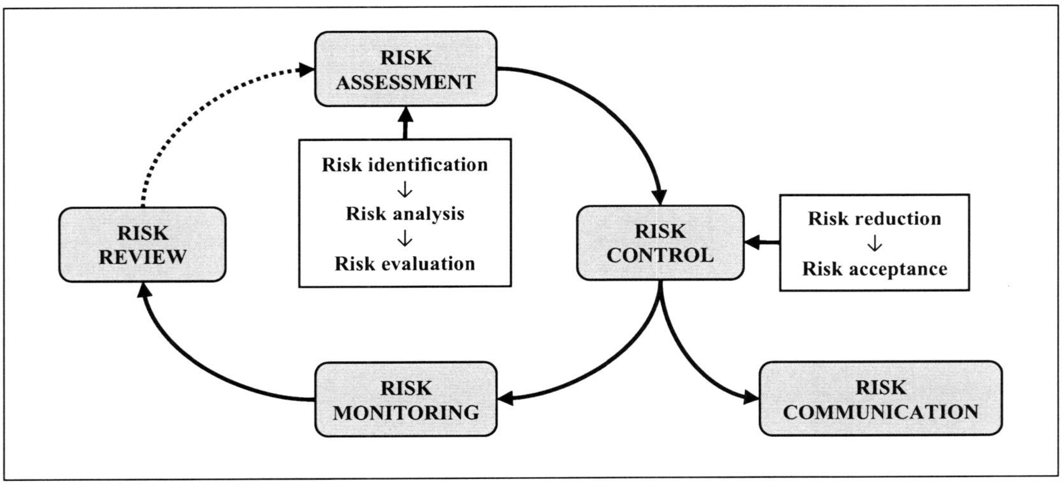

Fig. (2). Risk management stages.

Risk Assessment

Risk assessment is a systematic process of organizing information to support a risk decision to be made within a risk management process. It consists of the identification of hazards and the analysis and evaluation of risks associated with exposure to those hazards [6].

Before starting any risk assessment it is necessary to have a well-framed process, where its inputs, outputs and stages are well known. A detailed flowchart is essential for doing this. Then, in a first step, it is possible to detect the hazards and their causes and effects (harms) and, in a second one, risk can be assessed.

This is an important bottleneck, because there is not always sufficient information at disposal. If this is the case, it is evident that our assessment will just be tentative and subject to further improvement when more information will be available. It has to be born in mind that the accuracy of a risk assessment is directly related to the level of available information. Neither using the best analytical tools, nor being an expert in risk assessment will fill up this gap. Anyway, a teamwork with experts on different disciplines and some amount of experience will go a long way towards doing an accurate risk assessment (here accurate should be understood as "as best as possible").

In a practical way, it is possible to divide risk assessment into three activities:

Risk identification: *The systematic use of information to identify potential sources of harm (hazards) referring to the risk question or problem description.*

Risk identification addresses the "What might go wrong?" question, including identifying the possible consequences [7].

Risk analysis: *The estimation of risk associated with the identified hazards.*

Risk evaluation: *The comparison of the estimated risk to given risk criteria using a quantitative or qualitative scale to determine the significance of the risk* [8].

Risk Control

The purpose of risk control is to reduce the risk to an acceptable level. The amount of effort used for risk control should be proportional to the significance of the risk. Decision makers might use different processes, including benefit-cost analysis, for understanding the optimal level of risk control. Risk control might focus on the following questions:

- *Is the risk above an acceptable level?*
- *What can be done to reduce or eliminate risks?*
- *What is the appropriate balance among benefits, risks and resources?*
- *Are new risks introduced as a result of the identified risks being controlled?* [9]

Risk acceptance is the decision to accept risk, whereas risk reduction is defined as the actions taken to lessen the probability of occurrence of harm and the severity of that harm [10].

It is evident that what really matters is not just detecting hazards and evaluating their risk but deciding if they are acceptable or not and consequently, in the first case, controlling them and, in the second, attempting to reduce them. Risk reduction can be achieved by introducing changes in the process, in the product or in the monitoring strategy. These changes, however, may appear impossible, because of technical or regulatory reasons; then, the product or the process should be abandoned because risk is bigger than its advantages. See Fig. (**3**).

As we are going to see later in this chapter the determination of risk is not a straightforward process. Often the lack of precise information turns inaccurate the evaluation of risk. Then, it might be objected that its acceptance is inacceptable, but this is forgetting that the main advantage of risk management is less assessing accurately risk than knowing and appraising hazards and applying control measures for them. Again, the anecdote of the small city car that went to the mountain lake can be useful. Even if the exact estimation of the risk should had been difficult, it should had been possible to understand that the advantage of going independently to the lake was clearly outweighed by the sheer possibility of breaking the car and that paying for a Land Rover excursion was a practical and effective hazard control (and consequently, risk reduction) measure.

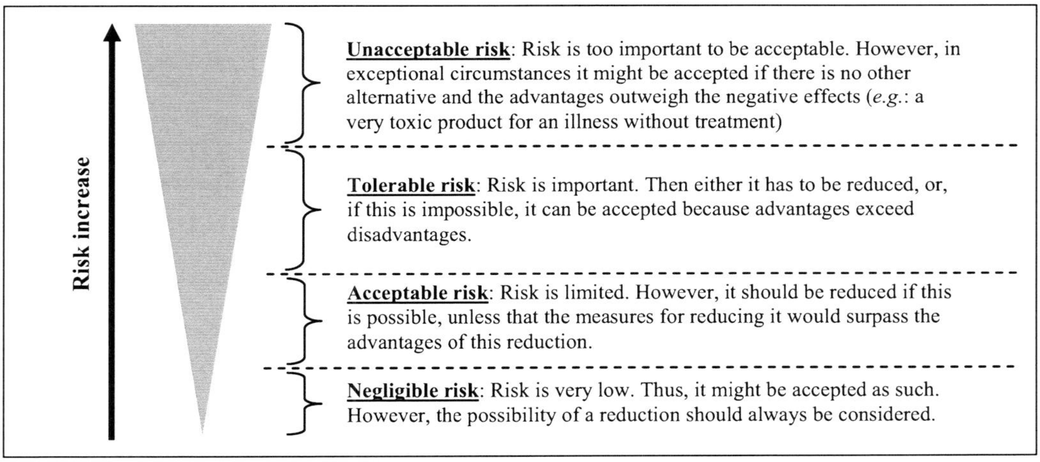

Fig. (3). Risk levels and their significance.

Risk Communication

Once risk is known and accepted it can be communicated. Risk communication is *the sharing of information about risk and risk management between the decision maker and other stakeholders. Parties can communicate at any stage of the risk management process. The output/result of the quality risk management process should be appropriately communicated and documented. Communications might include those among interested parties; e.g. regulators and industry, industry and the patient, within a company, industry or regulatory authority, etc. The included information might relate to the existence, nature, form, probability, severity, acceptability, control, treatment, detectability or other aspects of risks to quality* [11].

Risk Monitoring

Once a level of risk has been accepted and communicated, the corresponding process can be performed taking into account the necessary measures for keeping the hazards and their related level of risk under control. In fact usually is not the hazard itself which is monitored but the selected process attributes or parameters. While they remain within the established acceptance ranges and do not show tendencies towards a deviation, the process can be considered under control and this includes the hazards and their risk levels.

Risk monitoring supplies the necessary information to realize the risk review.

Risk Review

Risk management is a never-ending process. Manufacturing procedures may change because of voluntary controlled changes, but also because trends detected by monitoring dictate such changes or because new technologies can alter the suppositions under which the risk assessment was performed. This is precisely what we understand by "continual improvement", a better hazard control and the reduction of the risk associated to our process.

The output/results of the risk management process should be reviewed to take into account new knowledge and experience. Once a quality risk management process has been initiated, that process should continue to be utilized for events that might impact the original quality risk management decision, whether these events are planned (e.g., results of product review, inspections, audits, change control) or unplanned (e.g., root cause from failure investigations, recall). The frequency of any review should be based upon the level of risk. Risk review might include reconsideration of risk acceptance decisions [12].

PRACTICAL ORGANIZATION OF RISK MANAGEMENT

Fig. (**4**) summarizes the practical approach to risk management.

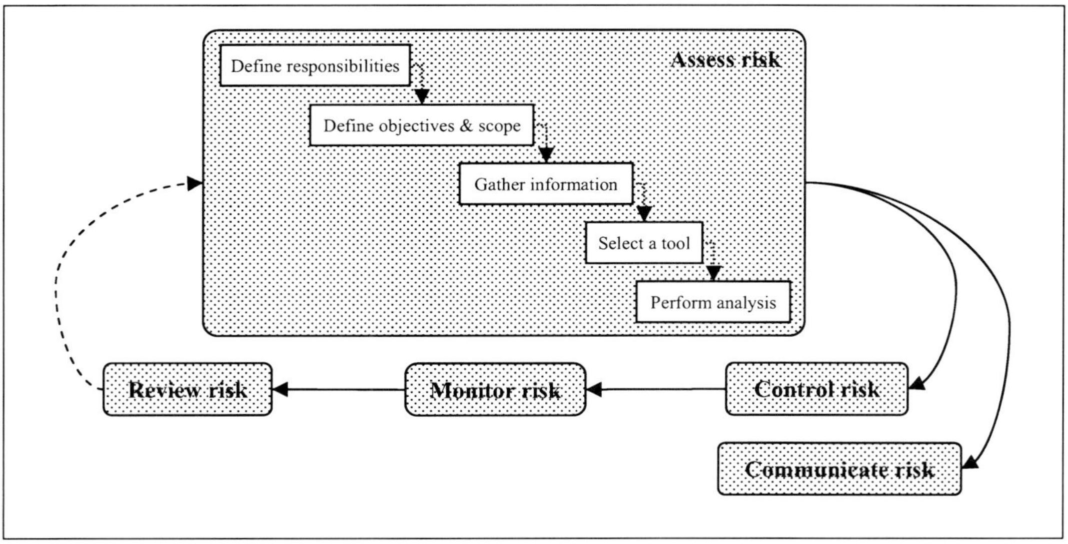

Fig. (4). Risk management implementation cycle.

Assess Risk

Define Responsibilities

This step could be described as "appointment of a task force" because risk assessment requires a good knowledge of the item being assessed and it is normally understood that this requires the intervention of several specialists. Although this is the desirable approach in most cases it is not possible and the responsibility for developing risk assessment is given to a single person. In this case the technician who is selected for this task requires a minimal amount of knowledge and experience. But even if there is not a task force it is always necessary consulting with other technicians, inside and outside of the unit, in order to improve knowledge.

Define Objectives and Scope

Everyone who has performed risk assessment knows of the menace of getting lost in a jungle of data. This can be avoided if before starting any assessment its objectives and scope are exactly defined.

It is necessary to know the limits, inputs and outputs of the item submitted to analysis and then decide what will be included in the assessment and what will not. It is also indispensable to state clearly which is the intent of the analysis (*e.g.* detect failure modes, detect quality hazards, quantify risks, *etc.*).

Gather Information

It is evident that in order to assess anything it is necessary to get acquainted with it. In practice as a baseline this usually means preparing a flowchart (or revising an already existing one). This flowchart should divide the process into manageable steps. Besides, any complementary information should be welcome (*e.g.* diagrams, use and maintenance instructions, procedures, *etc.*).

Select a Tool

Concerning the big question of how to perform risk assessment there are good and bad news. Good news is that there are several risk analysis tools, but bad news is that these tools are just effective if you possess all the necessary information and you do not consider them a kind of magic potion. Here, the analyzer is much more important than the analysis tool.

Admittedly, risk analysis tools are not wonder tools giving us unknown information, but they facilitate the structured arrangement and comprehension of the information that we already have.

What really matters with these tools is that they help in detecting and assessing the risks. This is why in most cases they can be freely used and adapted to particular needs. Remaining as close to procedures as officially described in technical literature may only be important for comparative purposes.

The selection of particular risk management tools is completely dependent upon specific facts and circumstances [13].

It is neither always appropriate nor always necessary to use a formal risk management process (using recognized tools and/or internal procedures e.g. standard operating procedures). The use of informal risk management processes (using empirical tools and/or internal procedures) can also be considered acceptable. Appropriate use of quality risk management can facilitate but does not obviate industry's obligation to comply with regulatory requirements and does not replace appropriate communications between industry and regulators [14].

There is no perfect tool; each one has its advantages and limitations. Therefore, it is possible and often desirable to combine different tools to achieve better results.

A tool is chosen taking into account the amount of information available, the goal to achieve and the level of formality desired. In case of possessing limited knowledge or performing a preliminary assessment unspecific tools may suffice, but usually a specific tool will be selected (Fig. **5**). Some remarks may help:

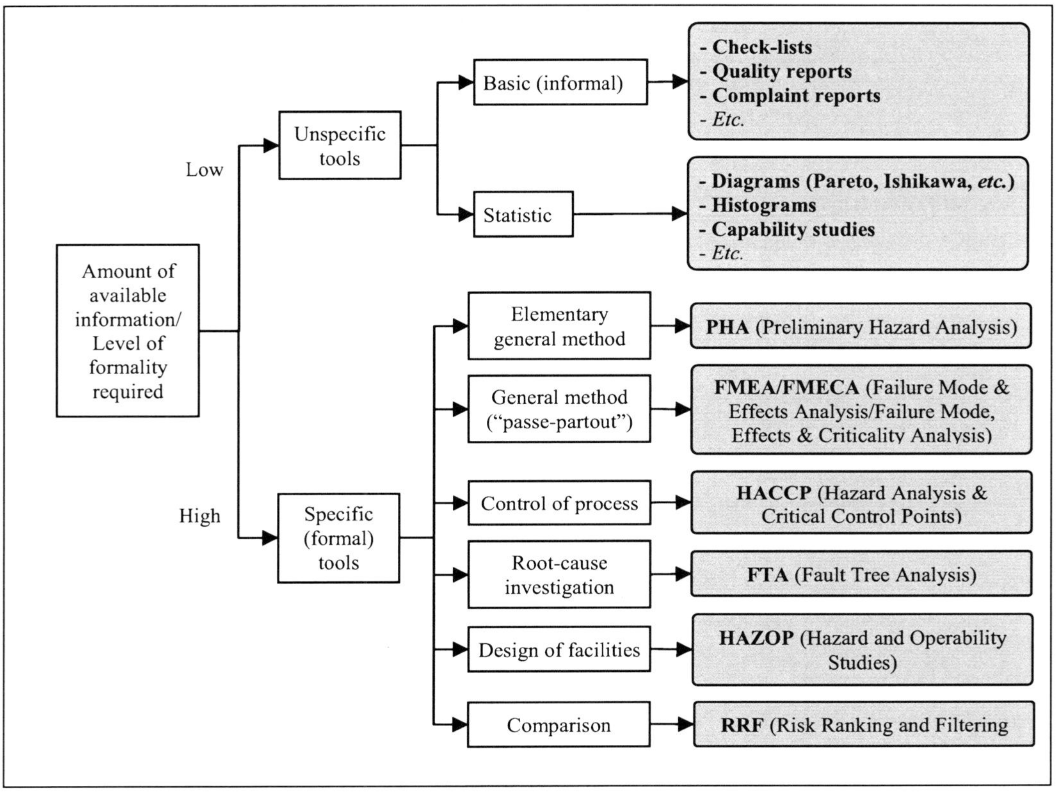

Fig. (5). Tentative classification of the most common tools used for risk assessment.

1st Unspecific tools are always useful as a complement of specific tools;

2nd Specific tools are not exclusive. As they use different approaches it is possible to use more than one tool at the same time in order to get a wider view.

3rd If, upon implementation, the tool which was chosen appears not very appropriate, it can be easily changed. In fact, usually a change of tool just supposes restructuring the information that had been gathered.

4th It has to be decided whether the assessment will be limited to the appraisal of hazards or risks will be estimated, either qualitatively or quantitatively.

Perform Analysis

Each tool has its own approach and way of handling data. See below.

Although experience in risk assessment goes a long way towards getting a proficient analysis, it is usually necessary to spare some reflection time. Once that a draft of the assessment is ready it is left for a certain time "lying fallow" (as far as this is possible) and then reviewed and modified until getting a fully satisfactory result. Review by other technicians is also highly advisable.

It has to be kept in mind that a risk assessment has to be logical (remember that tools just help in organizing information, but do not change it; thus, if information was correct the outcome should be right too). If it does not appear as such it means that there is something wrong with it and has to be carefully reviewed.

Control Risk

Once the existing level of risk in the process is known it is necessary to decide if it is sufficiently low and, thus, it can be accepted or if it has to be additionally reduced (by process modification, by introduction or improvement of the existing controls, by fostering personnel training, *etc.*). After any modification it is necessary to review the risk assessment taking into account the new situation and deciding again if the residual risk can be accepted.

Although each case is different and requires a particular study, it is possible to follow this approach:

- Final risk estimation: High. This risk cannot be accepted and has to be reduced.

- Final risk estimation: Medium. This risk can be only provisionally accepted supposing that it cannot be reduced. Additional control measures should be introduced and after a given period of time (*e.g.* six or twelve months) the risk assessment should be reviewed in order to find ways for reducing risk.

- Final risk estimation: Low. Risk can be accepted. However, in future revisions it should be intended to reduce risk as far as possible.

Then, once the risk assessment is finished and the residual risk is accepted a report can be prepared.

Communicate Risk

As described before, the outcome of the risk assessment can be communicated.

Monitor Risk

Risk should be one of the elements to be monitored routinely for ensuring that the rationale used during the risk assessment was correct and remains such.

Review Risk

This is both an element of risk management and of continual improvement. It is evident that if monitoring shows any problem it is necessary to think of reviewing risk. But even if monitoring follow-up does not show any problem a periodic risk review is necessary (*e.g.* 3-5 years, depending on the criticality of the process) in order to verify its correctness and diminish the risk level as far as possible.

RISK ASSESSMENT TOOLS

Unspecific Tools

As risk assessment is based on gathering and analyzing information, any type of structured information (*e.g.* check-lists, quality reports, complaint reports, *etc.*) can be used in order to improve the knowledge on the hazards of a process and their associated risks. The statistical treatment of data provides more information on the situation and is always welcome for a better appraisal.

Cause and Effect Diagrams

These diagrams analyze problems and causes systematically. They are also known as fishbone diagrams, due to their graphical form, and as Ishikawa diagrams in honor of Kaoru Ishikawa who developed them.

To build a cause and effect diagram it is necessary to define and determine the problem to be analyzed. The most relevant factors are then identified and finally the causes and sub-causes of the factors are named. See Fig. (**6**).

They are useful because they allow the association of multiple possible causes with a single effect.

Histograms

Histograms are diagrams that represent the relative frequency of data occurrence. Collected data on parameters can be converted into histograms by following these steps (Table **1**):

- Define the cell intervals by establishing their boundaries. Cell intervals have to possess equal width. Upper and lower limits of a cell should represent the maximal and minimal values for this interval. Boundaries should preferably lie between possible values and a given value can only be placed in a given cell.

- If there is a known target value then it should be placed in the middle of a cell interval.

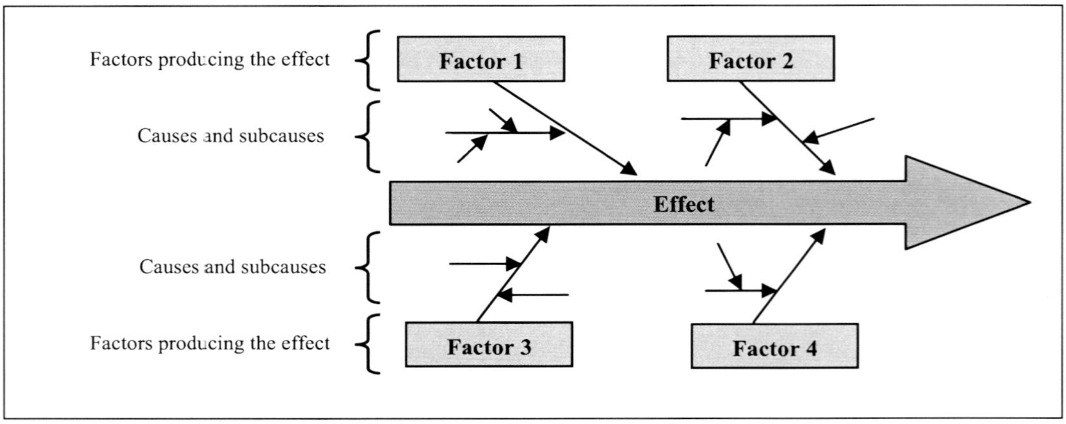

Fig. (6). Cause and effect diagram or Ishikawa diagram or Fishbone diagram.

- Determine the number of cells. There are different rules for determining it, for instance, the square root of the number of data (N) or 1 + log N/0.3.

- In practice, it is not usually convenient to have more than 10 cells.

- Group the data into intervals and determine their frequency (amount of data per cell interval).

- Draw cell boundaries on the horizontal X-axis. It is not necessary to take the origin as zero.

- Draw the scale of frequencies on the vertical Y-axis. In this case, it is necessary to take the origin as zero.

- Plot the cells.

Table 1. Histogram.

Cell boundary	**Middle point (U_l + L_l/2)**	**Tally**	**Frequency**	
30-34	**32**	**II**	**2**	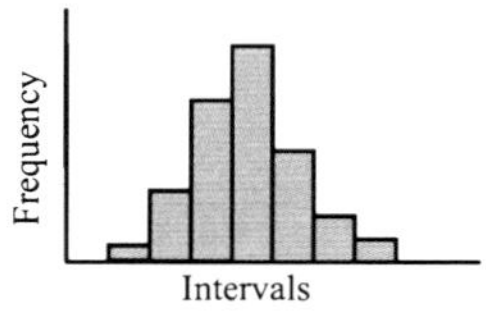
35-39	**37**	**HH II**	**7**	
40-44	**42**	**HHHHHHHH**	**15**	
45-49	**47**	**HHHHHHHHHHH**	**20**	
50-54	**52**	**HHHHH II**	**12**	
55-59	**57**	**HH**	**5**	
60-64	**62**	**III**	**3**	

Pareto Charts

Pareto charts are based on the 80/20 rule, established by the Italian economist Vilfredo Pareto, which states that in many distributions 80% of the situations arise from just 20% of the causes. Thus, by arranging the data according to priority or importance, it is easy to distinguish between the important few and the insignificant many. A Pareto chart (Fig. **7**) is prepared by (Table **2**):

(a) Listing all the elements (in the example, all the causes of failure) and determining their frequencies.

Table 2. Pareto chart.

(a) Listing			**(b) Ranking**			
Element (cause of failure)	**Tally**	**Frequency**	**Element** (cause of failure)	**Frequency**	**Cumulative frequency**	**% of total**
G	HHHHHHHH IIII	19	A	60	60	20.6
C	HHHHHHHHHHHHHHHHHHHHHHHHHH III	48	B	55	115	39.5
H	HHHHH II	12	C	48	163	56.0
D	HHHHHHHHHHHHHHHHHHHH IIII	39	D	39	202	69.4
F	HHHHHHHHHH IIII	24	E	28	230	79.0
A	HHHHHHHHHHHHHHHHHHHHHHHHHHHHHH HHHHHH	60	F	24	254	87.3
I	HH I	6	G	19	273	93.8
B	HHHHHHHHHHHHHHHHHHHHHHHHHHHHHH HH	55	H	12	285	97.9
E	HHHHHHHHHHHHHH III	28	I	6	291	100.0

(b) Ranking the elements and creating cumulative distributions.

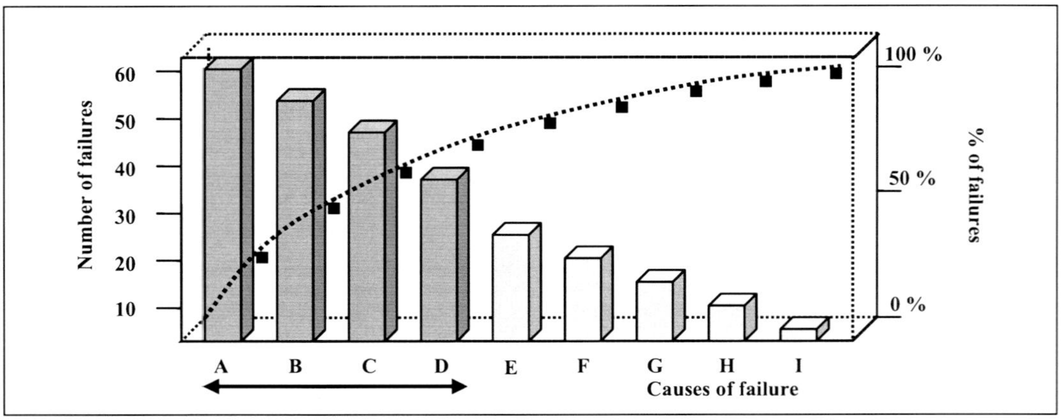

Fig. (7). Pareto chart.

Capability Studies

When measuring process variables, individual measures tend to differ one from another. This is why measurable variables should have a target value and an acceptance range, defined usually between two specification limits (upper and lower). These differences are known as variability, which is inherent to any process.

When a continuous variable is monitored, it will usually be distributed about a mean or average. If its values are plotted they will show a bell-shaped arc known as normal curve or Gaussian distribution. This curve is characterized by its mean value, which defines its centre, and by the standard deviation (σ – sigma), which defines its shape. The bell-shaped curve is wider as values are more scattered (standard deviation increases). For a normal curve 68.3% of values fall within ± 1 standard deviation of the average, 95.4% within ± 2 standard deviations and 99.73% within ± 3 standard deviations. See Fig. (**8**).

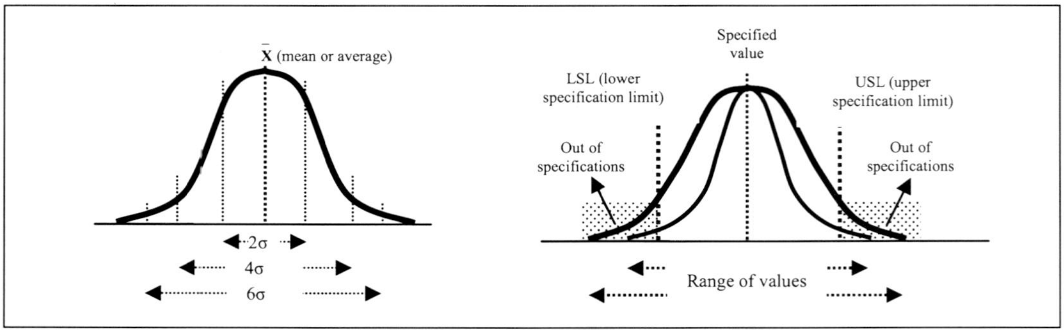

Fig. (8). Normal curve.

Ideally the average value obtained for a variable (parameter) of a given process should be centered, that is to say, close to the target value, and the scattering of its values should be less than the specified process range. This would ensure that the values of this parameter fall within the specified range. See Fig. (**9**).

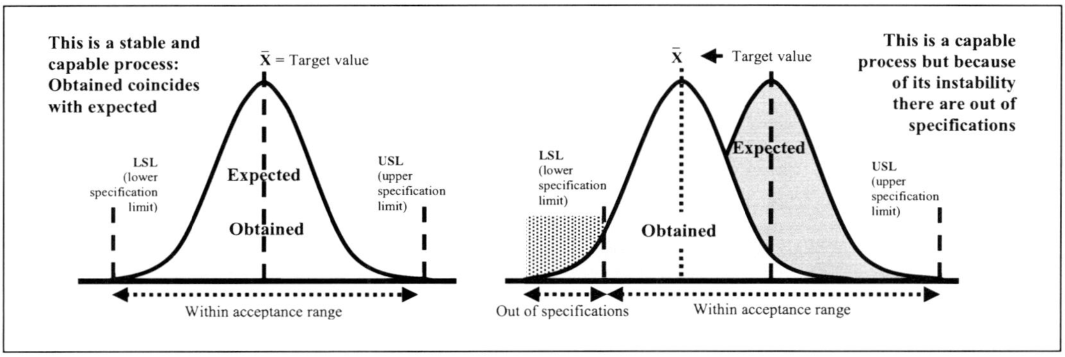

Fig. (9). Process capability.

Throughout the process, the average can shift (non-centered mean) resulting in an unstable (out of control) process. Besides, the variation around the average can be so great that some values exceed the specification limits (too scattered values) resulting in a not capable process. Therefore, it is necessary to achieve stable and capable processes, possessing a centered average on the target value and a reduced standard deviation or, in other words, processes showing a limited variation and therefore a consistent level of performance. Process capability is the repeatability and consistency of a process in relation to its requirements (specification limits). Thus, process capability is a measure of the degree to which a process is or is not meeting its requirements.

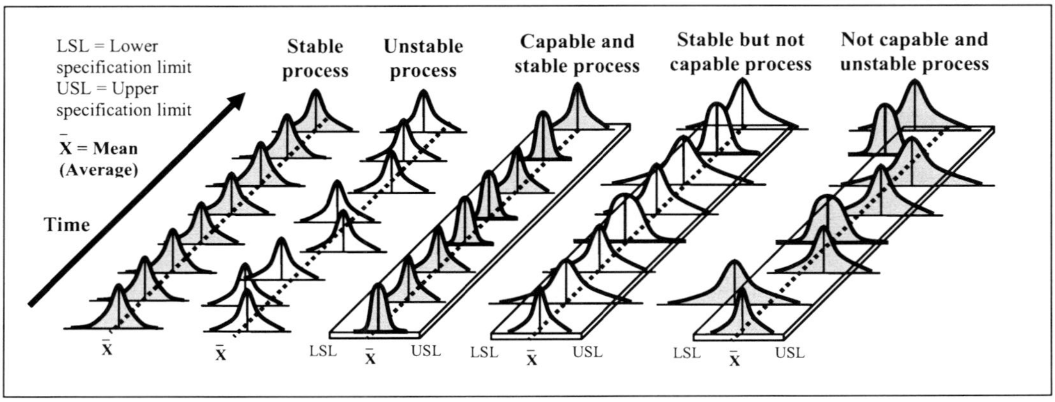

Fig. (10). Process stability and capability.

Process capability can be expressed with capability indices, which compare the distribution of a process in relation to the specification limits and they determine if the process is capable of meeting established specifications. The most commonly used capability indices are Cp and Cpk. If acceptable values are obtained, the process consistently produces a product that meets the specification limits. See Fig. (**10**).

Cp

If we take for granted that the mean of the process is centered on the target value, it is possible to use the Cp (process capability index). Cp is a simple process capability index that relates the acceptable distribution of the specification limits (range) to the measure of the variation of the process, represented by 6σ, where sigma is the estimated process standard deviation. The capacity index (Cp) indicates if 99.7% of the values of the studied characteristic are within the interval mean ± 6σ. This requires a Cp higher than 1. If the process is in statistical control, and the process mean is centered on the target, then Cp can be calculated as follows: Cp = (USL - LSL)/6σ. See Fig. (**11**).

$$C_p = \frac{\text{Allowable process spread}}{\text{Actual process spread}} = \frac{\text{USL - LSL}}{6\sigma}$$

Process mean (average) is centered on the target

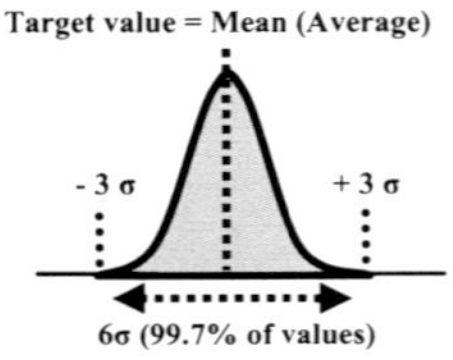

Fig. (11). Capability studies: Simple capability index (Cp).

Cp<1 means that the process variation exceeds specification, and therefore a significant number of out of specifications appear.

Cp=1 means that the process is merely meeting specifications. A minimum of 0.3% out of specifications will be made and more if the process is not centered.

Cp>1 means that the process variation is less than the specification, however, out of specifications might be made if the process is not centered on the target value. While Cp relates the spread of the process relative to the specified range, it does not take into account how close to the target value is the process average. This is why Cp is sometimes considered as process "potential"

Cpk

The Cpk index measures not only the process variation in relation to its specified limits, but it also considers the deviation of the process mean.

Cpl = (Mean – LSL)/3σ. Cpu = (USL – Mean)/3σ. Cpk is taken as the smaller of either Cpl or Cpu. See Fig. (**12**).

$$C_{pk} = \text{Minor of} \begin{cases} C_{pu} = \dfrac{USL - \bar{X}}{3\sigma} \\ C_{pl} = \dfrac{\bar{X} - LSL}{3\sigma} \end{cases}$$

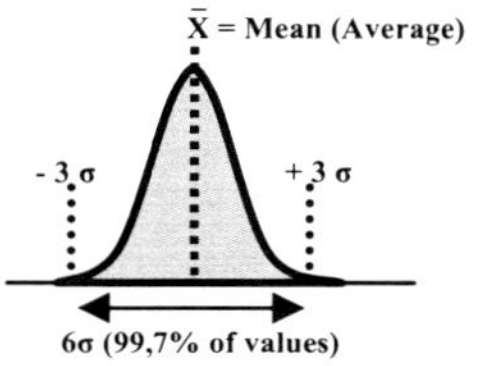

Fig. (12). Capability studies: Process capability index (Cpk)

Cpk values may start with 1.67 and have an expected goal of 2.0.

Process performance studies are performed to identify how well a process performs in the long run (at least one week). Two types of variation within the process are statistically measured: variation within subgroups and variation between these subgroups. They should include any likely factor of variability (*e.g.* different operators or materials, changes of configuration, machine adjustment, *etc.*). A successful evaluation of the performance of a process requires collecting data over an extensive period of time operating under normal conditions.

Specific Tools

These are tools specifically devised in order to perform risk assessment. They are very diverse as varied are situations and goals.

PHA

Preliminary Hazard Analysis (PHA) is a qualitative tool used to identify and reduce or control hazards in new or modified processes. It is mainly used to analyze a project during its initial phases, while there is limited information at disposal. PHA is developed by brainstorming of a group of experts who determine and analyze possible hazards and their causes and consequences, compare different options, and propose control measures. Although there is not a definite way of performing all this, it is possible to use checklists, lists with the characteristics of the product (quality, strength, purity, identity, *etc.*), lists with the stages of the process (mixing, granulation, *etc.*), or lists with the types of operation (starting, maintenance, normal/abnormal, cleaning, *etc.*) to facilitate analysis. When assessing production facilities or operations it has been very useful analyzing the causes and consequences of five possible types of quality hazards: (outer) contamination, cross-contamination, environmental contamination, error/mix up, and product degradation. In practice a

PHA brainstorming is realized by means of questions: Which are the hazards? What will happen if it appears this problem? What will happen if there is an alternative situation? *Etc.* [15]

In order to be able to ask questions it is necessary to have a flow chart of the process or a diagram of the concerned facilities. The goal of PHA is having a good understanding of the hazards which may jeopardize the quality of the products and either modify things in order to diminish or eliminate these hazards or provide methods for controlling them.

Results can be expressed as shown in Table **3**.

Table 3. Example of PHA table.

Stage	Hazard	Cause of exposition to hazard	Effect of exposition to hazard	Are control measures necessary?	Control measures implemented
				□ Yes/□ No	
				□ Yes/□ No	
				□ Yes/□ No	
				□ Yes/□ No	

It is worth commenting that in some cases it is not necessary to have a column describing effects because they are limited to something like "product out of specifications".

Results can also be shown in a flow chart with analysis of hazards (Fig. **13**).

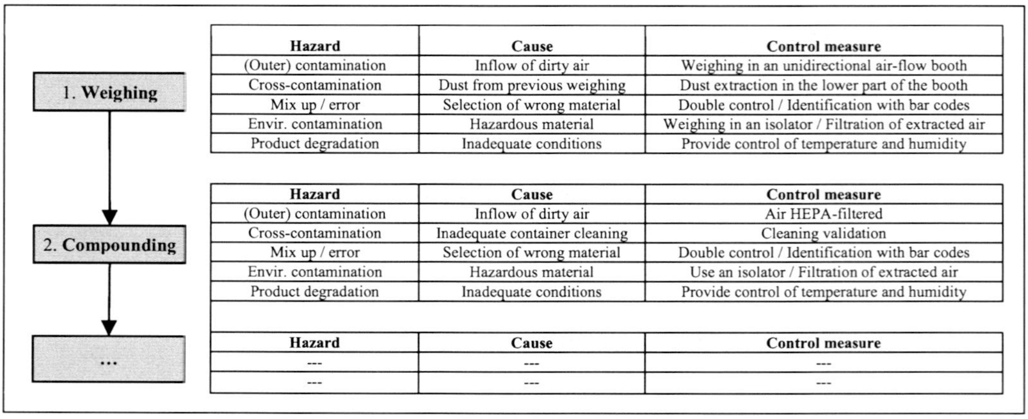

Fig. (13). Example of PHA flow-chart.

When hazards have been identified and analyzed and there is a better knowledge and understanding of the process or system it is possible to evaluate risk following the procedure described below for FMECA (assessment of probability, seriousness and detection in order to calculate the risk prioritization). In this case, instead of PHA it is spoken of PRA (primary risk analysis). See Table **4**.

Table 4. Example of PRA table.

Stage	Hazard	Cause	Effect	P	S	D	Risk prioritization

FMEA

Failure Mode & Effects Analysis (FMEA) is a tool that analyses a system or process to identify the potential failure modes, the causes of these failures and their probable effects [16]. FMEA can be extended to appraise risk and then it is known as FMECA. See below for information about how to use FMEA.

FMECA

Failure Mode, Effects and Criticality Analysis (FMECA) is a qualitative or quantitative tool that analyzes failure modes in terms of their severity, probability and ability to detect the malfunction mode (Fig. **14**). FMECA can be applied when the process to be analyzed is well known.

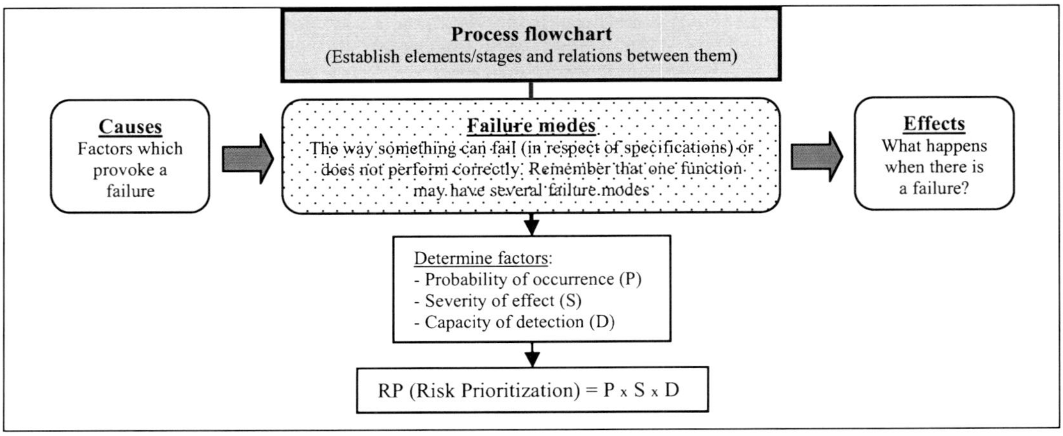

Fig. (14). FMECA approach.

The probability of occurrence (P) of a failure mode, also known as "frequency coefficient" (F), is in fact composed of two events, P_1 (probability of the cause that provokes the failure mode) and P_2 (probability of the event). Thus P (or F) = P_1 x P_2. The practical estimation of these probabilities is not an easy task, often they are given a certain value according to experience and then this value is adjusted as more experience is acquired. The severity of the effect (S) of a failure mode is an estimation of the damage caused by the appearance of the failure mode. That is to say, *a measure of the possible consequences of a hazard* [17].

The detectability or ability of detection (D) of a failure mode is an estimation of the capacity of discovering it when it occurs. It is important to point out that the ability of detection is an "inverse" factor, because the higher the detectability, the lower the score. It can also be expressed as "difficulty of detection", being then a factor like the others, the higher the difficulty of detection, the higher the score. That is to say, *the ability to discover or determine the existence, presence, or fact of a hazard* [18]. These three factors can be evaluated qualitatively or quantitatively in different levels or scales.

Qualitatively

A common qualitative estimation distinguishes three levels ("high", "medium" and "low"), as in Table **5**, but also more levels can be considered.

Table 5. Example of qualitative evaluation in three levels.

Evaluation	PROBABILITY	SEVERITY	DIFFICULTY OF DETECTION
High	The failure/accident occurs **frequently**	The consequences of the failure/accident are **important**	The failure/accident **will very likely not be detected**
Medium	The failure/accident occurs **periodically**	The consequences of the failure/accident are **moderate**	The failure/accident **might be detected**
Low	The failure/accident occurs **rarely**	The consequences of the failure/accident are **low**	The failure/accident **will very likely be detected**

Thus, adding "extreme" we would have four levels. And finally, a five level evaluation could be, for example (Table **6**), estimated as follows:

- Probability of occurrence (P) as "unlikely", "remote", "occasional", "repeated", and "inevitable";
- Severity of the effect (S) as "none", "minor", "low", "moderate", and "high";

- Detectability (D) as "almost certain", "high", "moderate", "low" and "remote".

Table 6. Example of qualitative evaluation in five levels.

Evaluation	PROBABILITY	SEVERITY	DIFFICULTY OF DETECTION
Very high	Almost always	Catastrophic	It cannot be detected
High	Often (probable)	Critical	It can only be detected when the process is already finished
Medium	Sometimes	Serious	It can be detected during one of the stages of the process
Low	Rare (improbable)	Minor	It can be detected during the stage in process
Very low	Non observable	Insignificant	It can be detected instantaneously

An important inconvenient of the qualitative evaluation of the factors appears when determining risk. Everybody would agree that low x medium x high = medium, but the score of low x low x high is not so evident (medium?). And this becomes even less clear if we consider more than three levels.

This is however less important that it might seem at first sight. As we have seen before, risk estimation is likely to be more a rough approximation than a very exact value. Thus, adding some more roughness might not be considered critical in most cases. This inconvenient, however, can be overcome by using a complementary table which would provide a homogeneous estimation (Table 7).

Table 7. Example of table for the qualitative estimation of risk.

RPR = Low x Low x Low = Low	RPR = Medium x Medium x Medium = Medium
RPR = Low x Low x Medium = Low-Medium	RPR = Medium x Medium x High = Medium-High
RPR = Low x Medium x Medium = Medium-Low	RPR = Medium x High x High = High-Medium
RPR = Low x Medium x High = Medium-Low	RPR = High x High x High = High
RPR = Low x High x High = Medium	----

Risk is estimated by integrating P, S and D to obtain the "risk prioritization ranking" (RPR).

<u>Quantitatively</u>

Quantitative estimations may use different scales:

- Linear: three-level (1, 2 or 3), five-level (1 to 5), ten-level (1 to 10).

- Exponential: 1, 2, 4, and 8.
- Logarithmic: 1, 10, 100, and 1000.
- Uneven or "enhanced": three-level (1, 3, 6), five-level (1, 3, 6, 10, 15), *etc.*

The approach to quantitative estimation follows suit, with the difference that instead of adjectives are used numbers. Thus, in a three level evaluation, instead of low, medium and high are used numbers (1, 2 and 3 – supposing that an even scale is being used).

Table 8. Example of quantitative evaluation in five levels with two options (linear and uneven).

Evaluation (two options)		PROBABILITY	SEVERITY	DIFFICULTY OF DETECTION
1st	2nd			
5	9	Expected >80% of times.	Batch is OOS and it is rejected.	No detection.
4	7	Expected between >50% and ≤80% of times	There are deviations and batch is investigated and rejected.	Detection but only when the process is finished
3	5	Expected between >10% and ≤50% of times.	There are deviations and batch is investigated but accepted.	Detection during a stage of the process, before finishing it.
2	3	Expected between >1% and ≤10% of times.	A trend is detected, but limits are not exceeded and the batch is not investigated.	Detection during the stage in process.
1	1	Expected ≤1% of times.	There is no trend and limits are not exceeded. Batch is not investigated.	Instantaneous detection.

The use of different levels for each one of the three factors (Table **8**) allows for a better differentiation of the scores obtained (*e.g.* P and S linear and D uneven). Nevertheless, it has to be kept in mind that the more complex is the evaluation of the factors, the more difficult becomes the evaluation of the outcome of the risk analysis. It is preferable to start by using the simplest possible approach and only when more knowledge and experience are acquired it is advisable to turn to more complex approaches. And in any case, it is particularly important to define appropriately which are the criteria used to determine the levels or scales chosen.

Risk is estimated by multiplying P, S and D to obtain the "risk prioritization number" (RPN).

Table 9. Example of table for the quantitative estimation of risk.

RPN = 1 x 1 x 1 = 1 > Low	RPN = 1 x 2 x 3 = 6 > Medium-Low	RPN = 2 x 2 x 3 = 12 > Medium-High
RPN = 1 x 1 x 2 = 2 > Low-Medium	RPN = 1 x 3 x 3 = 9 > Medium	RPN = 2 x 3 x 3 = 18 > High-Medium
RPN = 1 x 2 x 2 = 4 > Medium-Low	RPN = 2 x 2 x 2 = 8 > Medium	RPN = 3 x 3 x 3 = 27 > High

Quantitative evaluation of the factors (Table **9**) turns easier and more exact the estimation of risk. In the annexed table is provided an example of quantitative estimation in three levels (qualitative estimation is given for comparison purposes).

The results of an FMEA or FMECA are given in tables. See Table **10**.

Table 10. Example of FMEA/FMECA table.

FMECA								
FMEA								
Process stage	**Failure mode**	**Cause**	**Effect**	**Factors**			**RP**	**Comments**
				P	**S**	**D**		

Some prefer to use tables where factors are placed beside their related aspect of the failure (mode, cause and control) as this facilitates their fulfillment (Table **11**).

Table 11. Alternative example of FMECA table.

Process stage	**Failure mode**	**S**	**Cause**	**P**	**Control**	**D**	**RP**	**Comments**

FMECA can also be used as a tool for the improvement of processes (Table **12**).

Table 12. Example of FMECA table as a tool for improvement.

Process stage	Failure mode	Effect	Cause	Factors			RP	Corrective actions	Factors			RP	Comments
				P	S	D			P	S	D		

HACCP

The Hazard Analysis and Critical Control Points (HACCP) is an organized method used to detect hazards and keep them under control. It has long been used in the food industry. HACCP assumes that every process has critical points that can be controlled. A "control point" (CP) is a process stage where there is a point that can be controlled, whereas a "critical control point" (CCP) is a stage where it is possible to apply an essential control to prevent a hazard or reduce it to an acceptable level (Fig. **15**). A "control measure" is any activity performed to prevent, eliminate or reduce a significant hazard [19].

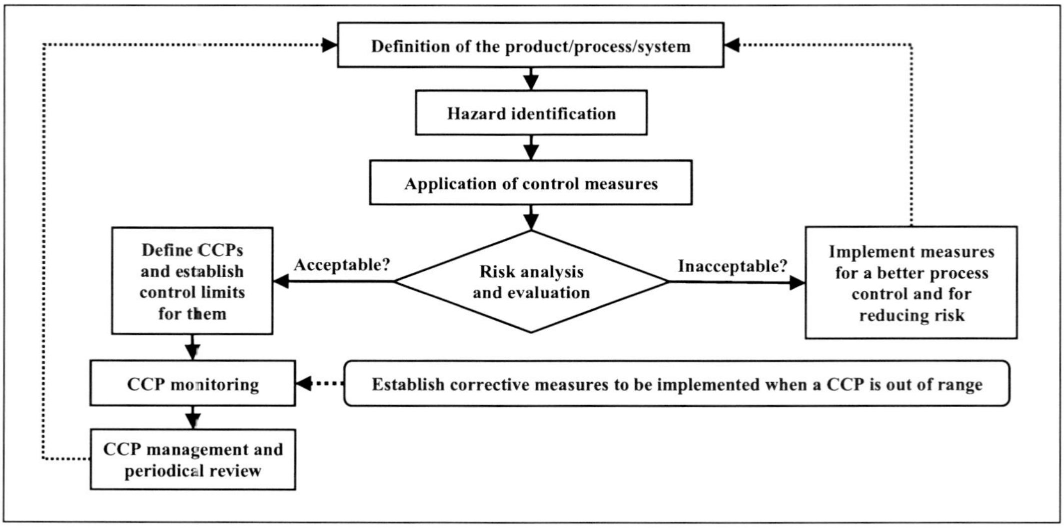

Fig. (15). HACCP rationale.

HACCP can be used to determine the scope of validation, but also to apply prevention measures and to program in-process controls.

As usual, to perform a HACCP it is necessary to have an updated flow-chart of the process to be analyzed. Each one of its operations/steps is assessed in order to detect potential hazards (Table **13**). This leads to the determination of the CCPs.

Table 13. Example of HACCP table I (establishment of CCPs).

Operation/Process stage	**Potential hazard**	**Is risk significant?**	**Why?**	**Preventive measures**	**Is it a CCP?**
Test for endotoxin in water	Presence of endotoxin in water	Yes	Presence of endotoxin is not acceptable	Monitoring	Yes
Measure of pH	pH outside range	Yes	Precipitation	Verify pH	Yes
Filter sterilization	Viable microbes in the filter	Yes	Product not sterile	Process validation and monitoring	Yes

In order to determine if the risk is significant it is possible to follow the approach used in FMECA, which can be synthesized in Table **14**.

Table 14. Example of CCP risk evaluation.

Potential hazard:		**Seriousness of hazard**				
		Insignificant	Minor	Severe	Critical	Catastrophic
Probability of hazard	Always					High risk
	Frequently (likely)					
	Sometimes			Medium risk		
	Rare (unlikely)					
	Non observable	Low risk				

Alternatively, the rationale exposed in Fig. (**16**) might be used to determine which hazards possess a significant risk to be considered as CCPs.

Once the CCPs have been recognized it is necessary to establish the strategy for keeping them under control. This includes defining their acceptable range (determined by the maximum and minimum values of the parameter that is controlled). A deviation is registered when the parameter is outside of the acceptable range.

It is necessary to define an HACCP plan describing the monitoring strategy and the corrective actions which will be developed in case of deviation (Table **15**).

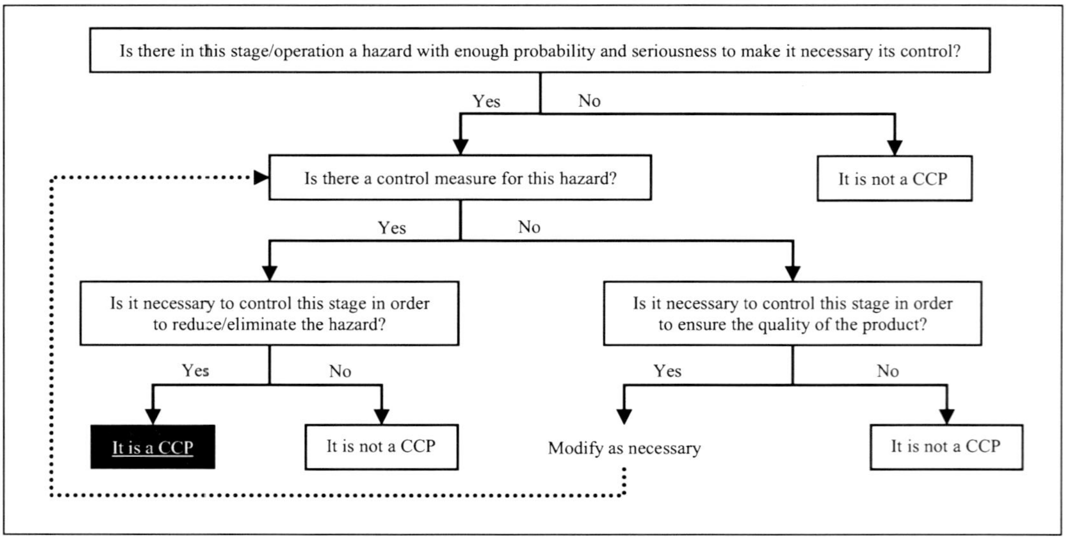

Fig. (16). HACCP rationale for CCP assessment.

Table 15. Example of HACCP table II (monitoring of CCPs).

CCP	Acceptable range	Monitoring			Corrective actions
		Who?	How?	When	
Endotoxin test in water	< 0,25 U.	QC technician	LAL test	Before starting the production	Stop production and call the supervisor
Measure of pH	pH = 6-7	Production supervisor	pH-meter	In process	Call the supervisor. Add more sodium hydroxide
Filter sterilization	Sterile	Production technician	Process parameters (P, T and t)	After sterilization	Stop production and call the supervisor

FTA

Fault Tree Analysis (FTA) is a deductive tool (*i.e.* from a problem to their causes) which is used after a fault or unwanted event (top event) has happened to determine the root causes (basic events) which led, or contributed to it. The result of an FTA is a pictogram of fault modes in the shape of a tree. This tree is drawn by means of logical operators (gates), which relate the top event with the basic event (a cause event which does not require further investigation), across intermediate events. Fault trees can be built vertically (with the top event on the upper side of the pictogram) or horizontally (with the top event on the right hand side of the pictogram) [20].

This tool evaluates system (or sub-system) failures one at a time but can combine multiple causes of failure by identifying causal chains. FTA can be used to establish the pathway to the root cause of the failure. FTA can be used to investigate complaints or deviations in order to fully understand their root cause and to ensure that intended improvements will fully resolve the issue and not lead to other issues (i.e. solve one problem yet cause a different problem). FTA is an effective tool for evaluating how multiple factors affect a given issue. It is useful both for risk assessment and in developing monitoring programs [21].

Symbols used in FTA can vary. In Table **16** are shown two types of symbols used to represent events. The pharmaceutical use of FTA most of times do not require using many of them. Besides, as these symbols are rather complex, it is always possible to substitute them by any type of figure. Then, the meaning is indicated in writing.

Table 16. FTA events.

Symbol		**Meaning**
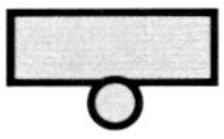	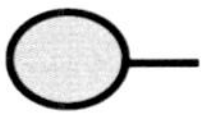	**Basic event**: Event that initiates a failure and does not need further development.
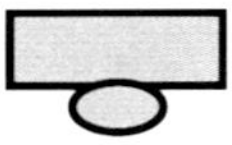	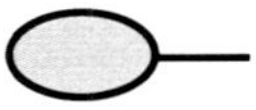	**Conditioning event**: Event that might condition a failure.
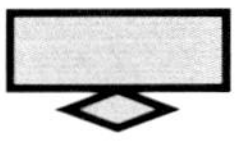	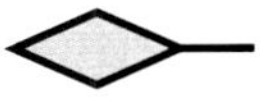	**Undeveloped event**: Event that is not developed, either because it cannot lead to a failure or because there is a lack of information.
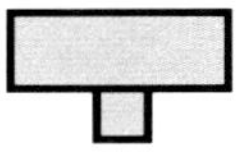	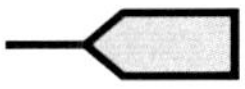	**House event**: Event that should normally occur.
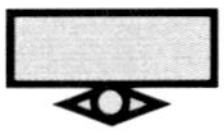	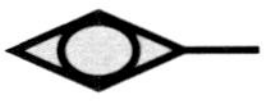	**Analyzed elsewhere**: Event which is studied in another part of the tree.
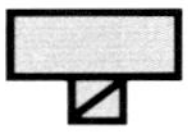	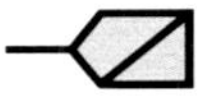	**Zero event**: Event that cannot happen.

The first step in a Fault Tree Analysis is to define the top event, its boundaries, and the level of resolution (usually determined by the level of information). The top event has to be concrete in order not to have a too vast tree.

Table 17. FTA "or" and "and" gates.

<table>
<tr><th>Gate</th><th>Symbols</th><th>Examples</th></tr>
<tr><td>OR
The event takes place when one of the entrance events appears alone or is combined.</td><td>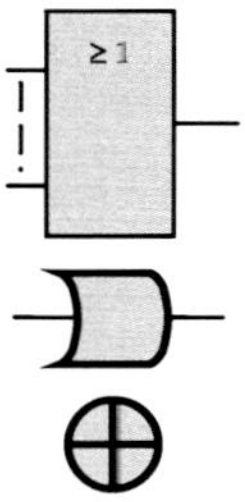
</td><td>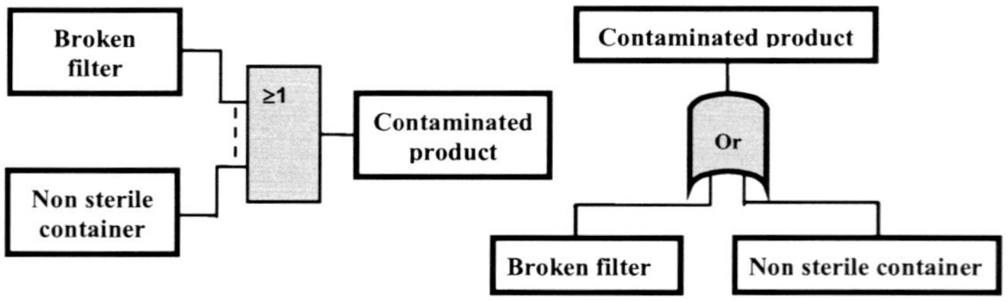
</td></tr>
<tr><td>AND
The event takes place only when all entrance events appear at the same time</td><td>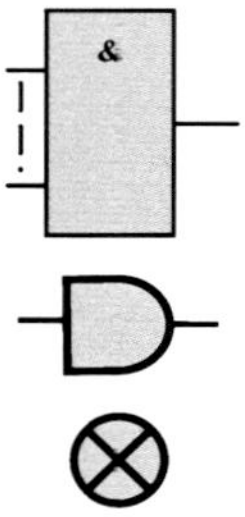
</td><td>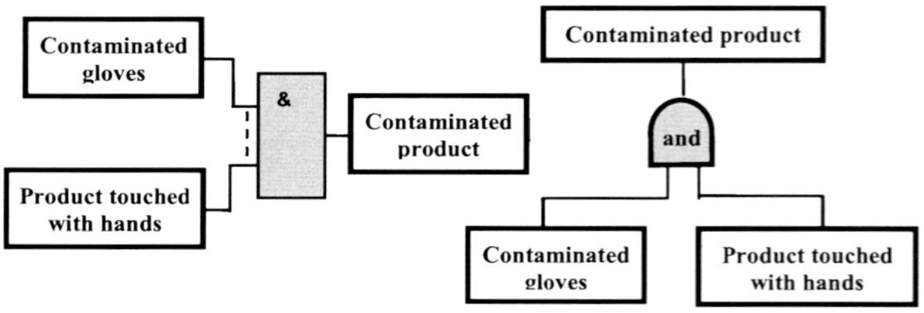
</td></tr>
</table>

Then, it is necessary to identify which immediate event or events are necessary and sufficient to produce the top event. The relationship between these events is shown by choosing the appropriate gate.

This process continues by looking for the chain of events and their relationship. One should not pass to a new gate before having completed all the entries to the gate being studied.

Although the two more common gates are the "**and**-gate" and the "**or**-gate" (Table **17**), other types of gates can be used to describe the relationship between the events (Table **18**).

Table 18. FTA: Gates.

Symbol	Meaning
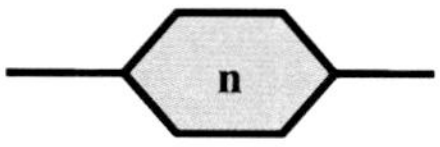	<u>**Combination gate**</u>: A result appears when a series of events occur at the same time.

Symbol	Meaning
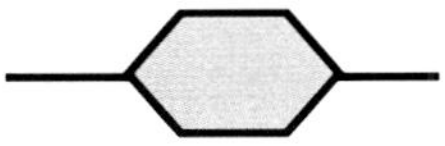	**Inhibition gate**: A result appears when a particular condition is fulfilled. This condition is indicated on the right of the door.
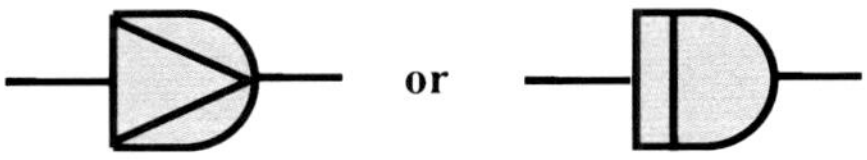	**Priority gate**: A result appears when a series of events occur following a given sequence. This sequence is indicated as a conditioning event on the right of the door.
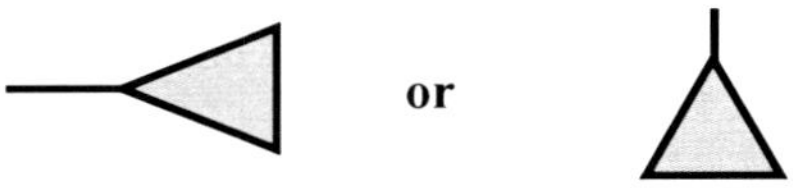	**Transfer in-gate**: The tree comes from another part of the pictogram.
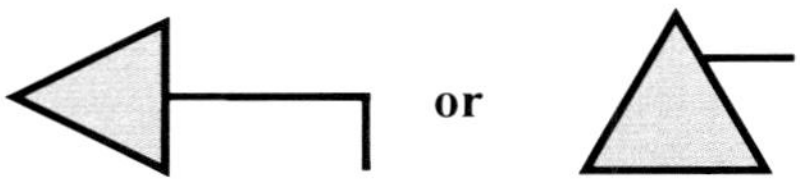	**Transfer out-gate**: The tree is continued on another part of the pictogram.
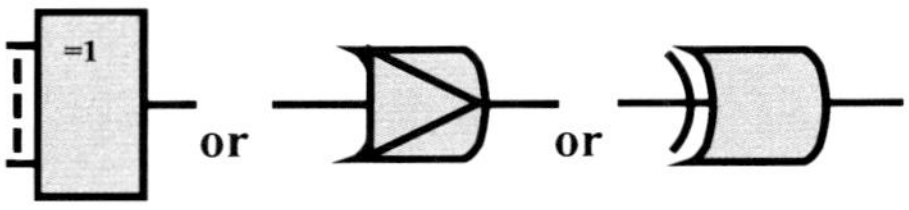	**Exclusive or-gate**: Event appears only when one of the two entry events takes place (normally used for two entry events).
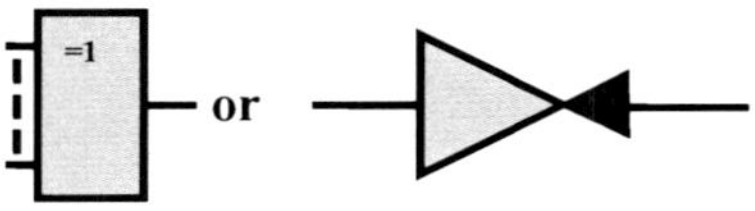	**Not-gate**: Event represents the opposite condition of the entry event.
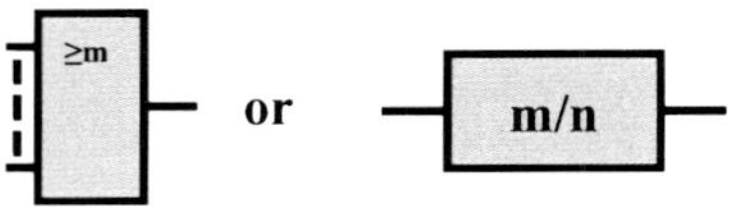	**Redundant structure**: Event appears only if at least m from the n entry events occur.
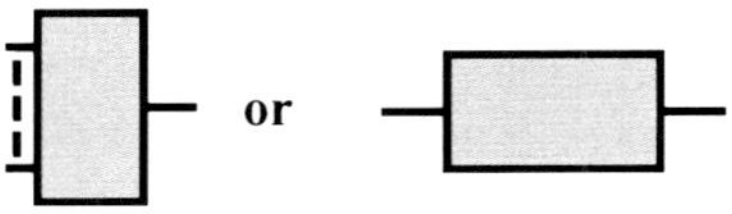	**General gate**: Symbol of a gate. Its function has to be described inside.

There is also a "general gate" that can be used to describe any type of relationship between events just by writing about it. As it was said before regarding events, different symbols are used to represent gates. Notwithstanding that, from a practical point of view, what matters is the understanding of the relationships between events, not how these relations are presented on the pictogram. This can be important for comparative purposes only or on formal reports to third parties.

Fig. (**17**) shows an example (using two types of symbols) of “common cause” and of “basic event”.

A fault tree can be considered complete, when basic events and intermediate events have been identified and appropriately connected by logic gates. Then a "cut set" can be defined as the minimal set of events that can lead to an incident.

A rule of thumb to see if a tree has been correctly solved is to invert it, that is, change it from failure to success. After doing this, the top event should still be correct. It should be kept in mind that gates are inverted too, thus "and-gates" become "or-gates" and *vice versa*.

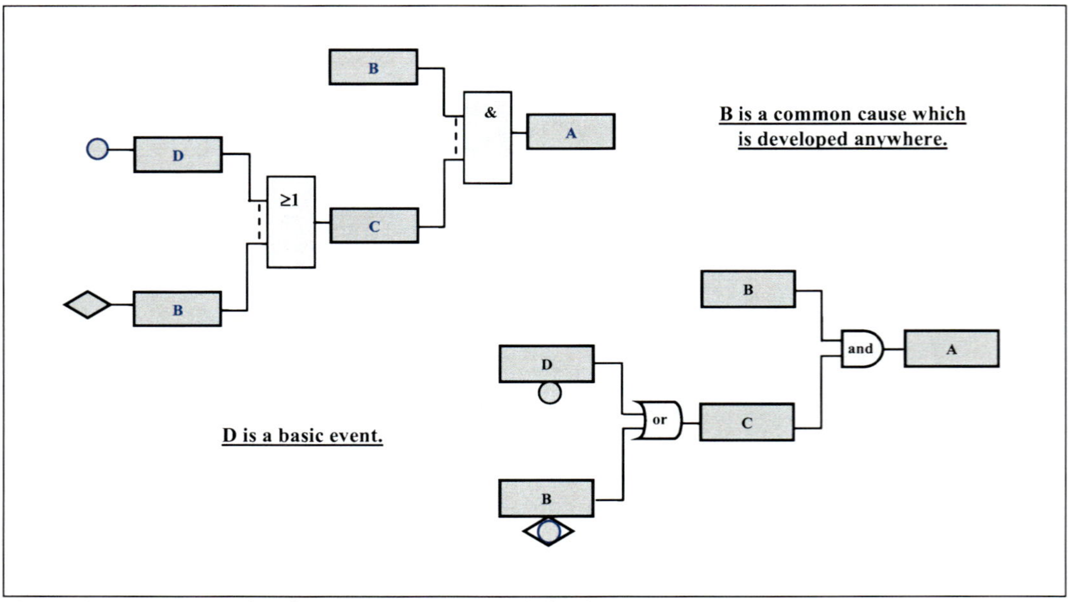

Fig. (17). FTA: Example of "common cause" and "basic event".

Although most fault trees do not contain any estimation of probability, it can also be included by taking into account that with or-gates probabilities are added, whereas with and-gates probabilities are multiplied. This is why sometimes on or-gates a + is written and on and-gates a dot or an asterisk is written (Fig. **18**).

The less basic events are, the more dangerous a cut set is. There is low redundancy protection when there are few and-gates.

HAZOP

The Hazard Operability Analysis (HAZOP) is a systematic inductive tool (*i.e.* from the causes to the problems) applied to systems in order to identify potential hazards or operational problems (Fig. **19**). HAZOP assumes that risk events are caused by deviations from the "intention of design or operation" [22].

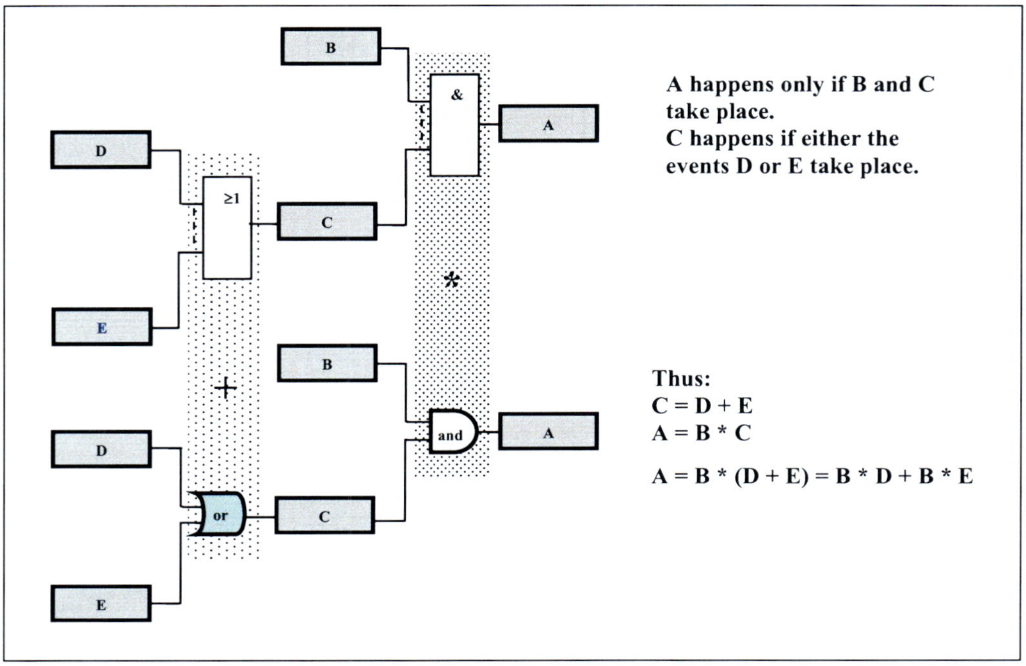

Fig. (18). Probability estimation in FTA.

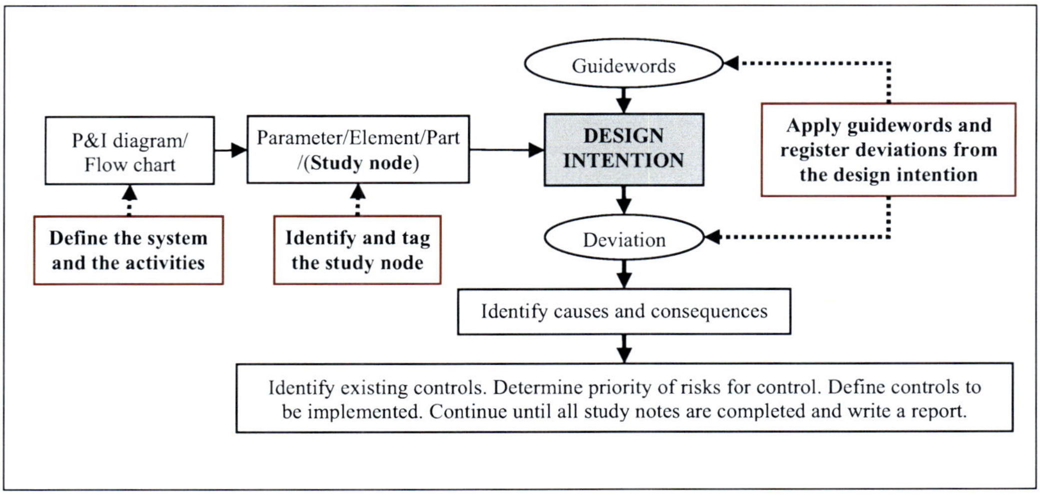

Fig. (19). HAZOP procedure.

Although HAZOP is mainly used during the development, it can be used at any lifecycle stage. The probability of each deviation is not estimated as a rule, but it is possible to include it.

HAZOP is particularly useful to identify the weak points of the systems. It can be used together with other methods, such as FTA (to discover the effect of multiple deviations) or FMECA (to quantify risk).HAZOP is a tool that uses "guide-words" to facilitate the identification of deviations (Table **19**).

On a practical side, it is possible to chose either guidewords and apply them to design intentions of the study nodes or the reverse (apply study nodes to guidewords). The result should be the same.

Table 19. HAZOP guidewords.

Type of deviation	Guideword	Meaning	Example of interpretation
Negative	No/not/none	Total negation of the design intention	There is no flow of liquid
Quantitative modification	More	Quantitative increase of the design intention	Higher temperature
	Less	Quantitative decrease of the design intention	Lower pressure
Qualitative modification	As well as	Qualitative increase of the design intention	Presence of impurities
	Part of	Qualitative decrease of the design intention	Partial discharge of liquid
Substitution	Reverse	Logical contrary of the design intention	Inverted flow
	Other than	Total substitution of the design intention	Different result of the operation
Time	Early	Before the design intention	Pressure increase before than intended
	Late	After the design intention	Flow later than intended
Sequence	Before	Action before the design intention	Operation before that intended
	After	Action after the design intention	Operation after that intended
Speed	Faster	Action faster than the design intention	Faster increase in temperature
	Slower	Action slower than the design condition	Slower increase in pressure

First of all, the system is divided into study nodes, which can be either elements (parts) or parameters. Then the design intention is defined for each one. Deviations are detected by applying guide-words. Thus, for instance, if the chosen parameter is “flow”, application of the guide-word “no” would mean “no flow” (*i.e.* tank is not filled). For each deviation, possible causes and consequences are determined. This allows for the identification of significant problems and, consequently, for their prevention (Table **20**).

Table 20. Example of HAZOP table.

Study node	#	Guideword	Deviation	Possible cause	Consequences	Implemented controls	Necessary action

It has to be pointed out that not all guide-words can be logically applied to each study node. Usually only a few of them make sense when applied to a given study node. Only those which logically identify possible situations are retained and written on the table. Those which make no sense are skipped.

Following is given a very simple example of HAZOP describing how guidewords can be used to analyze the operation of transfer of a product from one tank to another (Table **21**).

Table 21. Example of application of HAZOP.

Activity	Guideword	Deviation
Transfer of product A from the tank x to the tank Z. 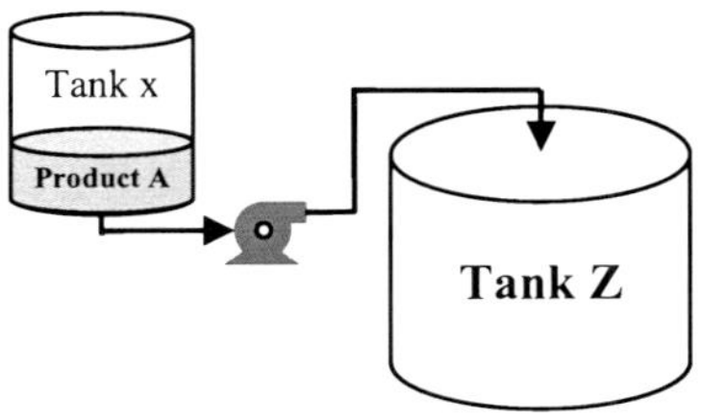	No/Not/None	No transfer of A
	More	More transfer of A
	Less	Less transfer of A
	As well as	Transfer of A and other product
	Part of	Partial transfer of A
	Reverse	Transfer from tank Z to tank x
	Other than	Transfer of other product than A
	Early	Transfer before the scheduled time
	Late	Transfer after the scheduled time
	Before	Transfer of A before other reactive
	After	Transfer of A after other reactive
	Faster	Transfer faster than planned
	Slower	Transfer slower than planned

As it can be seen in this example (Table **22**) some words make no sense (*e.g.* "as well as"; because there is only one product which can be transferred).

Table 22. Example of table of application of HAZOP.

#	Guideword	Deviation	Cause	Effect	Actions
1	No/Not/None	No transfer of product A	Tank x is empty	There is no reaction	Install level sensor in tank x
2	No/Not/None	No transfer of product A	Pump failure	There is no reaction	Install alarm
3	More	Transfer of a bigger volume of A	Operator error	Loss of product A	Provide an automatic system
4	Less	Transfer of a smaller volume of A	Operator error	Partial reaction	Provide an automatic system
5	As well as	Transfer of A and another product	N.a.	N.a.	N.a.
6	Part of A	Transfer of only a part of A	Operator error	Partial reaction	Provide an automatic system
7	Reverse	Transfer is from tank Z to tank x	Pump is broken	Backflow	Install a pump without possibility of backflow
8	Other than	Instead of A is transferred another product	Tank x is filled with another product instead of A	There is no reaction	Provide double control when filling tank x
9	---	---	---	---	---

RRF

RRF (Risk ranking and filtering) is a tool specifically devised for the comparison of different sets (units, processes, companies, *etc.*) possessing varied levels of risks. Once they are reduced to a common denominator they can be compared and this allows for the establishment of priorities [23].

As in any method, it is necessary to individualize first the hazards or problems and then the different attributes, components or elements, which make them up [24]. See Fig. (**20**).

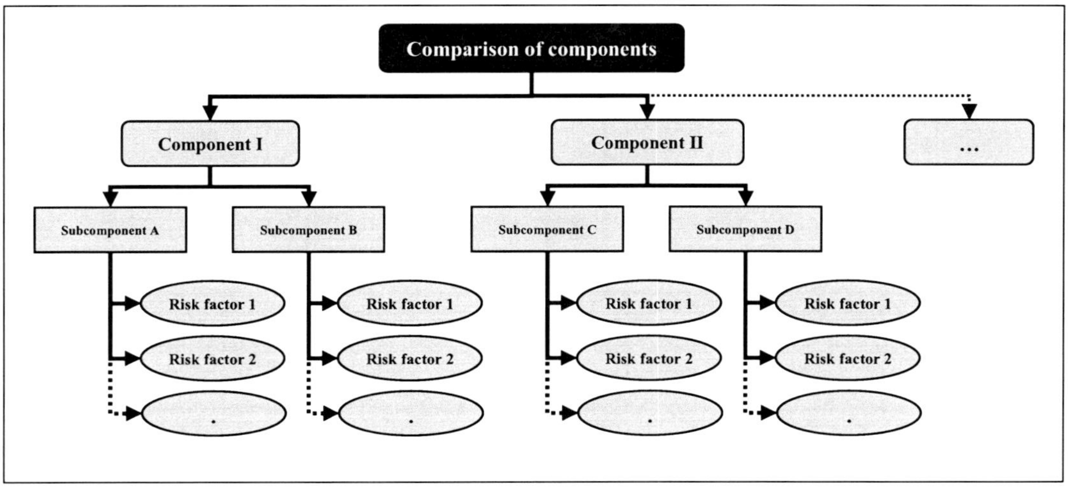

Fig. (20). Determination of risk factors in RFR.

Fig. (**21**) provides a practical example.

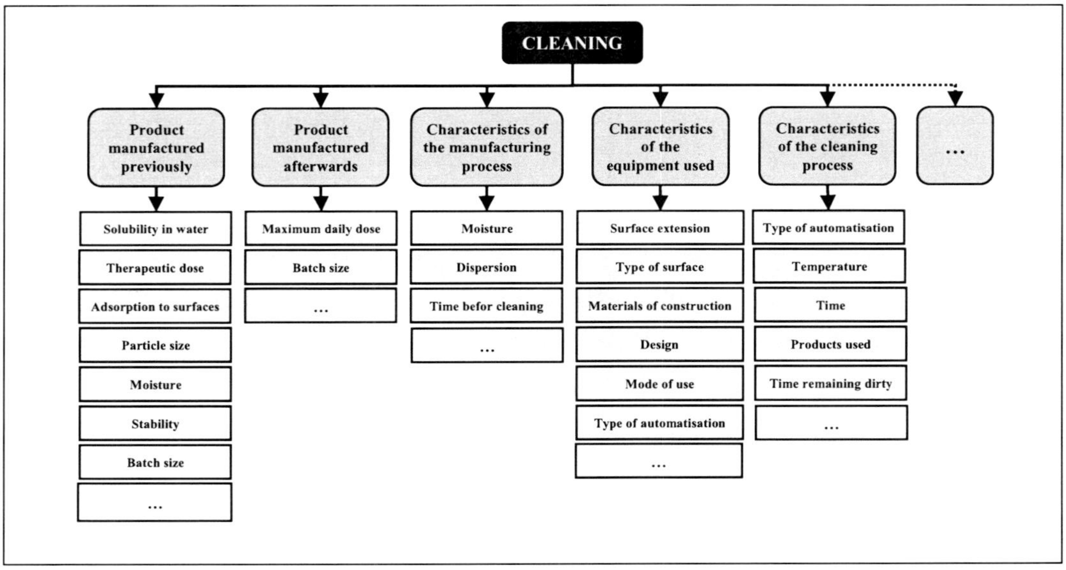

Fig. (21). Example of hazard or problem decomposition (factors intervening in cleaning) in RRF.

Then each component is evaluated in terms of risk. It is possible to get a comprehensive evaluation taking into account all the intervening factors. This allows for obtaining an overall risk for each one of them. Consequently, the components can be ranked according to their respective level of risk. Once that the components are ranked (*e.g.* classified in terms of risk level) they can be filtered (*e.g.* selected those who have lower risk score). See Fig. (**22**).

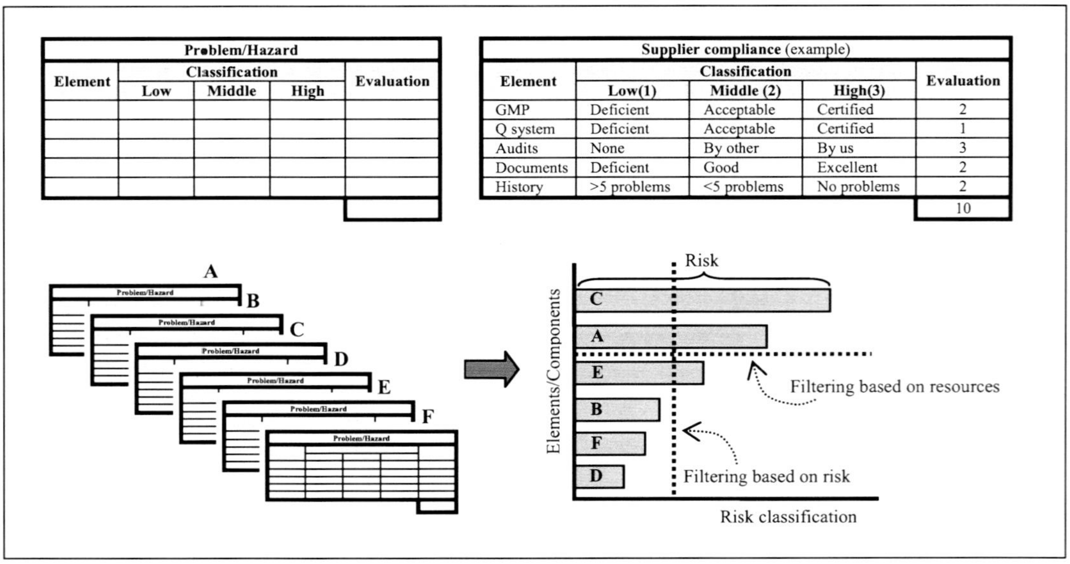

Fig. (22). Ranking and filtering of the problems or hazards in RRF.

It is also possible to rank and filter risks by using tables combining the three factors (probability, severity and difficulty of detection) which were previously described for FMECA (Fig. **23**). This allows for the establishment of priorities.

Risk classification		Severity		
		High	Middle	Low
Probability	High			Class 1
	Midd e		Class 2	
	Low	Class 3		

Risk filtration		Difficulty of detection		
		Low	Middle	High
Risk classification	Class 1			1st priority
	Class 2		2nd priority	
	Class 3	3rd priority		

Fig. (23). Risk estimation in RRF.

CONCLUDING REMARKS

The true problem in pharmaceutical manufacturing is not created by the existence of hazards, but by ignoring and not assessing them. This is why risk management is a key element for keeping processes and systems under control. Hazards are identified and their associated risk assessed and thus it is possible to ensure that the risk level will always be known and kept monitored. Improvement is obtained by a progressive reduction of the risk level.

CONFLICT OF INTEREST

The author confirms that this chapter contents have no conflict of interest.

ACKNOWLEDGEMENT

Declared None.

REFERENCES

[1] Vesper J. Risk assessment and risk management in the pharmaceutical industry: clear and simple. PDA Bethesda, MD, USA 2006
[2] WHO (World Health Organisation). WHO guidelines on quality risk management. In: WHO Expert Committee on Specifications for Pharmaceutical Preparations. Forty-seventh report (WHO Technical Report Series, No. 981). WHO, Geneva, Switzerland 2013. Annex 2.
[3] ICH (International Conference on Harmonisation of Technical Requirements for registration of Pharmaceuticals for Human Use). Quality Risk Management. Q9. ICH, Geneva, Switzerland 2005.
[4] PIC/S (Pharmaceutical Inspection Convention/Pharmaceutical Inspection Co-Operation Scheme). Assessment of quality risk management implementation. Aide-Memoire PI 038-1. PIC/S, Geneva, Switzerland 2012.
[5] Ibid. 7 (Glossary).
[6] Ibid. 7 (Glossary).
[7] Ibid. 7 (Glossary).
[8] Ibid. 4.3.
[9] Ibid. 7 (Glossary).
[10] Ibid. 4.4.
[11] Ibid. 7 (Glossary).
[12] Ibid. 4.5.
[13] Ibid. 4.6.
[14] Ibid. Annex II.
[15] Ibid. 1.
[16] IEC (International Electrotechnical Commission). Analysis techniques for system reliability – Procedure for failure mode and effects analysis (FMEA). International Standard IEC 60812:2006(E). IEC, Geneva, Switzerland 1985.
[17] ICH (International Conference on Harmonisation of Technical Requirements for registration of Pharmaceuticals for Human Use). Quality Risk Management. Q9. ICH, Geneva, Switzerland 2005. 7 (Glossary).
[18] Ibid.: 7 (Glossary).
[19] WHO (World Health Organisation). Application of Hazard Analysis and Critical Control Point (HACCP) method to pharmaceuticals. In: WHO Expert Committee on Specifications for Pharmaceutical Preparations. Thirty-seventh report (WHO Technical Report Series, No. 908). WHO, Geneva, Switzerland 2003. Annex 7.
[20] IEC (International Electrotechnical Commission). Fault tree analysis (FTA). Standard CEI/IEC 1025:1990. IEC, Geneva, Switzerland 1990.
[21] ICH (International Conference on Harmonisation of Technical Requirements for registration of Pharmaceuticals for Human Use). Quality Risk Management. Q9. ICH, Geneva, Switzerland 2005.
[22] IEC (International Electrotechnical Commission). Hazard and operability studies (HAZOP studies) – Application guide. Standard CEI/IEC 61882:2001. IEC, Geneva, Switzerland 2001.
[23] US FDA. Risk-Based Method for Prioritizing CGMP Inspections of Pharmaceutical Manufacturing Sites. A Pilot Risk Ranking Model. 2004.
[24] PIC/S (Pharmaceutical Inspection Convention/Pharmaceutical Inspection Co-Operation Scheme). A recommended model for risk-based inspection planning in the GMP environment. Recommendation PI 037-1. PIC/S, Geneva, Switzerland 2012.

Chapter 4: Quality Hazards in the Pharmaceutical Industry

CHAPTER 4

Quality Hazards in the Pharmaceutical Industry

Abstract: Pharmaceuticals are manufactured in purpose-build premises which are provided with controlled environment, with specialized equipment and with the necessary utilities. There, trained personnel following approved procedures transform inputs (materials) into outputs (pharmaceutical products). Therefore, the quality of these pharmaceuticals is linked to the quality of the above mentioned aspects. This was long understood and became the base of GMP: "keep the factors influencing quality under control and you will get quality". Nowadays it is possible, and necessary, to implement risk management to better recognize and control these quality factors. But, be that as it may, it is evident that without knowing and understanding the hazards which threaten quality, any quality assurance policy is doomed to failure. Thus, premises, utilities, equipment and personnel are analyzed in order to detect which hazards loom on the quality of pharmaceutical products. Then, these quality hazards are described and their causes determined with the aim of proposing measures for reducing their likelihood or keeping them under control. It is interesting to underline that changes in systems and equipment and in approaches to hazard handling have contributed in diminishing the risk, but most of the hazards remain basically the same. There is a wide coverage of the hazards linked to harmful products and microorganisms and the preventive measures, according to the risk level.

Keywords: Airlock, biohazard, BSC, clean area, contained area, contamination, cross-contamination, dust exhaust, environmental contamination, equipment, error/mix-up, degradation, HEPA filter, HVAC, OEL, personnel, PPE, premises, utilities, waste disposal.

QUALITY AT BAY

Long before the formal introduction of risk management in pharmaceutical manufacturing it was understood that the quality of the products depended on the elements which intervened in their fabrication, traditionally known as the 5 Ms (Machines-Medium-Men-Methods-Materials).

It was also perceived that often a single mistake might, perhaps, not be significant, but that the coupling of several mistakes could easily lead to an accident. Thus quality was seen as the result of having good procedures and then "doing things well", which excluded that a series of mistakes might constitute a chain of events leading to an accident (*e.g.* entrust a task to a new operator is, maybe, not very dangerous in itself, but if he is not adequately trained, supervised and has not a written procedure to follow, we would easily agree that it becomes very perilous indeed). This is, by the way, why GMP was born. GMP pointed out the main

Jordi Botet

quality mistakes affecting pharmaceutical manufacture and proposed "good procedures" to overcome or control them [1, 2, 3]. Nowadays we have advanced a step forward, as we use science-based approaches and risk management, but essentially quality hazards remain the same and have to be well known and understood prior to any quality management policy. This is why in this chapter the hazards linked to pharmaceutical manufacturing are described and analyzed in a systematic way. In fact, just five categories of hazards endanger product quality: contamination ("external", "crossed" and "environmental"), error/mix-up, and degradation. Once potential hazards are known it is necessary to identify the items which are going to be analyzed to see if these possible hazards did exist and then identify the possible causes and propose control measures. The items which are analyzed can be usefully classified using the method proposed in chapter 2 while describing the QMP (qualification master plan) and that can be summarized here by saying that manufacturing processes are performed in premises by means of equipment supplied with utilities and that in spite of the impressive progress of automation, the "human factor" still plays an important role.

Quality Hazards

Contamination

"Contamination" is defined as *the undesired introduction of impurities of a chemical or microbiological nature, or of foreign matter, into or on to a raw material or intermediate during production, sampling, packaging or repackaging, storage or transport. Whereas "cross-contamination" is the contamination of raw material, intermediate product or finished product with another raw material or product during production* [4].

Even accepting that starting materials meet specifications (yes, they can be already contaminated prior to its reception, but it is not considered here), within a pharmaceutical plant products can be contaminated by the most varied impurities. Although any contamination is, by definition, external to the substance which is contaminated, "contamination" by sand, dust, fibers, hair, pollen, pesticides, cleaners, lubricants, microorganisms, *etc.* can be dubbed "external contamination", whereas "cross-contamination" is produced by other materials or products. This distinction is important because, as we are going to see, both types of contamination involve different preventive approaches.

Besides, some materials and microorganisms manipulated in pharmaceutical plants are harmful for the operators and, if they break out from the premises, they cause pollution of the environment by their physico-chemical or biological toxicity and this can be called “environmental contamination”.

Error/mix-up

Although both words design the same fact (*i.e.* procedures were not followed), error is a more general term used to design that something is done in a wrong way, whereas mix-up refers usually that one thing is changed for another. Errors and mix-ups can affect different products, different batches of the same product or different stages in the production of a batch of a product.

Degradation

The quality of a material or product can be affected if exposed to inappropriate conditions (*e.g.* temperature, humidity, sunlight, illumination, radiation).

Pharmaceutical Plant Items

These above mentioned hazards threaten premises, utilities and operations (which include equipment and personnel), as shown in Fig. (**1**).

Premises

Pharmaceuticals are manufactured in premises which:

- Provide physical support to the production (installation of equipment, storage of products, setting for the operations, *etc.*) and adequate conditions for the products (temperature, humidity, illumination, *etc.*);
- Facilitate the development of processes and prevent mix-ups (separation of operations in different rooms, appropriate flows, delimitation of zones, *etc.*);
- Shelter products from contamination, coming from outside and generated inside (“cross-contamination”);
- Protect the environment from contamination by products manipulated inside.

A plant has different areas, which can be either service areas without GMP requirements or areas where GMP-regulated activities are developed. These latter can be subdivided into “gray” and “clean” areas (depending on the existence or not of environmental control). A plant contains the necessary facilities which are either utilities or production equipment. Personnel can intervene everywhere.

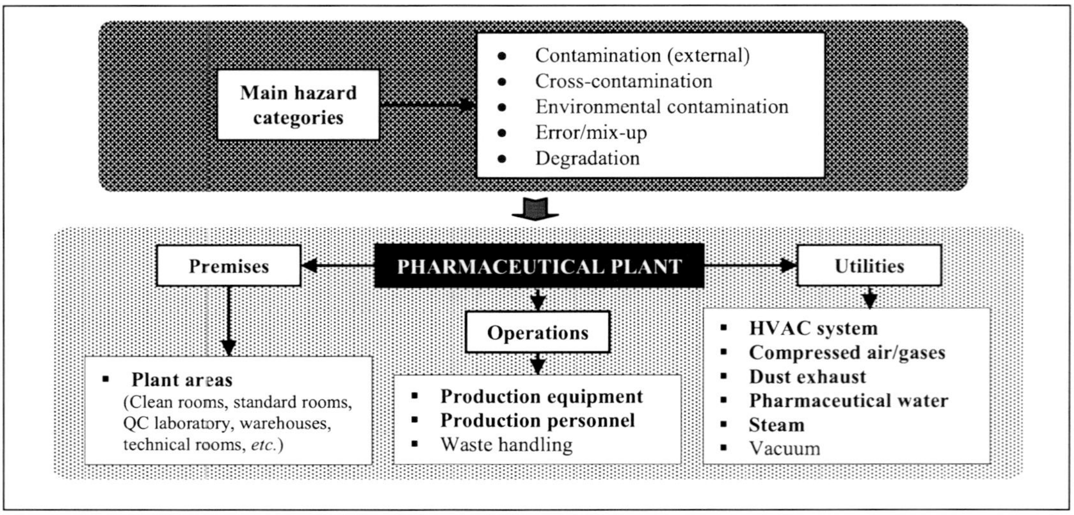

Fig. (1). Hazard analysis in the pharmaceutical plant.

Utilities

These are systems which provide the appropriate working environment and allow that production (in a strict sense) equipment works adequately:

- HVAC system: It controls the operational environment (climatization, ventilation and filtration of air);

- Compressed air/gases: Air is used either for the activation of valves or for displacing pieces (*e.g.* closures). Gases have different uses in manufacturing (*e.g.* nitrogen is often used to displace air and protect from oxydation).

- Dust collection system: When there is release of dust the system HVAC has to be strengthened with this specific system for dust extraction on the spot.

- Water for pharmaceutical use: Natural water is purified to obtain pharmaceutical quality water used in cleaning and production.

- Steam: It is mostly used as a calorific fluid (*e.g.* for sterilization, heating, *etc.*).

- Vacuum: Normally it is not considered because it has no GMP significance, but here it is included because of the threat of environmental contamination when manipulating harmful products or microorganisms.

Operations

The, properly speaking, manufacturing operations are performed with specialized equipment, staffed by trained personnel. *The correct manufacture and control of pharmaceutical products and active ingredients rely upon people* [5]. Appropriate waste disposal is key factor in tackling the problem of environmental contamination.

1st CATEGORY OF HAZARD: CONTAMINATION

Table **1** develops a PHA of contamination.

Table 1. PHA of contamination.

Concerned sphere	Hazard description	Hazard cause	Preventive measures
Premises/Plant areas	Entry of particles (dust, pollen, mist, *etc.*) from outside	Outside air can get in	(#1.1) Separation from outside
			(#1.2) Separation inside the plant (GMP/non GMP areas)
		Dirty air moves between different areas	(#1.3) Separation inside the plant (QC/Production)
		Untidy plant surroundings	(#1.4) Plant location
		Dirty incoming containers	(#1.5) Receiving areas
	Entry of vermin	No control of vermin	(#1.6) Vermin control
	Build-up of dust/dirt	Existence of points for the build-up of dirt	(#1.7) Design of premises
		Surfaces shedding particles and difficult to keep clean.	(#1.8) Sanitary room construction
		Inadequate cleaning	(#1.9) Room cleaning
Utilities/HVAC	Entrance of particles and inadequate air system	Air is not adequately treated and does not meet requirements	(#1.10) Air supply to classified areas (clean rooms)
			(#1.11) Air supply to non-classified areas
	Entry of contaminated air	Humidification with non pharmaceutical steam	(#1.12) Humidification with pure (pharmaceutical) steam

Table 1: contd...

Utilities/Dust exhaust	Entrance of particles (dust, pollen, *etc.*) from outside	External air gets into the rooms by the exhausting ducts	(#1.13) Protection against airflow inversion
	Diffusion of particles	Disruption of the pressure cascade	(#1.14) Protection against modification of ΔP
Utilities/Water for pharmaceutical use	Water not meeting requirements	Entry of contamination into the system	(#1.15) System design
		Inadequate water treatment	(#1.16) Water treatment
		Stored water is contaminated	(#1.17) Protection of the water
Utilities/Steam for pharmaceutical use	Steam not meeting requirements	Build-up of contamination	(#1.18) System design
		Passage of water contaminants to steam	(#1.19) Source of water
Utilities/Compressed air	Compressed air not meeting requirements	Air already contaminated	(#1.20) Source of air
		Air contaminated by the compressor	(#1.21) Compressor type
		Condensation of water	(#1.22) System configuration
Utilities/Compressed gases	Compressed gas not meeting requirements	Gas is not of pharmaceutical quality	(#1.23) Gas quality
Operations/equipment	Equipment contamination	Inadequate installation	(#1.24) Installation
		Inadequate cleaning	(#1.25) Cleaning
	Product contamination	Inadequate surfaces	(#1.26) Surfaces in contact with materials and products
		Access of contamination	(#1.27) Design
			(#1.28) Separation
Operations/Personnel	Product contamination	Persons act as carriers of contamination	(#1.29) Hygienic measures
			(#1.30) Wear appropriate clothing
		Tools and pipes act as carriers of contamination	(#1.31) Beware of tools and transfer pipes

Contamination Preventive Measures

Premises/Plant Areas

(#1.1) Separation from outside: The manufacturing areas of a pharmaceutical plant have to possess a controlled environment. As the outside environment is completely uncontroled it is necessary to separate inside and outside of the plant. The following measures contribute to this separation:

- Impracticable (fixed) windows, sealed walls, ceilings, and floors;

- Double doors communicating the plant with the outside in order to impede free direct communication. Entry to the clean areas should be across changing rooms and airlocks. Installation, as necessary, of physical hindrances to impede passage of dust or dirt (curtains, mats, *etc.*).

- Controlled way in/out of persons, materials and products.

(#1.2) Separation inside the plant (GMP/non GMP): Service non GMP areas should be separated from the GMP areas:

- Auxiliary areas for the personnel (canteens, lounges, *etc.*) should be separated from the manufacturing and control areas.

- Toilet areas should not communicate directly with the production, control or storage areas.

- Maintenance workshops should preferably be separated from the production and control areas. When the parts and tools of equipment are stored in the production areas, they should be kept separated in rooms or lockers reserved for that use.

- Animal houses should be well isolated from other areas, with separate entrance (animal access).

(#1.3) Separation inside the plant (QC/Production): QC laboratories should be separated from the production areas. Besides, areas assigned to biological, microbiological or radioisotope test methods should be separated from each other.

(#1.4) Plant location: Plants should not be located in contaminated areas and their immediate sorroundings should be kept clean and free from weeds and scrubs. Although this might seem contradictory with point (#1.1), it has to be born in mind that absolute plant separation is impossible (manufacturing requires inflows and outflows), consequently if the sorroundings of the factory are dirty and offer hiding and breeding grounds for vermin, this increases the possibility of entrance of dust, insects and animals into the plant.

(#1.5) Receiving areas: These areas should be planned and prepared to clean the containers of incoming materials, when necessary, before storage.

(#1.6) Vermin control: Active and passive measures should be implemented in order to impede the entrance of insects and other pests into the plant:

- Killing devices for flying insects close to gates/doors.
- Physical hindrances (doors, curtains, nets, *etc.*).
- Pest control procedures and programs (inside and outside the plant).

(#1.7) Design of premises: The layout and organization of the premises should hinder the build-up of dust or dirt, and in general, protect the quality of products.

(#1.8) Sanitary room construction: Starting materials, primary packaging materials and intermediate or bulk products should be exposed to the environment only in rooms possessing a "sanitary" character:

- Internal surfaces from floors, walls and ceilings should be smooth and free from cracks and unsealed joints. They should not shed particulate matter. They should allow for an easy and efficient cleaning and disinfection (if necessary).
- Utilities (*e.g.* pipework, ventilation points, light fittings, *etc.*) should be designed and sited to avoid the creation of recesses difficult to clean. Whenever possible the maintenance of the manufacturing areas should be performed from outside (from the technical areas).
- Drains should be of adequate size and designed and outfitted to prevent backflow. It is preferable not to have open channels, but if they are indispensable they should be shallow to facilitate cleaning and disinfection.

(#1.9) Room cleaning: Rooms should be cleaned according to approved procedures and labeled according to their state (clean, to be cleaned).

Utilities/HVAC System

(#1.10) Air supply to classified areas (clean rooms): They should be ventilated with HEPA-filtered air to meet the requirements concerning particles, humidity, temperature, microorganisms and differential pressure. Changing rooms have to be flushed with filtered air of the same standard than the zone where they lead.

A clean area is *an area with defined environmental control of particulate and microbial contamination, constructed and used in such a way as to reduce the introduction, generation, and retention of contaminants within the area* [6].

(#1.11) Air supply to non-classified areas: Other rooms, different from clean rooms, should be ventilated in order to ensure personnel confort and kept at a temperature adequate for the products being handled there (*e.g.* for secondary packaging). In warehousing areas temperature and, if necessary, humidity should be maintained within the approved range.

(#1.12) Humidification with pure (pharmaceutical) steam: If it is necessary to increase the humidity of the air supplied to the clean rooms, this can be obtained by injecting steam to the supply air. If steam is pure (pharmaceutical quality) it ensures that neither substances nor microbes will be introduced into the air. The injection of water droplets is not used because of the danger of microbial growth (in particular of *Legionella*).

Utilities/Dust Exhaust System

(#1.13) Protection against airflow inversion: The system has to be designed to ensure that when it is turned off there is not airflow inversion (with free penetration of outside air)

(#1.14) Protection against modification of ΔP: The system has to ensure that neither its connection nor its disconnection influences the differential pressure requirements of the room.

Utilities/Water for Pharmaceutical Use System

(#1.15) System design: Water systems should be protected from contamination by supplying water under permanent overpressure and by being free of defects.

(#1.16) Water treatment: Potable water (public supply or spring or well) is purified to obtain water of higher quality for specific pharmaceutical uses. The water treatment, storage and distribution system should be designed, constructed and maintained so as to ensure a reliable source of water of an appropriate quality. They should not be operated beyond their designed capacity and should be kept adequately by implementing a maintenance program.

(#1.17) Protection of the water: Water for pharmaceutical use cannot be protected by addition of chemicals (*e.g.* chlorine), therefore the growth of microorganisms has to be prevented during its production, storage and distribution. This is possible by keeping it under constant circulation at a range of temperature inadequate for microbial growth (temperature above 70 °C or not more than 10 °C), by addition of ozone (which has only oxygen as by-product) or by UV radiation.

Utilities/Steam for Pharmaceutical Use System

(#1.18) System design: Although steam is self-sterilizing in a bad designed system there could be points of water stagnation with possibility of microbial growth (if the system is left at room temperature for some time) and consequent passage of endotoxins to the steam.

(#1.19) Source of water: If using an inadequately purified water (*e.g.* containing substances and/or endotoxins) the obtained steam could be contaminated with volatile substances and/or endotoxins.

Utilities/Compressed Air System

(#1.20) Source of air: If the air supplied to the compressor is contaminated the compressed air will be contaminated too.

(#1.21) Compressor type: If the compressor is not oil-free (lubricated) the compressed air could contain oil.

(#1.22) System configuration: When air contains a high percentage of humidity there is a risk (depending on the dew point temperature and the room temperature) of water condensation. This water could support the growth of microorganisms and contaminate the air. This is why the system has to be well designed (*e.g.* without condensation points) and usually include a dehumidifier.

Utilities/Compressed Gases Systems

(#1.23) Gas quality: Gases are received in pressure-filled cylinders. If the gas has not the adequate quality (*e.g.* industrial gas) it might contain impurities and thus, contaminate products.

Operations/Equipment

(#1.24) Installation: Equipment should be installed in such a manner as to diminish any risk of contamination.

(#1.25) Cleaning: Utensils, equipment and materials entering into the plant could be dirty and become vectors of contamination.

- Containers of materials entering into production areas should be clean; they should be controlled in the entrance airlock and if necessary cleaned/sanitized;

  An "airlock" is *an enclosed space with two or more doors, which is interposed between two or more rooms, e.g. of differing classes of cleanliness, for the purpose of controlling the airflow between those rooms when they need to be entered. An airlock is designed for use either by people or for goods and/or equipment* [7].

- Equipment/utensils should be cleaned not to be a source of contamination, when introduced into the plant and after being subjected to maintenance.

- Service materials (*e.g.* cleaners, sanitizers, lubricants, pest control agents, *etc.*) should never come into contact with the products. Nevertheless, whenever possible, these materials should be of appropriate grade (*e.g.* food grade) to minimize health risks.

- Equipment used for washing, cleaning and drying should not be a source of contamination.

(#1.26) Surfaces in contact with materials and products: The quality of products should not be significantly affected by the parts of equipment that come into contact with them. The materials of construction of these parts should neither react with them nor be additive or absorptive.

(#1.27) Design: Closed equipment is usually preferable to control contamination. It is necessary to take appropriate measures when using open equipment and when opening closed equipment.

(#1.28) Separation: In order to impede the contamination by people production equipment is closed or separated from them by "restricted access barrier systems" (RABS) or isolators.

Operations/Personnel

(#1.29) Hygienic measures: Personnel act as vectors of contamination, either in/on them or on clothes. Human beings are symptomatic/asymptomatic carriers of microorganisms, on the skin surface, in the body or in injuries. Moreover, persons shed continuously great amounts of skin particles and these particles often harbor microorganisms. This is why operators have to be considered an important source of contamination.

- Personnel hygiene is important, because the amount of contamination on the body is inversely proportional to the level of hygiene. In some cases personnel should take a shower before entering the production premises.

- *All personnel, prior to and during employment, should undergo health examinations as appropriate. Personnel conducting visual inspections should also undergo periodic eye examinations* [8].

- Personnel shall report to supervisors any health condition that might contaminate the products (*i.e.* open lesions on the exposed part of the body or perceptible illnesses). These persons should not come in contact with materials or products.

- Personnel should wash hands (and use disinfectant) before entering the production areas. Materials and products should never be touched with bare hands. One should use gloves and even in this case avoid direct contact with the product, using instead a clean/sterile instrument.

- In clean areas neither jewels nor wrist-watches should be worn.

- Personnel should not use cosmetics that can shed particles.

- *Smoking, eating, drinking, chewing, and keeping plants, food, drink, smoking material and personal medicines should not be permitted in production, laboratory and storage areas, or in any other areas where they might adversely influence product quality* [9].

(#1.30) Wear appropriate clothing: On entering the premises personnel leave their outdoor clothes in the change room and put on clean plant clothing and shoes. Afterwards they have to change again clothing if they have to enter specific production areas. The type of operations realized in one area defines the type of clothing needed. The rule of thumb is that the higher the level of cleanliness required, the most covered the body should be (in order to retain inside the clothing the skin particles shed by the body). Garments, in this case, do not intend protecting the operator but the product.

(#1.31) Beware of tools and transfer pipes: Tools used in the production operations and pipes used for conveying water should be cleaned, sanitized and stored according to written procedures. These procedures should specify the action limits for microbiological contamination and describe the measures to be taken in case of excursion. It is necessary to keep in mind that any tool and, particularly a pipe, left with water inside is a potential breeding ground for microorganisms.

2nd CATEGORY OF HAZARD: CROSS-CONTAMINATION

Table **2** shows a PHA of cross-contamination.

Table 2. PHA of cross-contamination.

Concerned sphere	Hazard description	Hazard cause	Preventive measures
Premises/Clean rooms	Diffusion of dust within the plant	Communication between areas	(#2.1) Separation of areas
	Cross-contamination during sampling/weighing and production	Dust build-up/Poor separation and cleaning	(#2.2) Sampling & weighing areas
			(#2.3) Design
			(#2.4) Cleaning
Utilities/HVAC	Transfer of air with particles	Passage through the air-handling system	(#2.5) Separation of air-handling systems
		Recycled air is not adequately filtered	(#2.6) Evaluate advantages of recycling air
		Passive displacement of particles between rooms	(#2.7) Establish cascade pressures
	Cross-contamination during sampling/weighing	Liberation of dust during operations	(#2.8) Sampling & weighing booths
Utilities/Dust exhaust	Diffusion of dust	Communication between rooms	(#2.9) Protection against communication of rooms
		Disruption of the pressure cascade	(#2.10) Protection against modification of ΔP
Operations/equipment	Direct contamination of one product by another	Equipment is dirty	(#2.11) Adequate cleaning
		Different products side by side	(#2.12) Product separation
	Diffusion of particles	Liberation of dust during operations	(#2.13) Closed equipment:
Operations/personnel	Diffusion of particles	Passage from an area to the other with the same clothing	(#2.14) Specific area clothing

Table 2: contd...

		Clothing covered with dust	(#2.15) Air showers
	Direct cross-contamination	Direct passage of contamination by contact	(#2.16) Hygienic practices

Cross-Contamination Preventive Measures

Premises/Plant Areas

(#2.1) Separation of areas: The simplest way of hindering the passage of dust from one point to another is the separation of the operations into different rooms. This space separation is complemented with the environmental separation exerted by the HVAC system. Passage among different areas is performed through airlocks, where space and air are combined to separate the adjoining areas. In order to impede that doors remain opened they should preferably open towards the side of higher pressure and be self-closing. This is the strategy used in a plant where different products are manufactured (shared facilities in multi-product premises) and it is acceptable when no hazardous materials and products are handled.

Materials and products can be considered hazardous because of their very high pharmacological activity (*i.e.* very low quantities are sufficient for producing a pharmacological effect) or because of their adverse effects (genotoxicity, carcinogenicity, reproductive development toxicity or sensitization). Therefore it is of the outmost importance to be able to ensure that these materials and products will never contaminate other materials or products. This can be attained by three strategies:

(A) Manufacturing in multi-product plants but within clean rooms designed to provide appropriate separation (airlocks, air filtration, pressure cascades, *etc.*), working within closed systems and ensuring that no adverse effects will be caused by residual active substance on the surfaces of equipment (*i.e.* cleaning validation).

(B) Manufacturing in a multi-product plant but within a separated suit of clean rooms.

(C) Manufacturing in a dedicated segregated plant.

Each substance requires particularized study (*i.e.* risk analysis and validation) in order to determine which is the right strategy, that has to be approved by the regulatory authorities.

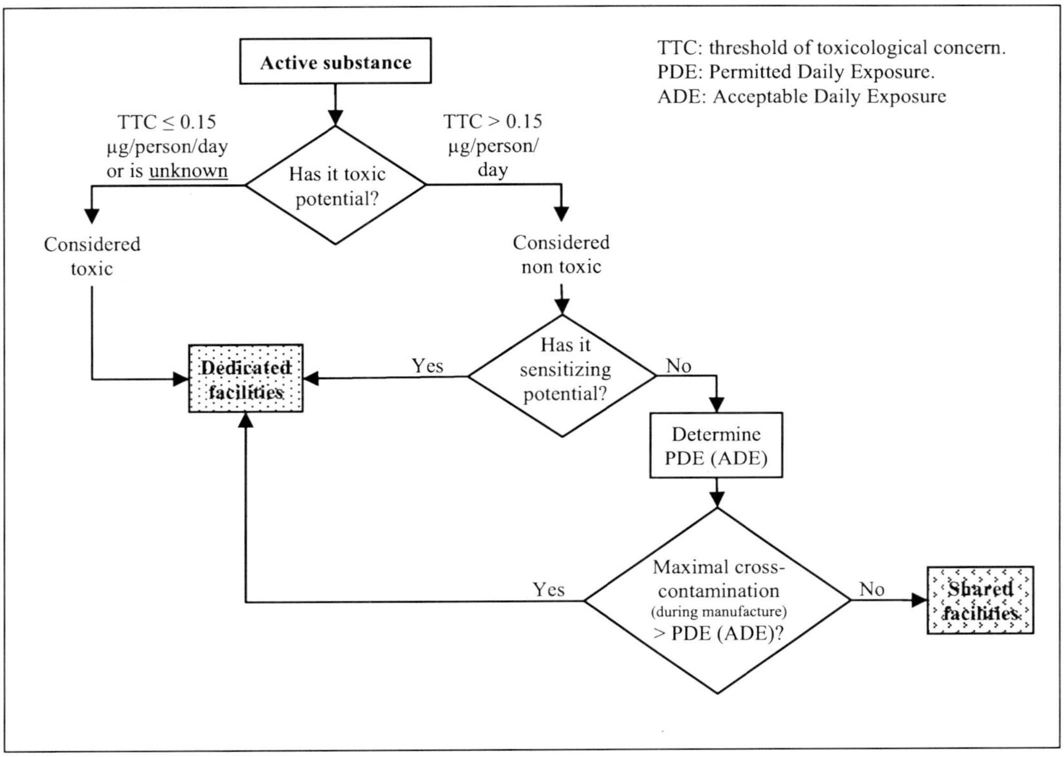

Fig. (2). Schematic rationale for determining the need of dedicated manufacturing facilities.

As it can be seen in Fig. (**2**) the first aspect to consider is "toxicity" (genotoxicity, carcinogenicity, reproductive development toxicity, *etc.*) which can be expressed by the "threshold of toxicological concern" (TTC), fixed at 0.15 µg/person/day for active substances (APIs). The second point to be taken into account is the sensitizing potential. And, finally, the effect on other materials or products because of cross-contamination is estimated by means of the PDE (Permitted Daily Exposure) or ADE (Acceptable Daily Exposure) [10].

The intended objective is always being below the "no observed effect level" (NOEL), defined as the highest tested dose of a substance or product at which no effect is observed, to wit: there is neither negative effect on the health (in a toxicological study) nor therapeutic effect (in a clinical study).

NOEL can be modified taking into account several security factors to obtain the PDE (Permitted Daily Exposure) or ADE (Acceptable) Daily Exposure) defined as the dose which is improbable that cause an adverse effect on a person exposed to it during every day of her/his life.

Therefore:

- Beta-lactam antibiotics are highly sensitizing and allergic reactions have been associated with penicillins and non-penicillin beta-lactams (Fig. **3**). This is why they have to be manufactured in dedicated and self-contained facilities to minimize the risk of a serious medical hazard due to cross-contamination [11].

Among the substances which possess in their molecule the beta-lactam ring are some antibiotics (i.e. beta-lactam antibiotics), which can be grouped in five classes according to their side-chains.

- Penicillins (e.g. ampicillin, oxacillin)
- Cephalosporins (e.g. cephalexin, cefaclor)
- Penems (e.g. imipenem, meropenem)
- Carbacephems (e.g. loracarbef)
- Monobactams (e.g. aztreonam)

Beta-lactam ring

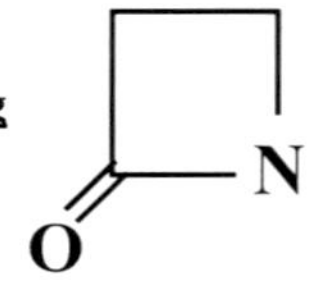

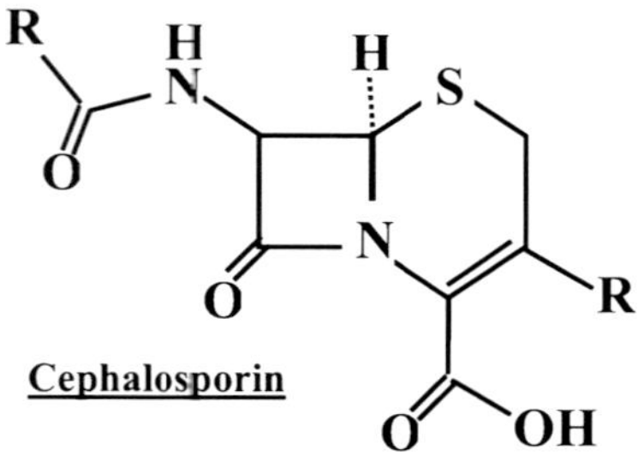

Cephalosporin

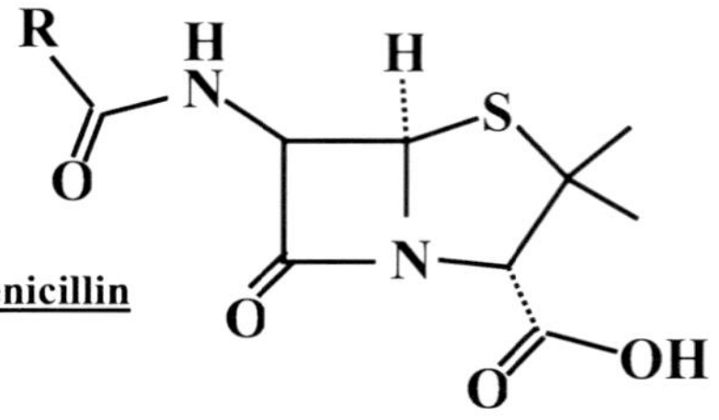

Penicillin

Fig. (3). Beta-lactam antibiotics.

- Biological preparations with live microorganisms and products with radioisotopes require dedicated and self-contained facilities for security reasons.

- Highly active products (like antibiotics, hormones, cytotoxic substances, *etc.*) should be manufactured ensuring that there will not be cross-contaminations by following the above described strategy.

- Technical agents of poisonous nature (*e.g.* herbicides, pesticides, *etc.*) should not be produced in the same premises where pharmaceutical products are manufactured.

(#2.2) Sampling and weighing areas: There should be specific sampling and weighing areas:

- Sampling of starting materials should be performed in a separated area and it should be carried out in such a way as to avoid any contamination. This area is usually located in or near the storage zone.

- Starting materials should be weighed in a separated weighing area. This area should be designed to prevent contamination by an adequate control of dust. It can be either a part of the storage zone or a part of the production areas.

(#2.3) Design: Premises should be designed with enough space for allowing appropriate working, cleaning and maintenance.

(#2.4) Cleaning: Cleaning procedures should be validated. Labels in the rooms should indicate if they are clean or to be cleaned.

Utilities/HVAC System

(#2.5) Separation of air-handling systems: Separated air-handling facilities for differenciated areas, usually with different requirements (*e.g.* animal houses).

(#2.6) Evaluate advantages of recycling air: If air in the production areas is recycled it is necessary to take measures to control the diffusion of dust. Air recycling means energy savings but also increased risk of cross-contamination (even if air is HEPA-filtered), thus the convenience of recycling should be evaluated. An alternative is recovering energy from the air instead of recycling it.

(#2.7) Establish cascade pressures: Particles can be easily displaced suspended in the air (depending on their size). This is why gradients of pressure, and their associated flows of air, allow for the control of cross-contamination:

- Clean rooms for production of liquid or semi-solid forms are usually kept at positive pressure respect the corridor (and the outside) to impede the entrance of particles.

- Clean rooms where solid forms are produced are usually kept at negative pressure respect the corridor to impede the exit of particles (but at positive pressure respect the outside of the plant).

- Clean rooms where toxic products are manufactured are kept at negative pressure respect the corridor and the outside to impede exit of particles.

There should be indicators of differential pressure when ΔP is critical. The ΔP values should be registered regularly. An alarm should warn of system failure.

(#2.8) Sampling & weighing booths: In sampling and weighing areas there is generation of dust. This is why operations are performed within booths, which allow manipulating under unidirectional airflow. Below, there is an extraction flow of air which ensures the exhausting of any dust produced during the manipulations (Fig. **4**). The estimation of yield by weighing when there is risk of dust release can be performed in the weighing area or in an especially dedicated area with the same characteristics.

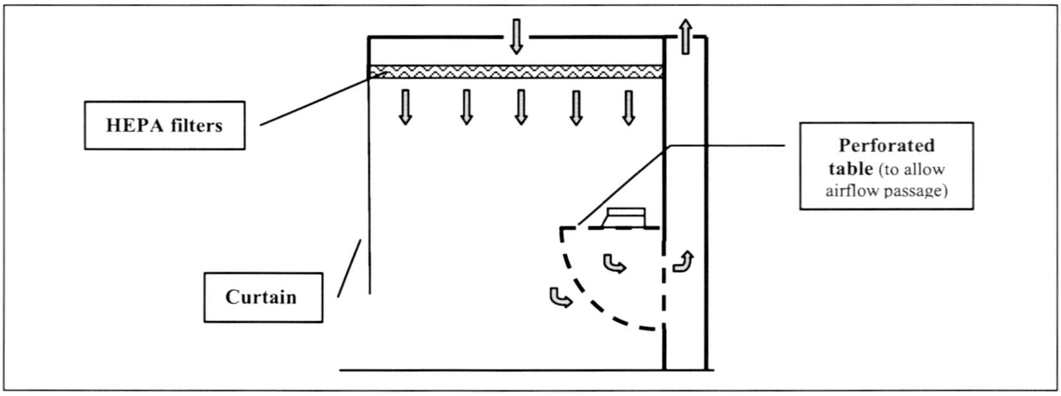

Fig. (4). Sampling/weighing booth.

Utilities/Dust exhaust System

During certain operations (*e.g.* when mixing, processing or packaging powders) there is an important generation of dust and it is necessary to supplement the HVAC system with a dust exhausting system.

(#2.9) Protection against communication of rooms: The system has to be designed to ensure that when it is turned off there will be not communication between rooms possessing use points of the dust extraction system.

(#2.10) Protection against modification of ΔP: The system has to ensure that neither its connection nor its disconnection influences the differential pressure requirements of the room.

Operations/Equipment

(#2.11) Adequate cleaning: Equipment should be cleaned following validated cleaning procedures. In multi-product equipment the intention is impeding the contamination of a batch by rests of the preceding one. In dedicated equipment the aim is impeding the contamination of a batch by degradation products of preceding batches and/or by microbial colonies developed on rests of product. The state of cleanliness of equipment should be indicated by attaching a label. It should be taken into account that dirty equipment or parts of equipment taken to the washing room are a likely source of contamination while moving.

(#2.12) Product separation: In a room, in principle, only one product at a time should be processed. The equipment and the room are labeled. In order to increase productivity it is possible to organize campaign productions, where multiple batches of the same product are produced in series.

(#2.13) Closed equipment: Closed equipment is preferable to impede cross-contamination.

Operations/Personnel

(#2.14) Specific area clothing: Change of clothing when changing of area,

(#2.15) Hygienic practices: Wash hands, put on new gloves and contact product with clean and sterilized instruments, as necessary.

(#2.16) Air showers: When there is liberation of dust during the operations the exit from the room across an airlock provided with an air shower can diminish the likelihood of contaminating other rooms.

3rd CATEGORY OF HAZARD: ENVIRONMENTAL CONTAMINATION

The word environment is used not only to design the people, air, water and land that surrounds the plant but also the people, air and surfaces within the plant.

Non harmful products, in principle, do not suppose a critical environmental problem, although it is evident that the uncontrolled liberation of any product is unacceptable. Completely different is the case of harmful products. They require a careful manipulation in order to avoid environmental contamination both inside and outside from the plant. Hazard can be originated by toxic substances [12] or by harmful microorganisms [13, 14].

The danger of a substance is evaluated by means of the "occupational exposure level" (OEL) defined as the concentration of substances in the air which is not likely to cause adverse effects on most healthy workers exposed 8 hours a day, 5 days a week. Dangerous substances should have "Material Safety Data Sheets" (MSDSs) which provide information on them.

The danger of microorganisms is assessed in four levels or risk groups (RG 1, 2, 3 and 4). To each one of these groups corresponds a required biosecurity level (BSL 1, 2, 3, 4) or protection level (P 1, 2, 3 and 4). See Table **3**.

Risk Group 1 *(no or low individual and community risk): A microorganism that is unlikely to cause human or animal disease.*

Risk Group 2 *(moderate individual risk, low community risk): A pathogen that can cause human or animal disease but is unlikely to be a serious hazard to laboratory workers, the community, livestock or the environment. Laboratory exposures may cause serious infection, but effective treatment and preventive measures are available and the risk of spread of infection is limited.*

Risk Group 3 *(high individual risk, low community risk): A pathogen that usually causes serious human or animal disease but does not ordinarily spread from one infected individual to another. Effective treatment and preventive measures are available.*

Risk Group 4 *(high individual and community risk): A pathogen that usually causes serious human or animal disease and that can be readily transmitted from one individual to another, directly or indirectly. Effective treatment and preventive measures are not usually available.*

Table 3. Summary of characteristics of the four risk groups of microorganisms.

Characteristic	RG 1	RG 2	RG 3	RG 4
Risk for the person	Minimal	Low	High	Very high
Risk of epidemic	No	No	Low	High
Therapy/prevention	Unnecessary	Available	Available	Non available
Manipulation	Bench	UDF bench/BSC II	In BSC II	In BSC III/ In BSC II + pressure suit/ In BSC III + pressure suit
Great quantities of RG 2 should be treated as RG 3				

Hazards are similar in all groups, but with an increase in risk. This is why, roughly speaking, although the approach is about the same, the measures which are put into practice are aligned with the level of risk. For the sake of simplicity, the preventive measures described in a general way are complemented with tables which detail its practical application according to the risk level.

Table **4** develops a PHA of environmental contamination.

Table 4. PHA of environmental contamination.

Sphere concerned	Type of hazard	Cause of hazard	Reference #
Premises/Clean areas	Unawareness of danger	Lack of warning	(#3.1) Identification
	Diffusion of hazardous organisms/products	Lack of separation	(#3.2) Separation
			(#3.3) Personnel flow
			(#3.4) Material flow
		Leakage	(#3.5) Isolation
		Lack of decontamination	(#3.6) Decontamination
		Inadequate lay-out and design	(#3.7) Ergonomy
		Inadequate storage	(#3.8) Safe storage
		Hands cannot be washed	(#3.9) Hand washing basins
		Doors are left open	(#3.10) Doors
		Lack of containment	(#3.11) BSC
		Liberation of viable organisms	(#3.12) Sterilizator
	Unsuitable cleaning	Inadequate surfaces and design	(#3.13) Sanitary design
	Loss of system control	Accident or emergency	(#3.14) Safety
Utilities/HVAC	Inadequate containment	Inappropriate system design	(#3.15) System configuration
	Liberation of hazardous organisms/products	Poor filtration/inactivation	(#3.16) Exhaust air
		Loss of integrity of HEPA filter	(#3.17) HEPA filter control
		Contaminated filters and ducts	(#3.18) Decontamination
		Staff unaware of HVAC failure	(#3.19) Alarm
	Energy loss	Full system work at all times	(#3.20) Save energy

Table 4: contd...

Utilities/Dust exhaust	Liberation of hazardous organisms/products	Dust is liberated while unloading the system	(#3.21) Safe dust collection
		Dust is liberated while unloading the cleaners	(#3.22) Vacuum cleaners
	Contamination by exhaust air	Exhaust air is supplied to the system	(#3.23) Dust exhaust
Utilities/Water	Liberation of hazardous organisms/products	Water is contaminated	(#3.24) Protection of water from contamination
Utilities/Vacuum	Liberation of hazardous organisms/products	Passage of organism/products to vacuum pipe	(#3.25) Protection against contamination
		Poor filtration of exhaust air	(#3.26) Vacuum exhaust air
Operations/equipment	Liberation of hazardous organisms/products to the environment	Spillage	(#3.27) Spillage retention
		Equipment used for different processes in different areas	(#3.28) Dedicated equipment
		Equipment permits diffusion of organisms/substances to the environment	(#3.29) Use of closed systems
Operations/personnel	Operator contact with the hazardous organism/product	Inadequate separation	(#3.30) Separation operator/product
	Liberation of hazardous organisms/products to the environment	Operator moves around with contaminated suit	(#3.31) Suit decontamination
Operations/waste disposal	Liberation of hazardous organisms/products to the environment	Inadequate handling of waste and effluents	(#3.32) Safe handling
			(#3.33) Disposal
			(#3.34) Exhaust air
			(#3.35) Effluent decontamination

When handling hazardous materials/products the protection requirements are usually three-fold:

- Protection of materials and products from the contamination and this requires isolation and separation, as seen before.

- Protection of the operators by product containment in closed equipment or in isolators and/or operator protection with personal protective equipment (PPE).

- Protection of the outside environment by product containment.

Environmental Contamination Preventive Measures

These measures are summarized in Table **5**.

Premises/Plant areas

(#3.1) Identification: "Biohazard" symbol should be placed at the entrance when manipulating microorganisms of RG 2 or higher. It should also be fixed on potentially contaminated equipment (refrigerators, freezers, containers, *etc.*). In case of other hazards it is also advisable follow suit providing an indication of the type of hazard and any practical information deemed necessary (Fig. **5**).

BIOHAZARD
Access limited to authorized personnel

- **Biosecurity level:** ....
- **Involved microorganisms:** ....
- **Responsible person:** ....
- **Emergency contact (1):** .... ☎ ....
- **Emergency contact (1I):** .... ☎ ....

Fig. (5). Biohazard warning at the laboratory entrance.

(#3.2) Separation: The contained area must be separated and provided with access restricted to authorized personnel. It should be placed in a separate building or in the same building, but in a well delimited and protected area. Rest, eating and drinking areas should be separated and located outside of the contained area.

(#3.3) Personnel flow: Access of personnel across a first changing room and exit across a separated second one. Both changing rooms are divided into inner and outer part, with an intermediate shower. Entrance supposes a complete change of clothes, consequently outdoor clothing and personal items should remain outside.

If the entrance changing room is not provided with a shower there should be a transversal bench to divide clearly the two parts of it. The way out changing room should be provided with a shower.

In case of using protective suits (*e.g.* P4) the operator has to pass a decontamination process before acceding to the way out changing room.

(#3.4) Material flow: Access of materials through airlocks/pass-through. In case of biohazard they should be provided with a disinfection system, as necessary, or consist of a double-door sterilizator. Doors should be interlocked to impede the opening of both doors at the same time and also the opening of one door before completing the disinfection/sterilization process.

(#3.5) Isolation: The area where dangerous products are manipulated should be a taut structure with air tight floors, walls and ceilings. Windows should be closed, sealed and break-resistant. The intention is to exclude the possibility of leakage through paneling joints, cracks, *etc.* It is important to exclude the possibility of leakage through service areas.

A "controlled area" is an area constructed and operated in such a manner that some attempt is made to control the introduction of potential contamination (an air supply approximating to grade D may be appropriate), and the consequences of accidental release of living organisms. The level of control exercised should reflect the nature of the organism employed in the process. At a minimum, the area should be maintained at a pressure negative to the immediate external environment and allow for the efficient removal of small quantities of airborne contaminants.

A "contained area" is an area constructed and operated in such a manner (and equipped with appropriate air handling and filtration) so as to prevent contamination of the external environment by biological agents from within the area [15].

(#3.6) Decontamination: Rooms should be sealable for performing decontamination.

(#3.7) Ergonomy: There should be sufficient space for the safe development of the laboratory work and for cleaning and maintenance:

- Laboratory furniture should be resistant; there should be open spaces that can be reached for cleaning under equipment, cabinets and benches.

- There should be adequate space for the storage of supplies for immediate use. There should be additional space for long-term supplies, placed outside the working areas of the laboratory. There should be space and facilities for the adequate handling and storage of specialized materials, such as compressed and liquefied gases, radioactive materials or solvents.

(#3.8) Safe storage: There should be areas for the safe and protected storage of special materials and products such as: radioactive and highly active items, substances presenting particular risk of misuse, narcotics and other dangerous medicines, and materials fire or explosion-prone.

(#3.9) Hand washing basins: Each laboratory room should have hand-washing basins, if possible near the exit door and provided with hands-free controls.

(#3.10) Doors: Doors should be provided with vision panels and be fire-resistant. They should be self-closing, if possible, and ensure a tight closing.

(#3.11) BSC: Biological safety cabinets should be protected from air currents by being placed away from walking areas, doors and ventilation points. See chapter 8 for detailed information on biological safety cabinets.

(#3.12) Sterilizator: The containment laboratory should be provided with an autoclave for the decontamination of contaminated waste material.

(#3.13) Sanitary design: The design of the laboratories should take into account the suitability of the materials of construction. The objective is having smooth, water-proof and resistant surfaces allowing easy cleaning and disinfection:

- Walls, ceilings, floors and working surfaces (bench tops) should be smooth, resistant and impervious, and without cracks or junctions for effective cleaning and disinfection.

- Floors should be slip-resistant.

- Fittings should be embedded in walls and sealed. Openings through surfaces for service pipes or cables should be sealed to ensure isolation.

- Chairs should be covered with non porous material which might be easily cleaned and disinfected.

- No floor carpets should be used.

(#3.14) Safety: There should be safety systems in place covering foreseeable emergencies (accident, fire, electrical failure, flood, earthquake, *etc.*):

- Emergency shower and eyewash facilities.
- Exit signs.
- The electricity supply should be reliable. There should be, whenever possible, a stand-by generator for supplying essential equipment, such as biological safety cabinets, incubators and freezers. It should also provide energy for the ventilation of animal cages and for keeping a negative ΔP.
- Emergency lights, fire detectors, fire extinguishers (dioxide of carbon/powder), gas detectors in the upper part of BSC (if there is use of gas), break-through panel for emergency exit use.
- Permanent communication with the outside by interphone and by visualization of critical operations.

Table 5. Characteristics of the premises according to the biosecurity level.

Feature		BSL 1	BSL 2	BSL 3	BSL 4
(#3.1) Identification	"Biohazard" sign	No	Yes	Yes	Yes
(#3.2) Separation	Workplace separated from other activities in the premises	No	Optional	Yes	Yes
	Controlled access	No	Optional	Yes	Yes
	Services within the controlled area	Yes	Optional	No	No
(#3.3) Personnel flow	Access by airlock	No	No	Optional	Yes
	Shower	No	No	Optional	Yes
(#3.4) Material flow	Equipment airlock/pass-through can be disinfected	No	No	Yes (if possible)	Yes
(#3.5) Isolation	Viable organisms handled in isolation from the environment	No	Yes	Yes	Yes
(#3.6) Decontamination	Controlled area sealable for fumigation	No	No	Optional	Yes
	Approved disinfection procedures	Yes	Yes	Yes	Yes
(#3.7) Ergonomy	Easy manipulation and cleaning	Yes	Yes	Yes	Yes
(#3.8) Safe storage	Safe storage of hazardous products/microorganisms	Yes	Yes	Yes	Yes (secure storage)

Table 5: contd…

(#3.9) Hand washing	Decontamination and cleaning fittings that operate without hand contact	No	Optional	Yes	Yes
(#3.10) Doors	Vision panels and tight closing	Optional	Yes	Yes	Yes
(#3.11) BSC	Manipulation in a BSC	No	Yes	Yes	Yes
(#3.12) Sterilizator	Double-door sterilizator	No	No	Optional	Yes
(#3.13) Sanitary design	Follow rules of "sanitary" design	No	Yes (bench)	Yes (bench and floor)	Yes (bench, walls and floor)
(#3.14) Safety	Emergency supply of energy	No	No	Yes	Yes
	Emergency exit	Door	One direction exit door	One direction exit door	Airlock
	Physical contention must be ensured in case of earthquake	No	No	Optional	Yes
	Contention must be ensured in case of fire	No	No	Optional	Yes
	In case of flood it is ensured that water will not carry away equipment/containers	No	No	Optional	Yes (equipment should maintain operativity)
	Operations can be seen from outside	No	No	Optional	Yes
	Phone communication or equivalent	No	Optional	Yes	Yes (hand free)
	Automatic fire alarm	No	Optional	Yes	Yes

Utilities/HVAC system

(#3.15) System configuration:

- Microbiological, biological and radioisotope laboratories require separated specialized HVAC systems provided with separate air-handling units.
- Air-handling units should be accessible from outside the controlled areas.
- It is possible to recycle air into the contained area after HEPA-filtration, but for a better operator protection no recycling is prefered. Contaminated recycled air should be filtered by prefilters and HEPA

filters located in a bag-in-bag-out case. If products are particularly harmful it should be recommended to use duplicated HEPA filters.

- Contained area should be kept at negative differential pressure (ΔP), with continuous monitoring and alarm. Pressure cascade should ensure containment. In every room there should be a ΔP indicator.

- The start and stop of impulsion and exhausting fans and other associated fans should be syncronized in order to ensure that ΔP and airflows are maintained when starting and stoping the system. These interconnection sequence should also operate in case of failure of a fan in order to prevent a inversion of airflow in the system.

- It is recommended to have an emergency system in case of failure. This is indispensable when there is a high level of hazard.

- It is recommended to have doubled air dampers as a safety measure.

- There are filtration systems water/air which allow for the elimination of particles in the air and thus, increasing filter efficiency.

- The supply of air to production areas and laboratories should be separated.

(#3.16) Exhaust air: Air before being exhausted has to be HEPA-filtered across HEPA filters that should be at least H13. Contaminated exhausted air should be filtered by prefilters and HEPA filters located in a bag-in-bag-out case. If products are particularly harmful it should be recommended to use duplicated HEPA filters. Exhaust air should be discharged to the outside of the buildings and dispersed away from the air intakes and from places with people.

The exhaust air from biological safety cabinets should be passed through HEPA filters and discharged outside. The exhaust system should not affect the air balance of the cabinets and the ΔP of the rooms.

(#3.17) HEPA-filter control: All filters should be provided with differential pressure gauges in order to evaluate their loading. These gauges should be adequately installed to ensure tightness and also to be easily removable for substitution or calibration. They should have a label indicating the pressure of the clean filter and the pressure showing need of change.

(#3.18) Decontamination: The system of air ducts should permit gaseous decontamination. HEPA filters should be installed in a way to permit both decontamination and testing.

(#3.19) Alarm: There should be an alarm system, in order to stop production in case of HVAC system failure.

(#3.20) Save energy: Contained areas may have two types of operation to save energy. During working hours systems operate normally, whereas outside working hours critical equipment operate normally and uncritical equipment can receive minimal energy (*e.g.* air-conditioning has broader ranges of temperature and illumination and airflow rates are reduced).

Utilities/Dust exhaust System

(#3.21) Safe dust collection: The dust collector should be in a contained room (closed, tight and with negative ΔP). When unloading the collector operators should be adequately protected.

(#3.22) Vacuum cleaners: They should be be provided with H13 HEPA-filters too and they should be opened, unloaded and cleaned in a room with negative ΔP. Personnel should wear protective equipment.

(#3.23) Dust exhaust: The system should send the exhaust air through bag-in-bag-out filters in order to protect the environment. The exhaust outlet points outside the building should be located as far as possible of inlets and be higher placed to diminish the possibility of intake of the extracted air. The prevalent wind directions should be taken into account when positioning the inlet/outlet points.

Utilities/Water for Pharmaceutical Use System

(#3.24) Protection of water from contamination: There should be a reliable supply of quality water. The system for supplying drinking-water should be separated from that of the laboratory. The laboratory system should be provided with anti-backflow devices in order to prevent contamination.

Utilities/Vacuum System

(#3.25) Protection against contamination: Vacuum lines should be protected from contamination (*e.g.* with HEPA filers or liquid disinfectant traps). This protection should be provided to alternative vacuum pumps too.

(#3.26) Vacuum exhaust air: The vacuum extraction system should send the exhaust air through bag-in-bag-out filters in order to protect the environment.

Table **6** summarizes the features of the utilities.

Table 6. Characteristics of the utilities (HVAC and dust exhaust systems) according to the biosecurity level.

Feature		BSL 1	BSL 2	BSL 3	BSL 4
(#3.15) System configuration	Environmentally classified area	No	Optional	Yes	Yes
	Dedicated air-handling unit (AHU)	No	No	Optional	Yes
	Air-handling units accessible from outside the controlled areas	No	No	Yes	Yes
	Entrance and exit of air interlocked	No	No	Optional	Yes
	Emergency system for HVAC	No	No	Optional	Yes
	Controlled area at negative ΔP	No	No	Optional	Yes
(#3.16) Exhaust air	Supplied/exhausted air HEPA-filtered	No	No	Yes (exhausted)	Yes
	Sure change of filters (bag-in-bag-out)	No	No	Yes	Yes
	Treatment of exhaust gases from the closed system	N. a.	Minimize release	Prevent release	Prevent release
(#3.17) HEPA filter control	Filter integrity and loading control	N. a.	Yes	Yes	Yes
(#3.18) Decontamination	Can ducts and filters be decontaminated?	No	No	Yes	Yes
(#3.19) Alarm	Alarm in case of ΔP alteration	No	No	Yes	Yes
(#3.20) Save energy	Working/rest system operation	Yes	Yes	Yes	Optional
(#3.23) Dust exhaust	Filtration through bag-in-bag-out filters	No	No	Optional	Yes
(#3.25) Protection against contamination	Vacuum system separated from the controlled area with filter	No	No	Optional	Yes

Operations/Equipment

(#3.27) Spillage retention: There should be measures to be able to retain the whole contents of the biggest container in case of spillage.

(#3.28) Dedicated equipment: It is evident that in case of hazardous materials or microorganisms it is much better avoiding displacements of equipment in/out of the contained area. Cleaning becomes easier and more reliable with dedicated equipment.

(#3.29) Use of closed systems: Material should be adequately designed and personnel appropriately trained for ensuring that harmful organisms or substances will not be released to the environment. Organisms should be kept within closed systems, unless they have been inactivated.

Table **7** summarizes the characteristics of the equipment and the operations.

Table 7. Characteristics of the operations/equipment according to the biosecurity level.

Feature		BSL 1	BSL 2	BSL3	BSL4
(#3.27) Spillage retention	Controlled area designed to contain the entire spillage of the container of the closed system	No	Optional	Yes	Yes
(#3.28) Dedicated equipment	Area contains its own equipment	No	No	Optional	Yes
(#3.29) Use of closed systems	Seals designed	to minimize release	to minimize release	to prevent release	to prevent release
	Operations performed	to minimize release	to minimize release	to prevent release	to prevent release
	Bulk culture fluids not removed from the closed system unless organism	N. a.	inactivated by validated means	inactivated by validated chemical or physical means	inactivated by validated chemical or physical means

Operations/Personnel

(#3.30) Separation operator/product: When there is potential risk of aerosol release it is necessary to establish a barrier between product and operator.

This is possible either isolating the product within a BSC, or protecting the operator with "personal protective equipment" (PPE).

In case of low or medium hazard level usually a BSC II suffices, but with high hazard level (RG4) it is necessary either use a BSC III or use a BSC II and don a protective positive pressure suit (or even use BSC III and pressure suit). Both approaches differ in facility design and requirements. See Fig. (**6**).

Personal protective equipment (PPE):

- Airline respirator (AR): The mask of the operator is connected with flexible pipes and rapid connectors to a central air supply system. It is necessary to ensure that there will not be intake of contaminated air when connecting and disconnecting. T and RH are controled.
- Self-contained breathing apparatus (SCBA)/Powered air purifying respirator (PAPR)]: These are autonomous respiration systems which are connected to the operator mask. Air is extracted from the room where operator is working and it is sent to the mask by a fan powered by a battery.
- Semi-mask respirator with HEPA filter (type N95)

AR is better than SCBA. PPE is selected taking into account the relation between accepted OEL and the protection factor (PF) certified for the equipment.For areas with lower contamination level a semi-mask respirator can suffice.

(#3.31) Suit decontamination: In case of risk of dust contamination on clothing, operators, when going out of the contention area, should pass through a decontamination system (air/mist shower), before entering the exit changing room. All dirty clothing should be adequately packed in tight bags before going out of the containment area. Washing should be performed in an appropriate way to protect people and environment.

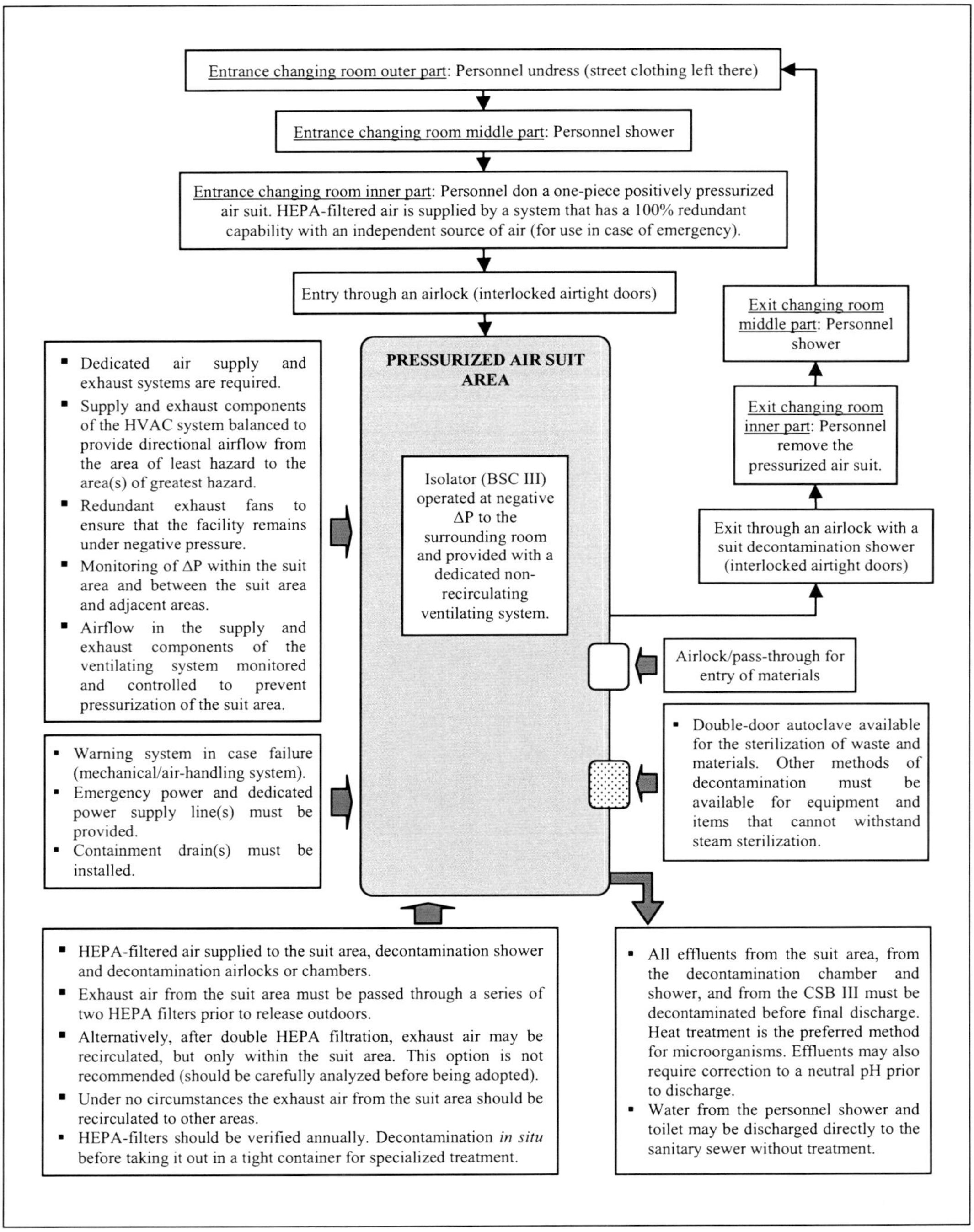

Fig. (6). Flow diagram of a P4 laboratory with operators using pressure suits.

Operations/Waste Disposal

(#3.32) Safe handling: The manipulation of liquid, solid and gas waste should not suppose a risk for the operators, for the products and for the environment. Neither the products manipulated in the plant nor their residues should be liberated to the atmosphere or be discarded directly to the drains.

All types of waste should be eliminated in a safe manner and this elimination should be documented. If this elimination is outsourced, the contract acceptor should be certified and authorised.

Laboratories should have fume hoods (cupboards) for the safe extraction of vapors and smoke. They have to be qualified to show that no fumes are liberated inside the laboratory.

(#3.33) Disposal: Infectious waste should be removed from the laboratory in a safe manner for decontamination and disposal. It should be transported according to applicable regulations in tight, sealed and unbreakable containers. If possible, it is advisable to have an incinerator in place.

(#3.34) Exhaust air: All the extraction systems of the equipment of the unit (fluid beds, coating drums, *etc.*) should send the exhaust air across bag-in-bag-out filters in order to protect the environment.

(#3.35) Effluent decontamination: If there are dangerous effluents they have to be treated before being sent to the sewer. See Table **8**.

Table 8. Characteristics of the effluent disposal according to the biosecurity level.

Feature		BSL 1	BSL 2	BSL3	BSL4
(#3.35) Effluent decontamination	System for the inactivation of biological effluents before their release	No	Yes, inactivated by validated means	Yes, inactivated by validated chemical or physical means	Yes, inactivated by validated chemical or physical means
	System for collection and inactivation of effluents of basins, showers and floor cleaning	No	No	Optional	Yes

4th CATEGORY OF HAZARD: ERROR/MIX-UP

Table **9** shows PHA of error/mix-up.

Table 9. PHA of error/mix-up.

Concerned sphere	Hazard description	Hazard cause	Preventive measures
Premises/Clean rooms	Mix-up of operations	Inadequate lay-out	(#4.01) Logical design
	Mix-up of materials/products	Inadequate flows	(#4.02) Material and personnel flows
		Lack of space	(#4.03) Storage space in the production areas
		Lack of separation between reception and dispatch	(#4.04) Warehouse separation of reception and dispatch
		Unclear identification and status	(#4.05) Warehouse storage areas
	Mix-up of samples/substances	Lack of space	(#4.06) Storage space in the QC laboratory
	Mix-up the state of quarantine/approved and of rejected/recalled/returned materials/products	Unclear identification and status	(#4.07) Warehouse quarantine
		Unsure segregation	(#4.08) Warehouse segregation
	Mix-up of printed materials	Unsafe storage	(#4.09) Warehouse storage of printed packaging materials
	Mix-up during production	Poor illumination	(#4.10) Illumination
Operations/equipment	Error during operations	Illogical installation	(#4.11) Design and installation
	Mix-up of fluids	Lack of identification	(#4.12) Identification of pipework
		Interchange of connections/adaptors	(#4.13) Non-interchangeable connections/adaptors
	Use of defective equipment	Unidentified faulty equipment	(#4.14) Removal/identification of faulty equipment
	Misuse of the facilities	Inadequate knowledge of the facilities	(#4.15) Drawings
Operations/personnel	Error	Double control	(#4.16) Independent check
	Wrong cloth donning	Lack of verification	(#4.17) Verification mirrors

Error/Mix-Up Preventive Measures

Premises/Plant areas

(#4.01) Logical design: Premises should be designed in order to minimize the risk of mix-ups and errors. Their layout should be appropriate to carry out the operations. This is why it is preferable the logical connection of the areas corresponding to the sequence of the operations and to the required levels of cleanliness.

(#4.02) Material and personnel flows: The arrangement of rooms following the logical order of operations, in order to prevent crossings of personnel or materials, contributes to diminishing the risks of mix-up. Any backward flow during operations must be avoided.

(#4.03) Storage space in the production areas: Working and in-process storage areas should minimize the risk of mix-up, cross-contamination and of incorrect control of the manufacturing steps (omission or erroneous implementation) by permitting the positioning of materials and equipment in a logical and orderly way.

(#4.04) Warehouse separation of reception and dispatch: Receiving and dispatch bays should be separated.

(#4.05) Warehouse storage areas: Storage areas should be of sufficient capacity to allow safe and orderly storage of the various categories of materials and products: starting and packaging materials, intermediates, bulk and finished products, products in quarantine, and released.

(#4.06) Storage space in the QC laboratory: Records, samples, solvents, reagents and reference standards should be appropriately stored in terms of space and, when necessary, of temperature (cooling).

(#4.07) Warehouse quarantine: If items under quarantine are stored in separate areas, they have to be clearly labeled and only authorized personnel should have access to them. It is possible to use other systems for quarantine (*e.g.* computerized systems) but they should provide the same level of safety.

(#4.08) Warehouse segregation: Physical or computerized segregation should be provided for the storage of rejected, recalled, or returned materials or products.

Computerized segregation should be validated in order to offer the same level of assurance than the physical one.

(#4.09) Warehouse storage of printed packaging materials: Printed packaging materials are critical because of the risk of mistake in the packaging of the finished product. This is why they should be carefully sampled and stored in a safe and secure manner.

(#4.10) Illumination: Production areas, especially where visual controls are performed, have to be well illuminated.

Operations/Equipment

(#4.11) Design and installation: The design, construction, adaptation, installation and maintenance should be adequate for the operations to be performed. Besides, their layout, design and location should minimize the risk of errors.

(#4.12) Identification of pipework: Fixed pipework should be visibly labeled to specify the contents and, where relevant, the direction of flow.

(#4.13) Non-interchangeable connections/adaptors: Gases and liquids should be provided with non-interchangeable connections or adaptors.

(#4.14) Removal/identification of faulty equipment: Defective equipment should be removed from the laboratories and from the areas of production. If this is not possible, equipment should be clearly labeled as out of order to prevent use.

(#4.15) Drawings: There should be maintained updated drawings of critical equipment and of the support systems.

Operations/Personnel

(#4.16) Independent check: The entry of critical data should be independently checked by a second person or by an automated system.

(#4.17) Verification mirrors: Changing rooms should be provided with mirrors to be able to check the appropriate clothing before entering the production area.

5th CATEGORY OF HAZARD: DEGRADATION

Table **10** develops a PHA of degradation.

Table 10. PHA of degradation.

Concerned sphere	Hazard description	Hazard cause	Preventive measures
Premises/Clean rooms	Degradation of materials/products during reception and dispatch.	Materials/products exposed to weather.	(#5.01) Warehouse bays protected from weather
	Degradation of laboratory instruments	Instruments exposed to inadequate conditions	(#5.02) Protection of laboratory instruments
Utilities/HVAC	Degradation of materials/products during production	Materials/products exposed to inadequate T/RH	(#5.03) Protection of materials/products during production
	Degradation of materials/products during storage	Materials/products exposed to inadequate T/RH	(#5.04) Protection of materials/products during production
Operations/equipment	Degradation of materials/products during production.	Sensitive materials/products exposed to light.	(#5.05) Light sensitive substances
Operations/personnel	Product kept at inadequate conditions	Non respect of the conditions of the product	(#5.06) Follow the approved production conditions

Degradation preventive measures

Premises/Plant Areas

(#5.01) Warehouse bays protected from weather: Receiving and dispatch bays should be designed to protect materials and products from the weather.

(#5.02) Protection of laboratory instruments: Instruments should be protected from damaging external conditions (*e.g.* electrical interference, excessive moisture, vibration, *etc.*) by isolation or installation in a separate room.

HVAC System

(#5.03) Protection of materials/products during production: This protection supposes keeping controled temperature and sometimes RH conditions in the production clean rooms. In the production rooms the HVAC system keeps a comfort temperature for the operators. This is usually an adequate temperature for the materials/products too, but if this is not the case they should be manipulated within special closed systems. If materials/products require particular RH conditions, then the HVAC system should be prepared to offer them (or special closed systems should be used)

(#5.04) Protection of materials/products during storage: The required storage temperature and sometimes humidity should be provided, controlled, monitored and recorded in the warehouse. For materials/products requiring particular conditions there should be cold chambers and freezers.

In the warehouse materials/products should be kept at adequate conditions of temperature (in the general storage racks, in refrigerators/cold chambers, or in freezers). Normally control of RH is not necessary because materials/products are protected within tightly closed containers or bags. Temperature is continuously monitored and deviations taken into account. Ensure adequate temperature conditions requires normally possessing a climatization system. The temperature probes for monitoring should be placed in the worst-case points (cooler and warmer). These points are determined by “temperature mapping” during the coldest and hottest months of the year.

Operations/Equipment

(#5.05) Protection of light sensitive materials/products: There are some materials which are degraded by light. During production they cannot be manipulated in rooms provided with standard illumination.

Operations/Personnel

(#5.06) Follow the approved production conditions: Personnel should be adequately trained and have procedures detailing under which conditions materials/products should be manipulated. These conditions should be respected and this should be checked by another person.

CONCLUDING REMARKS

The systematic analysis of quality hazards in pharmaceutical manufacturing is a very powerful means for becoming aware and understanding them and implementing a satisfactory quality managing system. A first general approach like the one shown in this chapter doesn’t require a detailed risk assessment. However, in a more advanced stage and with gained experience it might be possible evaluating it. And this supposes enhanced management and possibility of improvement by risk reduction.

CONFLICT OF INTEREST

The author confirms that this chapter contents have no conflict of interest.

ACKNOWLEDGEMENT

Declared None.

REFERENCES

[1] European Commission. Good manufacturing practices. Medicinal products for human and veterinary use. The rules governing medicinal products in the European Union. Volume 4. Brussels.

[2] US National Archives & Records Administration. Federal Register. Code of Federal Regulations (CFR). Title 21 (Food & drugs). Parts 210 and 211.

[3] WHO (World Health Organization). WHO Good manufacturing practices for pharmaceutical products: main principles. In: WHO Expert Committee on Specifications for Pharmaceutical Preparations. Forty-eighth report (WHO Technical Report Series, No. 986). WHO, Geneva, Switzerland 2014. Annex 2.

[4] Ibid. Glossary.

[5] Ibid. 9.1.

[6] Ibid. Glossary.

[7] Ibid. Glossary.

[8] Ibid. 11.1.

[9] Ibid. 11.1.

[10] EMA (European Medicines Agency). CHMP (Committee for Medicinal Products for Human Use), CVMP (Committee for Medicinal Products for Veterinary Use). Guideline on setting health based exposure limits for use in risk identification in the manufacture of different medicinal products in shared facilities. EMA/CHMP/CVMP/SWP/169430/2012. EMA, London 2014.

[11] U.S. Department of Health and Human Services. Food and Drug Administration. Center for Drug Evaluation and Research (CDER). Non-Penicillin Beta-Lactam Drugs: A CGMP Framework for Preventing Cross-Contamination. Guidance for Industry. Current Good Manufacturing Practices (CGMPs). FDA, Rockville, MD, USA 2013.

[12] WHO (World Health Organisation). WHO good manufacturing practices for pharmaceutical products containing hazardous substances. In: WHO Expert Committee on Specifications for Pharmaceutical Preparations. Forty-fourth report (WHO Technical Report Series, No. 957). WHO, Geneva, Switzerland 2010, Annex 3.

[13] US Department of Health and Human Services. Public health Service Centers for Disease Control and Prevention. National Institutes of Health. Biosafety in Microbiology and Biomedical Laboratories. HHS Publication No. (CDC) 21-1112. 5th edition revised. CDC, Atlanta, Georgia, USA 2009.

[14] WHO (World Health Organization). Laboratory biosafety manual. 3rd edition. WHO, Geneva, Switzerland 2004.

[15] European Commission. Good manufacturing practices. Medicinal products for human and veterinary use. The rules governing medicinal products in the European Union. Volume 4. Brussels: Glossary.

CHAPTER 5

The Pharmaceutical Quality System: The 21st Century Approach

Abstract: The Quality System is the nervous system of the GMP-body. The ruling brain is the Quality Manual, whereas the procedures which develop it are the nerves that control this GMP-body. The Pharmaceutical Quality System (PQS), as proposed by ICH Q10, has a slightly wider scope than GMP, as includes pharmaceutical development too. In terms of responsibility the senior direction of the company is a key factor of the quality system because determines its policy and objectives. The PQS is composed of two enablers and four elements. Enablers facilitate the attainment of the PQS objectives. A couple of elements were already in place relatively long ago (change management and CAPA system), whereas the other two are newcomers and focus on control on processes and products and on the PQS itself. The different approaches to the Quality Manual and its contents are described and commented. As a modern quality system is based on continual improvement it is necessary to identify and analyze the processes in the manufacturing plant. Processes can be kept in state of control by monitoring of variables/indicators. The latter can be monitored either during the same process (on-line or off-line) or after it by evaluation of data. Thus, improvement means variable/indicator improvement. The performance of the quality system itself must be reviewed by the management in order to ensure that it remains appropriate. The practical organization of the system is developed in documents known as general procedures of the system. The contents of these procedures are commented and their interrelations are analyzed.

Keywords: CAPA system, change management, continual improvement, document management, general procedures, incident management, knowledge management, management review, PAT, performance indicator, personnel management, PQS, Process manual, process map, Quality manual, quality objectives, quality risk management, quality policy, quality review, variable monitoring.

WHAT A QUALITY SYSTEM IS

In precedent chapters it has been analyzed why quality is a must for drug products and why different approaches to it have been adopted. Unfortunately, quality, as many other basic and evident concepts, is easier to describe and understand than to put into practice. We noticed that GMP is a basic tool to ensure quality (see chapter 1), but one thing is providing general orientation and another one very different is ensuring continual compliance. This is only possible by setting up a Pharmaceutical Quality System (PQS) which incorporates GMP. This could be expressed by a very simple equation: GMP + PQS = Ensured Quality.

Jordi Botet

GMP is well known and notwithstanding the fact that there are different texts it is something concrete, but then, what about the PQS?

For a long time there had not been a "pharmaceutical" quality system and general quality system models were adopted by the pharmaceutical companies and tailored to suit their needs. Most popular were the quality systems derived from the ISO 9000 family [1-3]. Consequently, many companies were accredited ISO. This meant that they were ISO audited on one side and GMP inspected on the other. The former was a company stake, whereas the latter was a requirement from the pharmaceutical competent authorities. In any case, the objective was ensuring continued GMP compliance.

This situation evolved at the beginning of the 21st century when, within the frame of the ICH, it was proposed a true and specific PQS model [4].

A "quality system" is *the sum of all aspects of a system that implements quality policy and ensures that quality objectives are met* [5].

In practical terms a PQS is the last step of a logical process that starts by defining the "quality policy", that is *the overall intention and direction of an organization regarding quality, as formally expressed and authorized by top management* [6].

This quality policy is then developed and implemented by the direction of the organization in what is functionally known as "quality management".

The basic elements of quality management are:

- *An appropriate infrastructure or "quality system", encompassing the organizational structure, procedures, processes and resources;*

- *Systematic actions necessary to ensure adequate confidence that a product (or service) will satisfy given requirements for quality. The totality of these actions is termed "quality assurance"* [7].

As for the rest, a quality system is compulsory (something not surprising because it is necessary for ensuring GMP compliance):

The manufacturer shall establish and implement an effective pharmaceutical quality assurance system, involving the active participation of the management and personnel of the different departments [8].

The restricting factor for the implementation of a PQS is the need of a good knowledge on materials, products and processes, but this can be overcome by understanding that it is better something imperfect than nothing (provided that weak points are well understood and continual improvement is envisaged).

CHARACTERISTICS OF THE PHARMACEUTICAL QUALITY SYSTEM

Objectives

The basic objectives of a PQS are three [9].

- **Achieve a quality product**. The system should allow the manufacturing of products meeting the specified quality attributes.
- **Establish and maintain a state of control**. The system should exert continued monitoring and control in order to ensure that products and processes are adequate ("continued suitability") and maintain their aptitude ("capability").
- **Facilitate continual improvement.** The system should identify and implement the improvement opportunities in order to increase the ability of meeting the quality requirements.

Organization

The PQS possesses a defined configuration and is based on essential principles. Two "enablers" help in building a structure based on the integration of GMP with a quality system. See Fig. (**1**).

(a) Basic Principles

1st <u>The PQS concerns the whole lifecycle of the product</u>

As seen in chapter 2, the quality of a product can only be controlled if previously it has been created. In other words, just a well known product (*i.e.* after an appropriate development), manufactured by a robust and well characterized process, can be effectively controlled regarding quality.

Quality depends not only on what is done in a phase of the lifecycle but also on what has been done in previous phases ("domino effect"). This is why in terms of quality lifecycle phases cannot be considered independently.

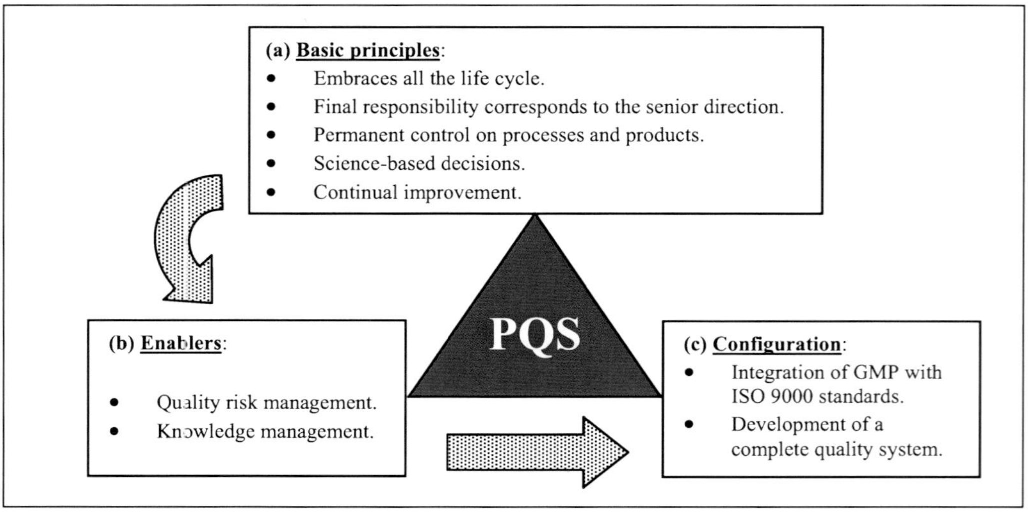

Fig. (1). Organization of the PQS.

2nd In the PQS the final responsibility corresponds to the senior direction

GMP describes the responsibilities of key personnel (see chapter 1). These technicians are all familiar with GMP. They are led by the high direction of the company and even if this direction is composed by technicians too, they often belong to other fields of science (*e.g.* economists or lawyers) and this supposes a potential risk of misunderstanding. All in all, although in the long run quality supposes always an economic boon, initially, it means expenses. Consequently, the high direction might be suspicious of activities curbing the productivity of the company. And it is evident than the lack of full support, not to mention of means, turns difficult the task of the technicians in charge of quality assurance. There is even worst, because if personnel perceive that their heads are not taken seriously by the direction it is evident that neither they are going to respect them.

This is why the PQS describes in detail the responsibilities of the direction in terms of supervision, support and by providing resources.

The responsibility for the development of the tasks described by GMP corresponds to key personnel, but the responsibility regarding the global performance of the PQS corresponds to the senior direction.

3rd The PQS requires permanent control on products and processes

Validation is performed on a limited number of batches and this is why it has to be complemented with a permanent concomitant validation. Thus, all batches are validated. Control is not focused on following the procedures, but in remaining within the design space or within the approved ranges for the critical parameters. Application of process analytical technology (PAT) to an operation supposes that it can be exactly monitored in real time by control of its critical parameters. This permanent control is not only required for the manufacturing processes, but for any process performed within the frame of the PQS.

4th Within the PQS frame decisions should be science-based

The simple mention of this point might be surprising, because it is evident that pharmaceutical activities are within the scope of science. However, not infrequently some activities (*e.g.* in the development of new products) have been done on an empirical base. Trial and error played an important role in the conception of new products and processes. The goal was to have a batch processing instruction in order to prepare a product possessing defined analytical characteristics. Whereas science-based development means that the process critical variables are known and that their acceptable ranges have been studied and established.

5th The PQS requires continual improvement

Improvement was a well-known practice outside from the pharmaceutical industry, but not within it. The protection of patients was based on a strict control of pharmaceutical products by the responsible authorities and this meant that any modification had to be authorized. Because of this, and also because of the previously mentioned strategy of control based on the exact repetition of the procedure, the pharmaceutical industry does not applied formally continual improvement.

Although it is evident that improvement in the pharmaceutical industry has to take into account the regulatory requirements and this means that innovation and process changes are not as free and simple as in other industrial branches, it is evident that does not affect most of quality improvements (*e.g.* variability reduction, better PQS organization and procedures, more accurate parameter control, *etc.*).

Any element of the PQS supplies information which might drive system improvement (Fig. **2**). This is why it is necessary to possess a systematic procedure for the study of the improvement opportunities and develop an implementation program for those considered appropriate. It is also necessary to reduce and control variation, thus increasing process capability (see chapter 4).

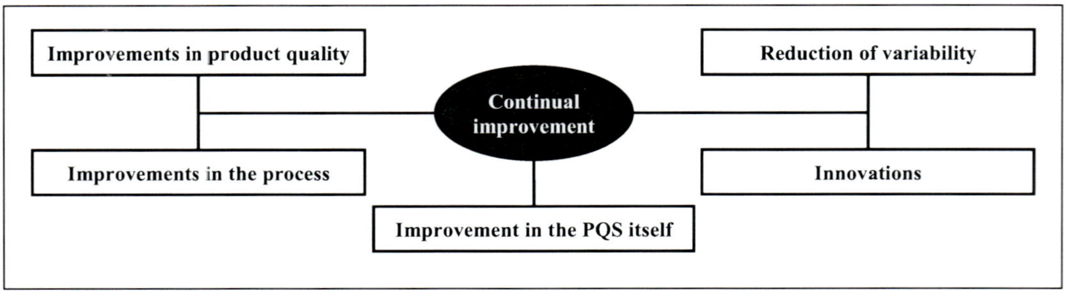

Fig. (2). Continual improvement.

(b) Enablers

Guideline ICH Q10 considers two "enablers" which are defined as tools or processes which supply the means to attain an objective.

1st Quality risk management

This is another important change. It was taken for granted that quality was an on-off value and, as we wanted it, we were bound to work perfectly in order to obtain a quality product, because imperfect work would lead to lack of quality. This apparently faultless rationale had, in fact, a flaw. Quality might be considered an absolute value, because products should posses it, but the perfection of our work cannot be an absolute value, because this is unattainable (*e.g.* if we decided to build a bridge capable of resisting all known earthquakes, floods and tsunamis – provided that this could be technically possible – how much would it cost? would the ratio cost/benefit be acceptable?). See chapter 3.

Risk management is the meeting-point of quality and work. If we accept that our work cannot be perfect and there is no alternative to this, we have to study which "perfection level" (or in other words which "risk level") we can attain and this has two important consequences. Firstly, we are going to know if our work provides a minimal quality baseline and secondly, improvement will be possible. If we accept that our work is not perfect and we can estimate its quality risk then we acknowledge that improvement means reduction in the quality risk (or increase in our level of perfection).

2nd Knowledge management

"Knowledge management" is *a systematic approach to acquire, analyze, store and diffuse information linked to products, manufacturing processes and components* [10].

The aim of knowledge management is capturing facts and data, understand them, filter them, put them at disposal of personnel to whom they might be useful and keep them for future uses. Knowledge management should be applied from data acquisition to information distribution all along the lifecycle of products.

The diffusion of knowledge within a company is not easy. Often there are important amounts of knowledge, but which are not useful because they remain the exclusive property of isolated persons, and like terrestrial animals living in islands in the middle of the ocean cannot spread out. And yet, in order to attain the above-mentioned goals of science-based decisions and continual improvement knowledge should be acquired and shared by all relevant personnel.

It is also necessary to fight against a common practice, according to which, when products are transferred from the development center to the manufacturing site all knowledge has been acquired and only validation is necessary (if a process is well-established, then production means following verbatim the procedures, and speaking about an increase of knowledge is out of place). Nowadays it is recognized that knowledge on processes and on products is a never ending course of action. Exactly as personnel receive continuous training, processes and products are subject to continuous increase of knowledge. In fact this progressive increase in product knowledge starts during development and goes on throughout its commercial live (*e.g.* see pharmacovigilance in chapter 12).

(c) Configuration

As exposed in the annexed figure, shown in guideline ICH Q10 [11], the PQS is a wide frame which manages quality in all the stages of the lifecycle. This is consistent with the concept that all these stages are interconnected and thus, should be globally managed. All the same, this creates a significant difference, because pharmaceutical development, the first stage of the lifecycle, is not covered by GMP. See Fig. (**3**).

This figure is also interesting because it highlights the relation between GMP and the PQS. GMP is practice and it deals on how to operate, which precautions to take and which points should be checked. Instead, PQS is management and explains how to attain and ensure GMP compliance. It is worth commenting that the exclusion of pharmaceutical development from GMP is just the consequence of admitting that the world of development is very different from the world of manufacturing in terms of organization and modus operandi, but this explains too why GMP was extended to investigational products. Even if the product development may not be performed within the GMP frame, the preparation of the dosage forms to be used in the clinical assays should be equivalent to the production of any other standard dosage form.

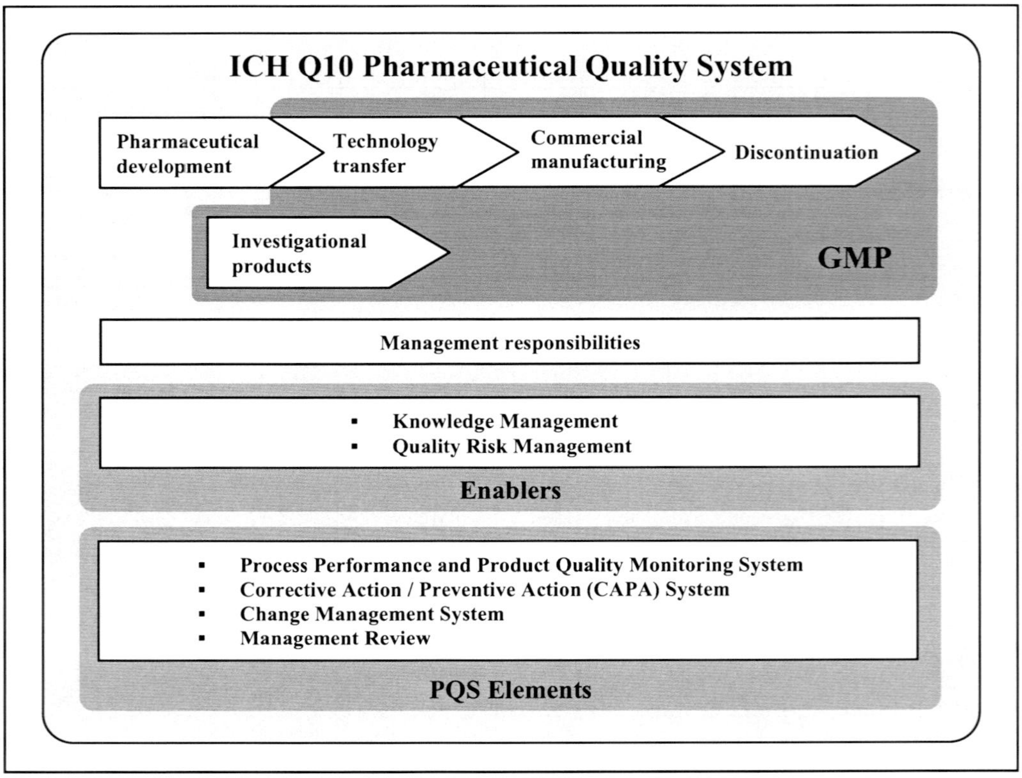

Fig. (3). Structure of the ICH Q10 PQS.

Enablers facilitate the attainment of the three above-mentioned main objectives of the PQS (quality products, state of control and continual improvement).

Let us consider the four elements or constitutional parts recognized in the PQS:

- Process Performance and Product Quality Monitoring System
- Corrective Action/Preventive Action (CAPA) System
- Change Management System
- Management review

Note: It is worth pointing out that the three first elements are considered systems because they are in fact composed of sub-elements.

To these four elements it could also be added "self-inspection" and "product quality review" which interact with them and are also considered in this chapter.

Process Performance and Product Quality Monitoring System

The purpose of this system is ensuring that the state of control, that is, a situation in which the ensemble of control measures warrants the appropriate performance of the process performance and the specified quality of the product, is maintained.

This system should choose and apply instruments in order to measure and analyze critical variables (parameters and attributes) and identify the sources of variation which affect the process performance.

Besides controlling variables, other performance indicators (deviations, non-conformities, rejects, recalls, complaints) and the results of internal audits and inspections should be taken into account.

The intent is increasing the degree of knowledge of the product and process and consequently diminishing the risk level and thus ensuring that the system operates in a state of control.

Validation is a never ending process. Before starting commercial manufacturing the process is validated ("prospective validation") with the aim of verifying that the variables are well identified and their acceptance ranges are adequately set. The approach used for this initial validation is manufacturing a certain number of batches and checking that by variable monitoring it is possible to keep the process under control and obtain a product meeting requirements.

From this moment on, critical variables are routinely monitored. This overcomes the main shortcoming of validation which is the limited number of controlled batches. Continuous process control means in fact "concurrent validation or continuous validation". On-going and off-line measurements ensure the maintenance of the validated state of control of the process during regular production. Control of critical parameters within acceptance limits, shown during validation, is maintained throughout. Thus, each manufactured batch is validated.

The aim of monitoring is double, on one hand verifying that critical variables meet specifications and therefore that the finished products possess the expected identity, strength, purity, and quality; and on the other detecting significant trends and unanticipated variables.

The objective of PAT is to ensure the quality of the products by performing real-time analysis, while reducing or eliminating final product testing. Manufacturing equipment is provided with devices (sensors, probes, *etc.*) to obtain timely process data on critical quality parameters and performance attributes of the operations.

Monitoring is performed by means of indicators such as:

- Critical attributes of starting and packaging materials;
- Critical attributes of intermediate, bulk and finished products;
- Critical process parameters;
- Deviations, non conformities and rejects;
- Complaints, devolutions and recalls.

Critical variables (attributes and parameters) should be within their specified ranges and do not show neither particular trends nor significant variability. Quality indicators should not get worse.

Product Quality Reviews

The intent of these reviews, as described by WHO and European GMP, is showing that a given company consistently manufactures products with the required quality and which meet their specifications, and ensuring that all modifications have been duly communicated to the regulatory authorities.

Regular periodic or rolling quality reviews of all licensed medicinal products, including export only products, should be conducted with the objective of verifying the consistency of the existing process, the appropriateness of current specifications for both starting materials and finished product to highlight any trends and to identify product and process improvements. Such reviews should normally be conducted and documented annually, taking into account previous reviews.

The manufacturer and marketing authorization holder, where different, should evaluate the results of this review and an assessment should be made whether corrective and preventative action or any revalidation should be undertaken. Reasons for such corrective actions should be documented. Agreed corrective and preventative actions should be completed in a timely and effective manner. There should be management procedures for the ongoing management and review of these actions and the effectiveness of these procedures verified during self-inspection. Quality reviews may be grouped by product type, e.g. solid dosage forms, liquid dosage forms, sterile products, etc. where scientifically justified.

Where the marketing authorization holder is not the manufacturer, there should be a technical agreement in place between the various parties that defines their respective responsibilities in producing the quality review. The Qualified Person responsible for final batch certification together with the marketing authorization holder should ensure that the quality review is performed in a timely manner and is accurate [12].

Holders of pharmaceutical Marketing Authorizations are obliged to carry out and document regular quality re-examinations of their manufactured products. These product reviews should include an analysis of the data collected during the manufacturing and of the implemented process improvements (Table **1**).

Table 1. Contents of the product quality review [13].

Item		Action
I	Starting and packaging materials	*A review of starting materials and packaging materials used for the product, especially those from new sources.*
II	In-process and finish product controls	*A review of critical in-process controls and finished product results*
III	OOS batches	*A review of all batches that failed to meet established specification(s) and their investigation.*
IV	Deviations and non-conformances	*A review of all significant deviations or non-conformances, their related investigations, and the effectiveness of resultant corrective and preventative actions taken.*
V	Changes in processes and analytical methods	*A review of all changes carried out to the processes or analytical methods*
VI	Marketing authorization variations	*A review of Marketing Authorization variations submitted/granted/refused, including those for third country (export only) dossiers*
VII	Stability monitoring	*A review of the results of the stability monitoring program and any adverse trends.*
VIII	Complaints, returns, recalls	*A review of all quality-related returns, complaints and recalls and the investigations performed at the time.*
IX	Adequacy of corrective actions	*A review of adequacy of any other previous product process or equipment corrective actions.*

Table 1: contd…

X	Post-marketing commitments	*For new marketing authorizations and variations to marketing authorizations, a review of post-marketing commitments.*
XI	Qualification program	*The qualification status of relevant equipment and utilities, e.g. HVAC, water, compressed gases, etc.*
XII	Technical agreements	*A review of Technical Agreements to ensure that they are up to date.*

(I) Starting and packaging materials: A review means verifying if the source specified in the Marketing Authorization is still being used, if there have been changes in their specifications, if they are adequate to guarantee the quality of the final product, and if the suppliers have been audited to ensure that they comply with GMP. It is also necessary to look for problems with incoming batches (faults or rejections).

(II) Critical in-process controls and finished product results: It is necessary to assess if there have been changes in relation to those specified in the Marketing Authorization and if those controls ensure that the finished product is of suitable quality. A review includes verifying that all test methods are appropriately validated.

(III) OOS batches: A review should include rejected batches. This means assessing which batches were rejected, which actions were taken to discover the causes and which corrective and preventive actions were implemented.

(IV) Deviations and non-conformances: It is necessary to review deviations and non-conformances. Describe them and indicate how they were investigated, which corrective and preventive actions were implemented and how effective they were in preventing their recurrence. It has to be verified if any of these actions meant a change in the Marketing Authorization.

(V) Changes to processes or analytical methods: The review includes the verification of changes to see if they have been duly authorized according to the change control procedures and validated as appropriate. If there have been changes it is necessary to check that they have been incorporated into the Marketing Authorization and that equipment has been qualified and the processes validated.

(VI) Marketing Authorization variations submitted during the review period: The review should describe all the Marketing Authorization variations which have been submitted (including both those approved and those refused). It is necessary to assess if the granted Marketing Authorizations reflect the actual manufacturing process and its quality control. If there have been variation refusals, it is necessary to indicate the reasons.

(VII) Stability testing results: Describe the results from routine stability testing of production batches (do they meet the shelf-life stated in the Marketing Authorization?). Provide data on any adverse trend that might be detected. Indicate if the controls in place are adequate to ensure the stability of the product and if the influence of changes in materials or manufacturing processes has been assessed and new tests carried out.

(VIII) Returns, complaints and recalls: Report any return, complaint or recall and describe how they have been investigated and which corrective and preventive actions have been implemented. Indicate if these actions have been effective.

(IX) Adequacy of previous process or equipment corrective actions: Review the effectiveness of the CAPA (corrective and preventative action) programs.

(X) Post marketing commitments: Verify if there is any information relating to Marketing Authorizations, such as samples or stability data, awaiting to be sent to the competent authorities and indicate when they will be available.

(XI) Qualification status of relevant equipment and utilities: Describe if process monitoring or evaluation have shown any failure or negative trend in the performance of critical equipment and utilities. Explain how they have been investigated, which corrective and preventive actions have been implemented and how they have effectively prevented recurrences. It has to be verified if any of these actions has meant a change in the Marketing Authorization or the need for re-qualification.

(XII) Technical Agreements: Review if there are updated technical agreements with all suppliers and contractors, if the description of the activities and responsibilities of each party is appropriate, and if they meet GMP requirements.

The Product Quality Review can be used as a tool for continuous improvement, as it contributes in diminishing the risk of out-of-specification results (and consequently the need of reprocessing or recall), in increasing of productivity and as well in meeting regulatory requirements. It also fosters communication and coordination among the different areas of the organization (production, engineering, quality and regulatory).

Corrective Action/Preventive Action (CAPA) System

The objective of this system known internationally as "CAPA" is ensuring that deviations are corrected and that preventive actions are established too in order to impede a recurrence of a problem. The CAPA system can be defined as a systematic method of operation that embraces the necessary actions to correct and prevent recurrences ("corrective action") and to eliminate the cause of potential quality problems that might lead to the non conformity of the product ("preventive action").

The situation that arises when procedures are not followed is termed deviation. Whereas changes are voluntary modifications, deviations are unwanted and unexpected modifications from the required situation. Deviations pose a threat to the state of control of the system and, consequently, they have to be adequately handled by the CAPA procedure.

Traditionally GMP has mainly underlined the correction of deviations in a reactive approach. Whereas modern quality systems focus on the prevention of deviations with the intention of being proactive. These latter measures require a deep product and process knowledge and a risk management approach.

CAPA system focuses on investigating, understanding, and correcting discrepancies while attempting to prevent their recurrence. Quality system models discuss CAPA as three separate concepts.:

- *Remedial corrections of an identified problem.*
- *Root cause analysis.*
- *Preventive action to avert recurrence of a similar potential problem* [14].

When problems (deviations, complaints, non conformities, *etc.*) appear, corrective actions must be taken to put everything right again. However, it is evident that, in quality, technical and economical terms, it is better to prevent the occurrence of problems by detecting and controlling them beforehand.

As problems will always exist, a documented CAPA program is necessary, both from the regulatory point of view and from the organization performance.

Corrective Action is a reactive tool for system improvement to ensure that significant problems do not recur. It is essential to determine what actions will reduce the likelihood of a problem recurring [15].

Preventive Actions. Being proactive is an essential tool in quality systems management. Preventive actions. will help ensure that potential problems and root causes are identified, possible consequences assessed, and appropriate actions considered [16].

A CAPA program is composed of different logical stages:

1st Problem identification

Any program has to start by identifying and defining the problem. Problems may be detected in different ways: following self inspections, trend data analysis, risk analysis management, complaints, QA observations, *etc.*

2nd Problem evaluation

Once the problem has been identified it is necessary to appraise its impact. Evaluate a problem means establishing its potential impact to the quality of products, its risk and the remedial action required.

3rd Problem investigation

Once the impact of the problem has been appraised, an action can be planned. It is necessary to determine its contributing and root causes, and then, clearly establish the objectives, strategies, resources and responsibilities.

4th Action plan

Once the problem and its cause or causes are known, a plan should be established to correct the situation or preventing its future occurrence. This plan has to be well defined and responsibilities clearly assigned.

5th Action implementation

The devised plan has to be carried out.

6th Follow-up

This is a stage of the utmost importance. What has been done must be revised by comparing it with what had been planned. It is also necessary to verify that implemented actions have not created any new problem. The action is then completed.

Change Management System

Processes are dynamic and consequently changes are inevitable. These changes, however, should be known, registered and be applied in a controlled manner in order not to affect the state of control on processes (Fig. **4**). Changes should be managed during the whole lifecycle, although with different characteristics and functions according to the stage.

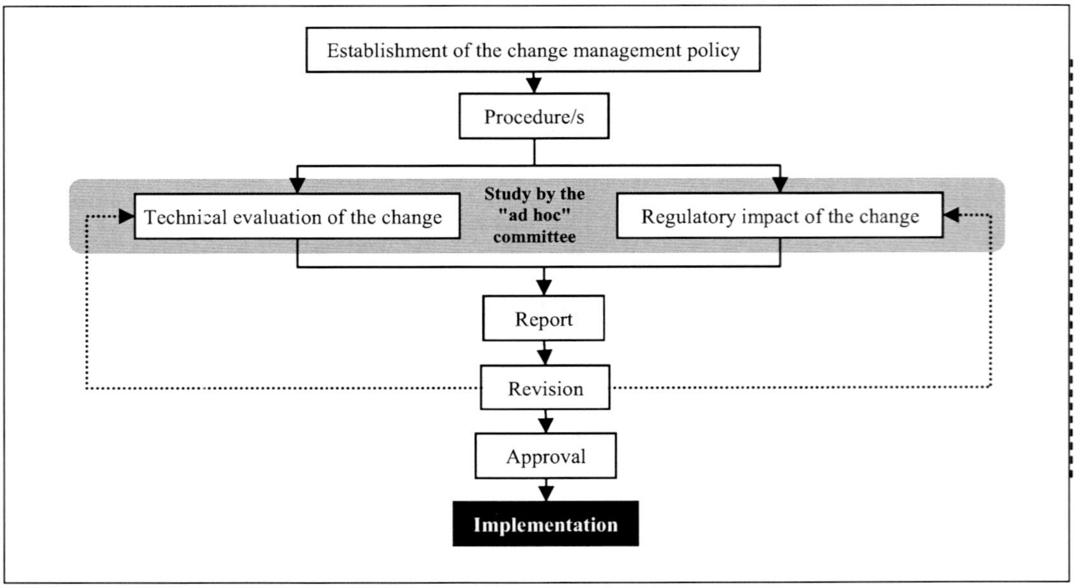

Fig. (4). Change management.

The evaluation of the possible impact on the registration documents handed to the authorities should be included in the study. Modifications after product discontinuation should also follow this procedure.

Although not a long time ago change management was just associated to facilities, equipment or processes after having been qualified/validated, nowadays this system has a very important role in the evaluation, approval and implementation of the modifications derived from performance monitoring and continual improvement. The proposed changes should be studied by a team of experts, using an approach based on risk analysis (Fig. **5**).

Management review

This review is chaired by the high direction of the company and its objective is evaluating all data regarding the quality system in order to detect anomalies or dysfunctions. The result of this review is the identification of improvement and training needs. This can result in the assignment of new resources or in the redistribution of those already existing. It is also an opportunity for the identification of knowledge to be preserved and diffused (Fig. **6**).

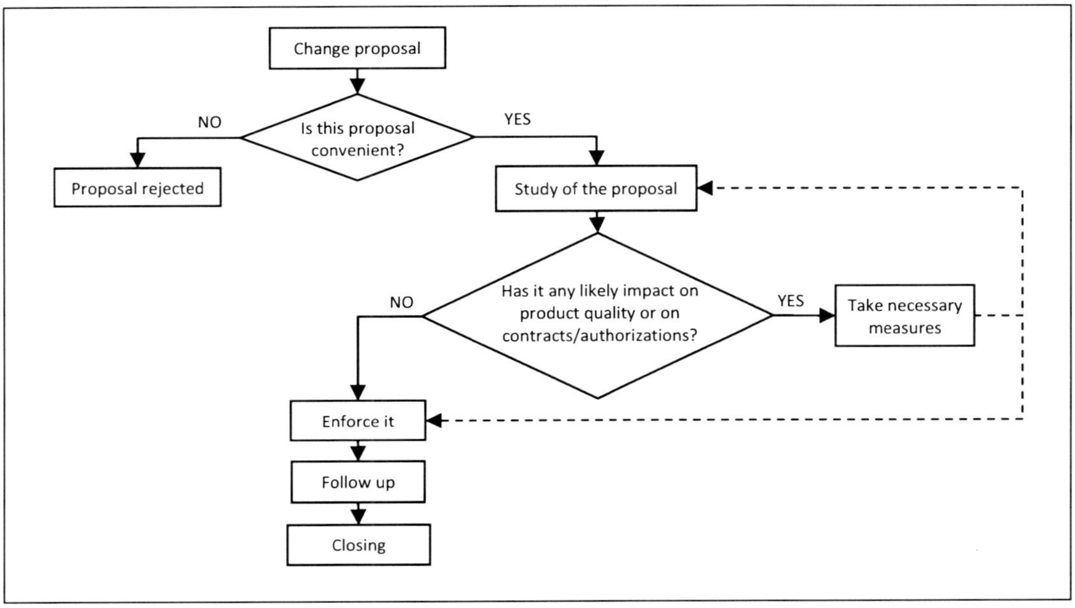

Fig. (5). Change management rationale.

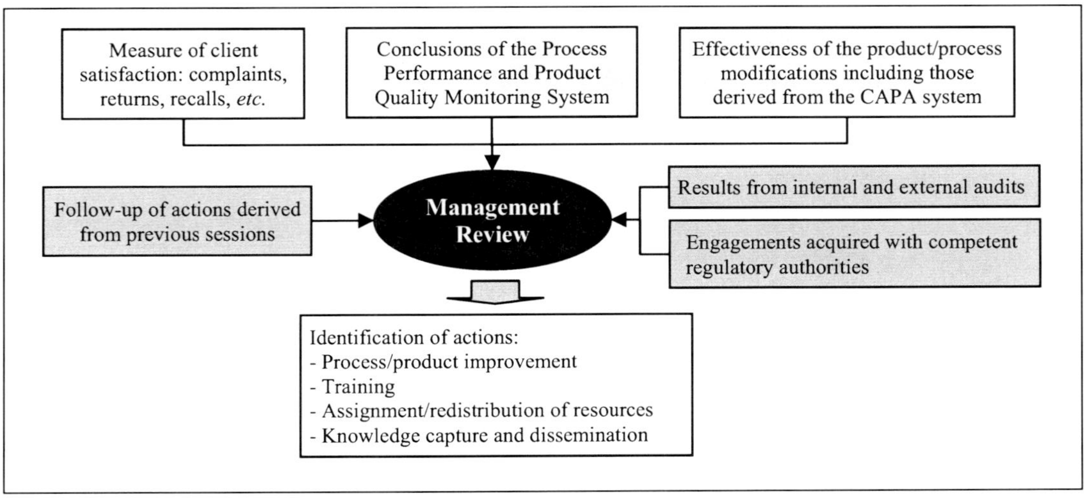

Fig. (6). Management review.

The objective is ensuring that processes keep their level of performance and that products maintain their quality throughout their lifecycle. Depending on the complexity and size of the company reviews may be subdivided to be performed at different organizational levels, always warranting, however, that relevant information will attain the high direction timely and effectively. In these reviews all information susceptible of providing knowledge on processes and products is considered, as shown in the annexed figure.

PRACTICAL IMPLEMENTATION OF A PQS

Having described the characteristics and organization of a PQS, following it is described how a system of this type could be practically implemented.

Prerequisites

Direction Support

Before implementing a PQS it is necessary to bear in mind what was said before: although in the long run a PQS fosters quality by diminishing non compliance and this has undoubtedly economical benefits, at the beginning it requires important investments in time and resources. As it has been described, the high (or senior) direction of the company has the ultimate responsibility in quality and thus is deeply implicated in many tasks, like approving high rank documents, communicating the quality policy of the company to all the employees, or leading system reviews. This is why if the company's direction is not wholly aware of its signification and is not really interested in implementing the PQS the chances of success are very low.

Employees Support

Although this is self-evident and it is supposed that by having the support of the direction the support of the employees is guaranteed, often this is not so simple. If a company lacks a real "quality soul" and employees are not motivated, they might see just "more work" in the implementation of the PQS.

"Cunning" Approach

Implementation of the ICH PQS represents an essential turning-point in the organization of the company and thus this requires patience and time. It is better starting little by little than trying to be too perfect and blocking everything. An imperfect procedure (*e.g.* limited number of variables, reduced frequency of sampling, *etc.*) is preferable to nothing. What counts is having a good understanding of what we are looking for, and then advancing towards this goal as much as possible. Any improvement should be welcome and understood as a move forward.

The soul of a 21st century GMP inspection is not finding "perfect" companies. This does not exist. Companies which admit their weaknesses and limitations but have a reasonable quality handling and a plan for improving it steadily can be relied upon. Whereas a company that says that does everything but in practice does almost nothing cannot be trusted.

This is why it is proposed to start with a restricted number of products (*e.g.* those more critical or selling) and then extend the amount of products which are monitored by critical variables. It is recognized that for many legacy products the amount of information is limited (in the past there was no "knowledge management"!). See chapter 11.

Organization

The practical realization of a PQS starts by preparing the documents which define the system and its organization.

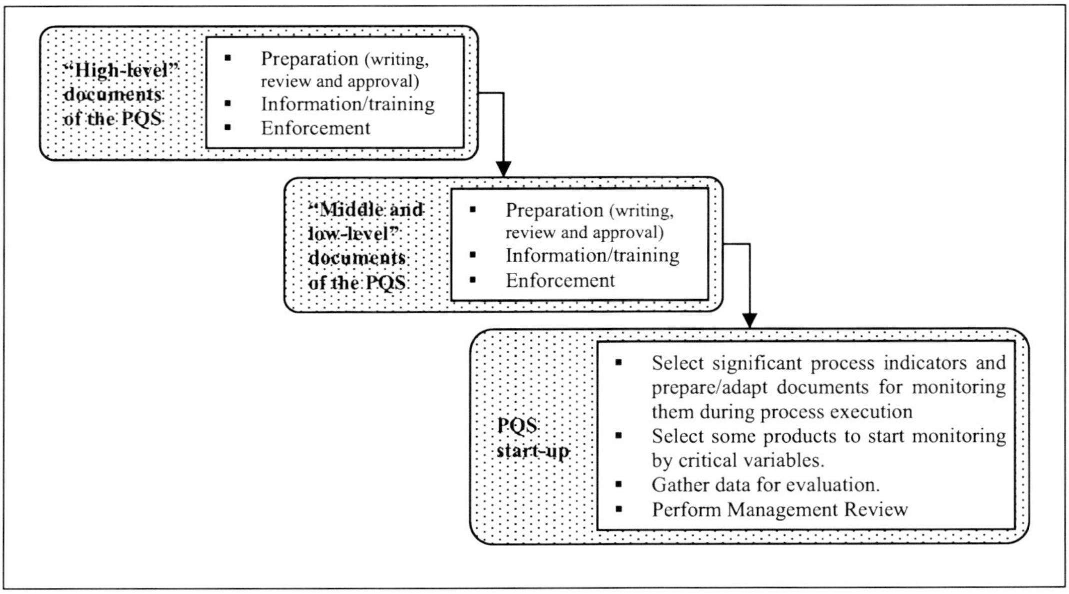

Fig. (7). PQS implementation roadmap.

The necessary documents belong to three different levels: high level documents outlining the system, the middle-level documents describing how to perform the tasks and the low-level documents gathering data (Fig. **7**). See chapter 6 for detailed information on documentation management.

PQS documents are prepared in two stages. First of all are written the high-level documents which establish the scope and rules of the game and then follow the general procedures which describe how this game is going to be played. Afterwards the rest of documents describe practically how to perform the necessary managing and manufacturing operations, and how to gather data.

Preparation of the PQS "High-Level" Documents

The key document of a PQS is the Quality Manual which describes the system and its organization. The Quality Manual is complemented with a "Declaration of the policy of quality" and with a Process Manual. The former is a very short document, usually a single side of a sheet, where the senior direction of the company formally declares the quality objectives of the company and the compromise with them. The latter is a document where the different processes which compose the PQS are described. If so decided, these documents could be easily gathered in a Quality Manual provided with the necessary annexes. What counts is not the number of documents but the contents.

Quality Manual

The Quality Manual (QM) presents the PQS system, its organization, documentation and responsibilities (Table **2**). It can be written following different approaches which stretch from a very simple document that will be developed in detail by other lower level documents, to a much more complex and detailed document requiring less detail in the lower level documents. The first approach is usually more popular because a simple Quality Manual can be easily delivered to third parts as a kind of presentation card of the company, because sensitive information is contained in other documents which remain in the company.

The Quality Manual should describe the responsibilities of the high direction, the handling of resources, the control of production and the evaluation activities. The high direction has the ultimate responsibility in ensuring that the PQS is effectively in place, that the quality objectives are met and that in the organization the respective roles and responsibilities are defined, communicated, understood and implemented.

Responsibilities of the high direction regarding the PQS:

- Provide an adequate structure (chart, job description, key personnel);

- Define scope, aim and procedures;
- Show commitment to quality and define quality objectives;
- Review the system (improvement in the PQS, in the products and processes and modify the distribution of resources).

<u>Responsibilities of the high direction regarding the resources:</u>

- Ensure that facilities, equipment and materials are adequate;
- Ensure that there is sufficient amount of adequately trained personnel, that individual responsibilities are clearly understood, and that all personnel know GMP.
- Ensure that the characteristics of the manufacturing plants (situation, design, construction and maintenance) correspond to the operations, minimize the risk of mix-up and impede cross-contamination. This should be defined and periodically reviewed.
- Ensure that outsourced operations possess the same quality level, and of control, than those developed in the own plant. This requires defining in a contract all matters which might affect the quality of the products.

<u>Responsibilities of the high direction regarding production:</u>

- Conceive, develop and document products and processes. It is necessary possessing adequate procedures regarding facilities, equipment and materials.
- Control inputs in order to ensure that only materials delivered by approved suppliers might be used in production.
- Define, apply and revise procedures for controlling operations.
- Establish and apply a procedure for handling of non-conformances.

<u>Responsibilities of the high direction regarding evaluation activities:</u>

- Analyze data in order to detect tendencies and improve systems.

- Perform internal audits at planned intervals.
- Use quality risk management assessing and controlling risks;
- Apply corrective actions to ensure that there will not be recurrence of significant problems;
- Identify potential problems and their root causes and apply preventive actions;
- Foster continual improvement.

Table 2. Example of contents of a QM.

Part		Contents summary
1. Company introduction		Information on the company, situation, purpose, activities and objectives.
2. Characteristics of the document	2.1. Glossary	Meaning of the main words/expressions used in the QM
	2.2. Purpose	Ensure GMP compliance as stated in ICH Q10.
	2.3. Scope	All the stages of the life-cycle.
	2.4. Approach	Use of enablers as per ICH Q10.
	2.5. Copy control	Distribution and control of QM copies.
	2.6. Modifications	Following the "change management" procedure
	2.7. Responsibilities	Written by QA and approved by the senior direction
	2.8. Binding character	For all personnel.
3. Quality management system requirements	3.1. General	The PQS is continuously checked and as necessary improved. Processes are identified and their performance followed by means of indicators. Necessary resources are allocated. Information ensured.
	3.2. Documentation	Description of the document levels of the PQS and of their life-cycle.
4. Responsibilities	4.1. Management responsibilities	Senior management commitment Internal communication Management reviews Management of outsourced activities and of suppliers Management of changes in product ownership
	4.2. Personnel responsibilities	Abstract of responsibilities of key personnel
5. Resource management	5.1 Resource assignment	Direction evaluates needs and assigns the necessary resources.
	5.2. Human resources	Short description of the personnel policy stressing their training and their knowledge of the quality policy.

Table 2: contd...

	5.3. Infrastructure	Short description of the policy regarding premises, facilities and equipment.
	5.4 Work environment	Measures are taken to identify environmental hazards and the necessary measures are applied.
6. Production and process control	6.1. Development	Critical variables and product profiles are determined.
	6.2. Technology transfer	Establishment of the monitoring strategy. Qualification and validation.
	6.3. Manufacturing	Description of the measures taken to ensure quality (documents, batch manufacturing records). Product control. Process control. Purchase control. OOS control. Identification and traceability. Storage and distribution. Control of measure and monitoring instruments. Outsourcing. Product quality review.
	6.4. Discontinuation	Managed as required by ICH Q10.
7. Measure, analysis and improvement	7.1 Self inspections	According to GMP.
	7.2. Process performance and product quality monitoring system	Monitoring and follow-up of the processes. Monitoring and follow-up of the products.
	7.3. CAPA system	Brief description of its organization. Corrective actions. Preventive actions
	7.4. Change management system	Brief description of this system.
	7.5. Management review	Brief description of how it is performed.
Annex		Organization chart

Declaration of the Quality Policy of the Company

A copy of this document is often framed and fixed to a well-exposed wall of the company. The objective is to show both to the personnel of the company and to visitors the engagement of the company in matters regarding quality and also which are the values of the company (usually expressed in a few not very long sentences with highlighted key words).

Process Manual

This document, after a brief introduction explaining the purpose and approach followed, is composed of sketches showing the process map of the company and of the existing processes. A process is any activity or series of activities which use resources in order to transform inputs into outputs and it is characterized by its function, its responsible/s, its inputs and outputs, its resources, its documentation, and its indicators or objectives. In a practical way processes can be classified as:

- Operational, when they are directly linked to production;
- Supporting, when they back up operational processes;
- Strategic, when they define the organization and operation of the company.

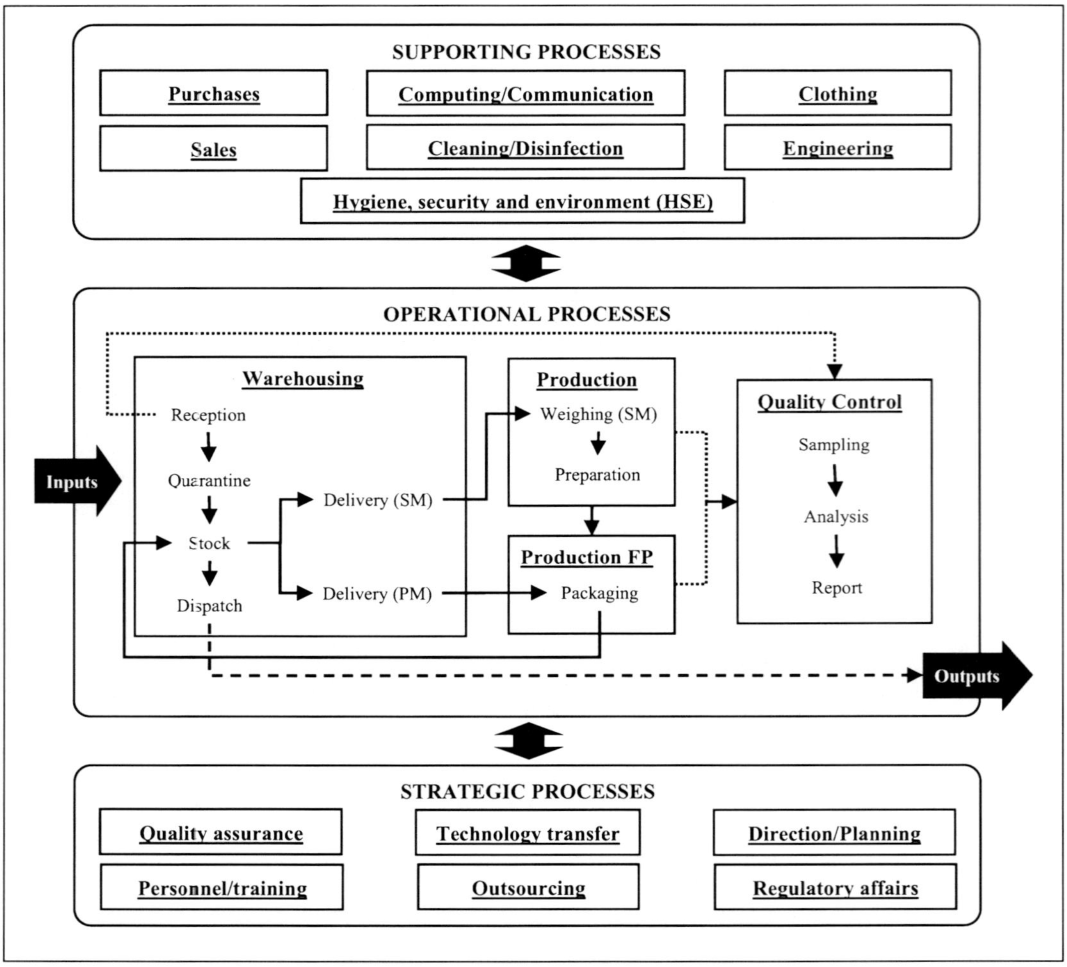

Fig. (8). Example of a process map.

Fig. (**8**) shows just a rough example of a process map of a laboratory. In fact although any laboratory would have a map of this kind, the number of processes may change (in relation to the scope of activities of the company) and also their complexity and interrelations. Each one of the identified processes has to be examined to determine how it can be monitored by means of indicators or objectives. Let us take, for instance "production of the finished product":

Function: Packaging of the bulk product with packaging materials in order to obtain the finished product

Inputs: Liberated batches of bulk products and packaging materials.

Outputs: Batches of finished products.

Responsible: Head of production.

Resources: Clean rooms with equipment for primary packaging. Conventional rooms with equipment for secondary packaging and complementary elements (pallets, transpallets, bins, drums, *etc.*).

Documentation: Set-up, checking and operational instructions for equipment or instruments; cleaning instructions for equipment or tools; packaging instructions and report. Reconciliation in packaging. Sampling and monitoring.

Indicators/Objectives: Packaging of the programmed batches, number of deviations, number of non conformities.

Approval and Information/Training on the PQS "High-Level" Documents

These high-level documents have to be approved, dated and signed by the senior direction. Then they have to be distributed to the heads of department and all personnel participating in the above mentioned processes have to be acquainted with them. Besides the normal training activities usually performed by departments it is also interesting to have a global meeting (or several according to the size of the company) where the direction presents and supports them.

Preparation of the Other Documents of the PQS

If the PQS high-level documents might be assimilated to the brain, which manages the whole body, the other documents could be seen as peripheral nerves. Between both we could consider an intermediate stage represented by the spinal cord. This is the approach we propose for documentation too. After the high level documents centered on the QM, we could distinguish middle level documents known as general procedures of the PQS and finally we would have the low level documents (batch records, procedures, instructions, *etc.*) with their associated registers. Whereas general procedures have a wide scope of application, the low level documents concern just a department, a process or operation, a product, a system or piece of equipment, *etc.*

Only the middle level documents (*i.e.* general procedures) are analyzed in this chapter, whereas the low level ones are considered in chapter 6.

The aim of the general operating procedures (GOPs) is to describe the practical company-wide development of the QM (*i.e.* concerning all or several departments). Generally speaking, the following documents can be considered:

- Document management
- Personnel management
- Change management
- Risk and knowledge management
- Incident, deviation and OOS management
- CAPA system
- Process performance and product quality monitoring system
- Management review
- Audits
- Product quality review
- Qualification/Validation policy
- Outsourcing

Document Management

This is a very important procedure which describes in detail how documents will be managed in the company (formatted, written, approved, distributed, updated, *etc.*). See Table **3**.

Documents play a significant role in the image of a company. This is why not only their contents is important, but also their format and aspect.

For more details on documentation see chapter 6.

Table 3. General Procedure of the PQS: Documentation. Example of contents.

Part		Contents summary
01	Document identification	Description of the types of documents, their outline, parts and format.
02	Document lifecycle	The different stages in the life of a document.
03	Writing	Short instructions about how better writing a document (following the brief directions contained in GMP).
04	Review	Responsibility for reviewing the document (who and how).
05	Approval	Responsibility for approving the document (who and how).
06	Diffusion and archiving	How and to whom are distributed the documents. How are handled the copies and where the originals are kept.
07	Training	How involved personnel are trained on documents.
08	Application and updating	The enforcement of documents and how they should be updated.
09	Discontinuation	What to do when a document is not necessary anymore.
10	Register management	Description of the GMP requirements concerning the filling of data (corrections. type of ink, fill-up blank spaces).
11	Annex: Lists of documents	It is necessary to have an updated list of existing documents. This list (usually classified by types of documents and by departments) is annexed to this document, because annexes are dated and can be changed at any time.

Personnel Management

This is clearly a very important document because it defines how personnel will be selected and appointed in order to ensure its capacity to develop the entrusted tasks and also how continual training will be handled. See Table **4**.

Table 4. General procedure of the PQS: Personnel management. Example of contents.

Part		Contents summary
01	Post descriptions	Which types of posts are recognized in the company, how they are organized and to whom corresponds this management.
02	Personnel selection and appointment	How personnel is chosen, tested and appointed.
03	Training	How training is managed, who is responsible and how training needs are assessed.
04	Entrance training	New personnel (or old personnel getting a new post, as necessary) should receive an admission training on general company and GMP subjects and on more specific subjects related to the post.

Table 4: contd...

05	Post assignment	Description of the formal procedure for assigning a post to a given person and how it is registered.
06	Continual training	How annual training plans are set-up and how new training needs are assessed and met.
07	Temporary personnel	Personnel might be temporary but their operations are not temporary. It is necessary ensuring that they will not affect quality.
08	Organization and maintenance of a personnel archive	A personnel archive with the professional CV, the training and the posts held in the plant.
09	Annex: Posts descriptions	The posts description indicating responsibilities, necessary training/experience, *etc.* can be annexed to this document

A company-wide general procedure is usually very practical, although it is evident that in big companies with differentiated areas of activity it might be complemented with other specific low level procedures. See chapter 7.

Change Management

This document describes the practical handling of changes in order to ensure that they do not affect the state of control and assure traceability (Table **5**).

Table 5. General procedure of the PQS: Change management. Example of contents.

Part		Contents summary
01	Change proposition	How and by whom a change can be proposed.
02	Classification of the change	Types of change: minor, major, like for like, *etc.*
03	Study and approval	Which the persons who should judge on the proposal of change are and how they should proceed.
04	Application	Once the change is approved it can be applied. It is necessary to indicate who and how does this. There are changes which require secondary actions (regulatory, qualification, validation, *etc.*).
05	Follow-up	After the implementation of the change it is necessary to check that it didn't affect the state of control.
06	Conclusion	How the change is considered satisfactorily implemented and its possible consequences are mastered.

Risk and Knowledge Management

This document defines the practical approach of the company towards the two enablers proposed by guideline ICH Q10. It describes which tools the company will use and how they are going to be applied. Here both enablers are gathered in the same document, but they can be separated in two documents according to the needs of the company. See Table **6**.

Table 6. General Procedure of the PQS: Risk and knowledge management. Example of contents.

Part		Contents summary
01	Quality risk management	Definitions of hazard, harm and risk. Risk management cycle (analysis, risk acceptance, risk communication, risk revision). Existing tools and how they are used. Company policy regarding risk management (approach, uses, tools, responsibilities) Determination of risk (severity, probability and detection). Risk estimation (qualitative or quantitative).
02	Knowledge management	Definition of knowledge management and its phases and functions. Description of the approach chosen by the company.
03	Annex: tools	It is possible to annex practical descriptions of the tools used by the company explaining when they should be used and how they should be implemented practically.

Incident, Deviation and OOS Management

This is a company-wide document which summarizes how incidents, deviations and cases of non compliance are going to be dealt with. It is useful because it determines which specific procedures are needed to treat the different situations that might appear. In order to provide a complete picture of the matter it considers not only the problems that appear during the manufacturing process but also those detected when products have already been distributed. This general procedure is closely related to the procedure dealing with the CAPA system, as all the problems should be recorded, investigated and, as necessary, followed by corrective/preventive actions. See Table **7**.

This document describes how "incidents" within the PQS (an event differing from normality, like, for instance, a breakdown) should be handled. Incidents may turn into "deviations" (an incident which implies separation from the approved procedures) and deviations into "OOS" (out of specifications) or "non compliances". Each one of these can be treated separately, although the three concepts are linked and can be handled together in a reactive chain (Fig. **9**). Each company chooses the approach that suits better its organization.

Table 7. General procedure of the PQS: Incident, deviation and OOS management. Example of contents.

Part		Contents summary
01	Incident detection	What an incident is and how it should be detected and handled.
02	Deviation detection	What a deviation is and how it should be detected.
03	Incident management	Recording, investigation and application of measures (if necessary).
04	Deviation management	Recording. Classification (critical, major, minor) and cause investigation. Application of measures (products being manufactured or products already distributed). Follow-up.
05	Conclusion	The whole process is reviewed and if everything is found correct the incident/deviation is considered closed.
06	Annexes: Register models	- Record form for incidents. - Record form for deviations.

The advantage of having a global procedure like this one is making people aware of the fact that all these problems are interrelated and as such have to be handled.

It is important to bear in mind that problems may appear in any of the activities realized within the PQS and as such constitute very important indicators of the adequate performance of the system. Many problems, in general, and frequent reproduction of the same problems, in particular, are indisputable indications that the PQS is not working as purported and that adequate measures are urgently required.

CAPA System

This document describes how the company will develop its policy of corrective and preventive actions. The CAPA system is the logical extension of the previous procedure, because incidents, deviations and OOS start actions (Table **8**)

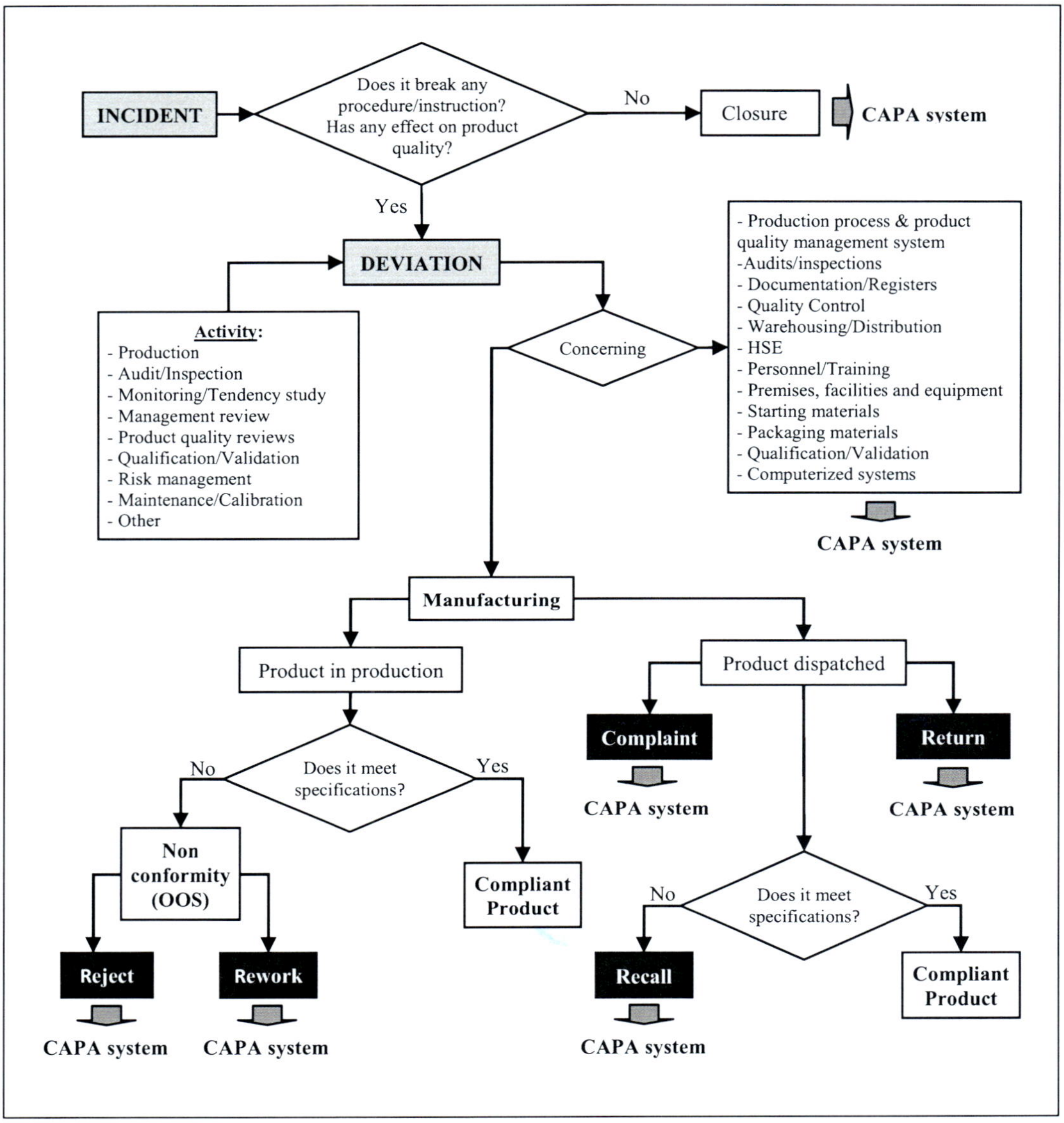

Fig. (9). Incident, deviation, OOS flowchart.

Table 8. General procedure of the PQS: CAPA system. Example of contents.

Part		Contents summary
01	Inputs	Description of the PQS aspects which may start CAPA actions
02	Management	The aspect requiring actions is analyzed and these actions are detailed (description, responsible, delays)

Table 8: contd...

03	Follow-up	The implementation of the corrective/preventive actions is followed to confirm that they are adequately implemented and to detect any unforeseen result.
04	Conclusion	The whole process is reviewed and if everything is found correct the CAPA plan is considered closed.
05	Annex: Register models	- Record form for corrective actions. - Record form for preventive actions.

The PQS of the 21st century emphasizes preventive activities (Fig. **10**). A good quality system should focus more in preventing problems than in correcting them.

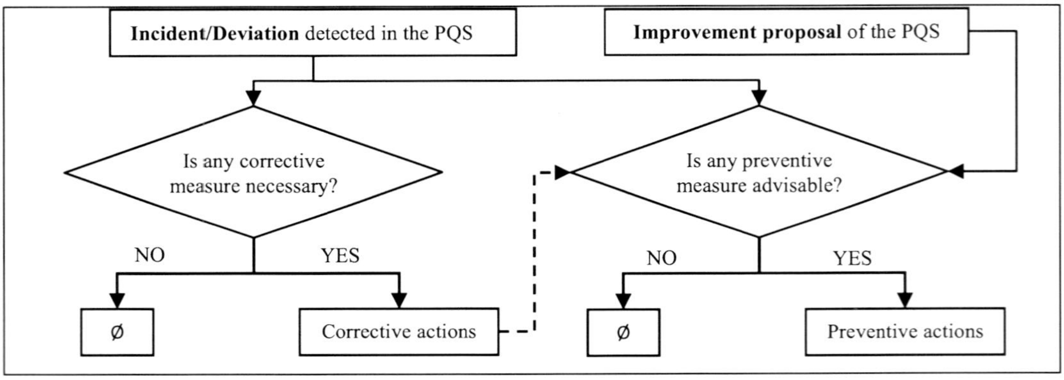

Fig. (10). CAPA system.

Process Performance and Product Quality Monitoring System

This document describes how the company will develop the monitoring of its processes and the quality of its products. See Table **9**.

Table 9. General procedure of the PQS: Process performance and product quality monitoring system. Example of contents.

Part		Contents summary
01	Performance indicators	How process indicators will be chosen and acceptance ranges determined.
02	Material and product attributes	How attributes for starting and packaging materials are going to be determined.
03	Process parameters	How operational process parameters will be determined and their acceptance ranges established.

Table 9: contd...

04	Annex: Indicators and variables	The above mentioned indicators and variables are listed including ranges, responsibilities and methods.

Management Review

This document describes how the company will handle the requirement of follow-up and evaluation of the PQS in order to keep it adequate and improve it, as necessary. An annex can provide a model of form to be filled during the management reviews. See Table **10**.

Table 10. General Procedure of the PQS: Management review. Example of contents.

Part		Contents summary
01	Periodicity and organization	How management reviews will be organized, who will take part in them and how often they will be hold.
02	Inputs	Detailing of all the data which should be analyzed in order to evaluate the performance of the PQS.
03	Outputs	After evaluating the inputs different improvement measures will be proposed, as necessary, including resource management
04	Annex: Management review form	Model of form to fill-in during the review. It details inputs, outputs, resources and their rationale.

Audits

This document describes how to perform audits, both internal and external. In any case every company should decide if it is better to have a single procedure or separated procedures for self-audits and external audit to suppliers or contract acceptors. This general document can establish the main lines of auditing and then other procedures can deal with the exact details of each type of audit. As in the other cases a company-wide document describing the main lines of a subject is usually very useful. See Table **11**.

Table 11. General procedure of the PQS: Personal behavior and clothing. Example of contents.

Part		Contents summary
01	Types of audits	Objective and scope of the audits and who starts them up. Classification of audit findings (critical, major, minor) and how they are going to be evaluated.

Table 11: contd...

02	Responsibilities	Who performs the audits (own personnel/external consultants, members of the team) and, as usually it is QA, then who audits QA. External auditors.
03	Periodicity	How audits are scheduled and how the subjects of audit are divided in order to facilitate inspection.
04	Preparation	How an audit is started (who is informed, how, with which time in advance, objectives and scope, *etc.*)
05	Realization	How the audit will be performed (personnel taking part in it, schedule, final meeting, *etc.*)
06	Report	After the audit a report should be prepared indicating the results and the findings.
07	Follow-up	The departments concerned by the findings should propose corrective measures with responsibilities and delays.
08	Annex1: Audit report	Form to be used for the preparation of the report.
09	Annex2: Aide-memoire	Check-lists to facilitate auditing and contributing to a homogeneous approach when audits are performed by different personnel.

Product Quality Review

As it was discussed earlier in this chapter the contents of the product quality review is well specified by GMP. Thus, this procedure is bound to follow the list of items indicated in the GMP guide and to provide, if necessary, remarks addressing particular aspects of the company. See Table **12**.

Table 12. General procedure of the PQS: Product quality review. Example of contents.

Part		Contents summary
01	Responsibilities	Who are responsible for this review and how they are going to gather the necessary data.
02	Schedule	When the data should be handled and the way they are going to be managed and prepared for the review.
03	Elements to be reviewed	Information to be included in the review (refer to the details provided in this chapter)
04	Annex: Form	A form with all the company elements to be filled in order to show homogeneity in the report.

Qualification/Validation Policy

As it was discussed in chapter 2, qualification and validation are applied to different items and thus they show marked differences. This is why it is often advisable to prepare separated Qualification and Validation Master Plans. Therefore, this procedure is just a general introduction to the qualification/validation policy of the company and a kind of introduction to the mentioned master plans. See Table (**13**).

Table 13. General procedure of the PQS: Qualification/validation policy. Example of contents.

Part		Contents summary
01	Approach to qualification/validation	Policy of the company regarding qualification and validation.
02	Scope	Brief description of the plant and the different systems and equipment to be qualified and processes to be validated.
03	Personnel	Personnel composing the qualification and validation teams.
04	Documentation	Documents which compose qualification/validation (protocols, reports) and their organization.
05	Change control	How changes are going to be managed
06	Training	The requirements of training for the teams.
07	Calibration	The requirements of calibration for instrumentation used in the tasks of qualification/validation.

Outsourcing

This document describes how the company will handle the contracts in order to outsource either production or analysis (Table **14**). GMP specifies the contents of these contracts in order to ensure that the level of quality assurance is the same in the contract giver than in the contract acceptors. See chapter 2 for more details.

Table 14. General procedure of the PQS: Outsourcing. Example of contents.

Part		Contents summary
01	Outsourcing	What can be outsourced and under which conditions.
02	Contract giver	Responsibilities of the company.
03	Contract acceptor	Responsibilities of the outsourced company.
04	Annex: Contract form	Model of contract to be used as an aide-memoire when preparing an outsourcing contract.

Start-up of the PQS

Once that the documents of the PQS have been approved and diffused and personnel are aware of the quality policy of the company and have received the adequate training the implementation of the PQS can start.

Fig. (**11**) summarizes the practical application of the PQS.

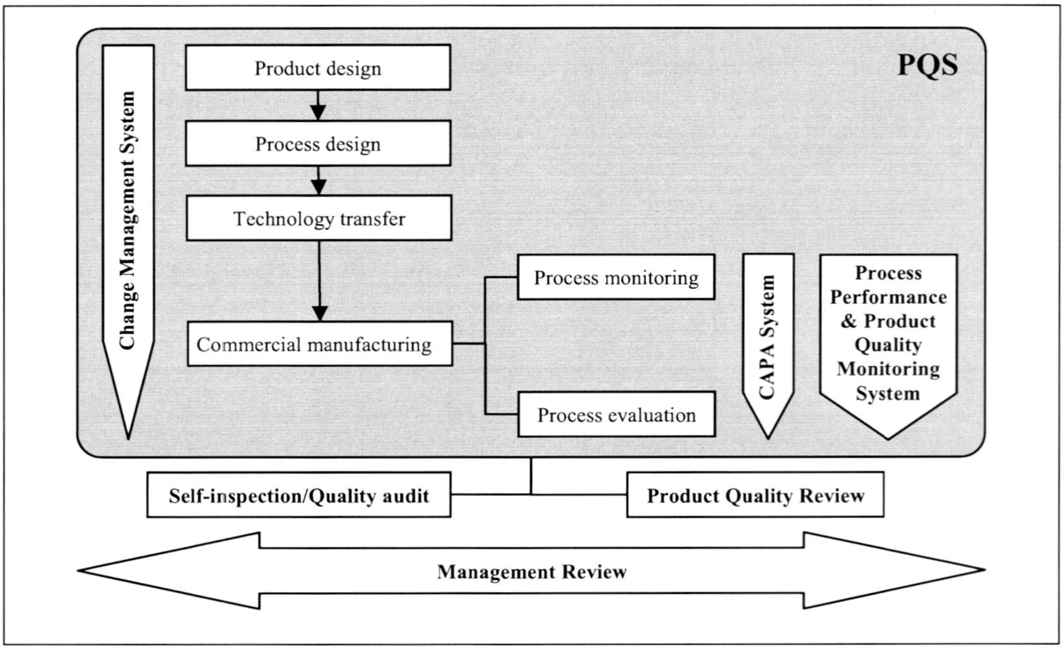

Fig. (11). Practical application of the PQS.

In practice it is possible to distinguish eight stages in the implementation of a PQS:

1st The four elements of the PQS should be implemented. From these elements two are GMP requirements and thus, they should be already in place ("Change management" and "CAPA system"). The other two belong particularly to the PQS ("Process Performance & Product Quality Monitoring System" and "Management review") and consequently require particular attention.

2nd Outside from the above-mentioned PQS elements, there are two GMP elements which are very useful instruments for controlling the performance of the PQS. The first one is constituted by the "Self-inspections" or "Internal Audits". The second one consists of the "Product Quality Reviews".

Self-inspections are an old instrument to control GMP-compliance, but they can easily be extended to PQS-compliance.

Product Quality Reviews are a more recent instrument and although primarily focused on the requirements of the regulatory authorities it can be secondarily easily turned into an instrument for the evaluation of process performance.

3rd Process monitoring, in general, requires identification (and setting of acceptance ranges) of indicators. For general processes, as it was described before, it is not very difficult and in the beginning it may be tentative just for gaining experience, but for production processes it is a more complex issue.

New products developed bearing in mind guideline ICH Q8 (see chapter 11) are transferred to the manufacturing site with an important amount of experience which includes critical variables and their acceptance ranges. Then, validation allows for their confirmation and for adjusting ranges and monitoring procedures. Once a product is validated it is ready for a well-monitored production process.

Unfortunately this is (usually) not the case with legacy products and as knowledge management did not exist in the past it is possible that there is a sensible lack of information on the product attributes and process parameters. In this case it is clear that it is not possible to take full advantage of the ICH quality approach.

4th As we are interested (and obliged) to adhere to the PQS approach it is possible to take a pragmatic intermediate approach with legacy products (see chapter 11).

- First step: Choose a limited number of products to start with (as we said before, for example, either those more important or those more critical).

- Second step: Gather all available information (and experience) on the chosen products. With these data and applying HACCP (see chapter 3) it should be possible to determine critical variables for monitoring the process and the product.

- Third step: Use a limited number of commercial batches (at least three) of the chosen products to perform a kind of revalidation consisting in showing that the critical variables can effectively be used to monitor a process which allows for yielding a product meeting specifications.

5th It is possible to start using the PQS model with the products and processes being monitored by critical variables. The critical variables allow for the process monitoring, but also for the process evaluation as it has been discussed before.

6th The statistical analysis of the data can be used both for the Product Quality Review to be handled to the regulatory authorities, but also as inputs to the Process Performance & Product Quality Monitoring System.

7th All the before mentioned data and, besides, the outcome of internal audits and of the CAPA system are shown to the high direction and evaluated during the Management Review.

8th The outcome of the Management Review is a list of aspects to be modified or added in order to improve the PQS.

CONCLUDING REMARKS

Exactly like the state, that has laws but needs the executive for making certain that they are put into action, GMP needs a PQS for ensuring compliance. And just like laws are modified to keep on with reality, the PQS system has to be regularly assessed to ensure its adequacy.

The 21st century PQS system is rather complex. Its organization and implementation requires an important amount of work and its maintenance supposes a never ending monitoring of processes to keep them under control. But notwithstanding that, the PQS is an adequate tool for ensuring a low risk level (or, to be more positive, a high quality level). In fact, currently it is the best way we have for ensuring GMP compliance.

CONFLICT OF INTEREST

The author confirms that this chapter contents have no conflict of interest.

ACKNOWLEDGEMENT

Declared None.

REFERENCES

[1] ISO (International Organization for Standardization). Quality management systems – Fundamentals and vocabulary. International standard ISO 9000:2005(en). ISO, Geneva, Switzerland 2005.
[2] ISO (International Organization for Standardization). Quality management systems – Requirements. International standard ISO 9001:2008(en). ISO, Geneva, Switzerland 2008.
[3] ISO (International Organization for Standardization). Managing for the sustained success of an organization — A quality management approach. International Standard ISO 9004:2009. ISO, Geneva, Switzerland 2009.
[4] ICH (International Conference on Harmonisation of Technical Requirements for registration of Pharmaceuticals for Human Use). Pharmaceutical Quality System. Harmonised Tripartite Guideline. Q10. ICH, Geneva, Switzerland 2008.
[5] Ibid.
[6] WHO (World Health Organization). WHO Good manufacturing practices for pharmaceutical products: main principles. In: WHO Expert Committee on Specifications for Pharmaceutical Preparations. Forty-eighth report (WHO Technical Report Series, No. 986). WHO, Geneva, Switzerland 2014. Annex 2.
[7] Ibid.
[8] The Commission of the European Communities. Commission directive 2003/94/EC of 8 October 2003 laying down the principles and guidelines of good manufacturing practice in respect of

medicinal products for human use and investigational medicinal products for human use. Official Journal of the European Union L 262/22 of 14.10.2003. Article 6.
[9] ICH (International Conference on Harmonisation of Technical Requirements for registration of Pharmaceuticals for Human Use). Pharmaceutical Quality System. Harmonised Tripartite Guideline. Q10. ICH, Geneva, Switzerland 2008. 1.5.
[10] Ibid. Glossary.
[11] Ibid. Annex 2.
[12] European Commission. Good manufacturing practices. Medicinal products for human and veterinary use. The rules governing medicinal products in the European Union. Volume 4. Brussels. Part I. 1.10 and 1.11.
[13] Ibid. 1.10.
[14] U.S. Department of Health and Human Services. Food and Drug Administration. Center for Drug Evaluation and Research (CDER). Center for Biologics Evaluation and Research (CBER). Center for Veterinary Medicine (CVM). Office of Regulatory Affairs (ORA). Quality systems approach to pharmaceutical CGMP regulations. Guidance for industry, Pharmaceutical CGMPs. Rockville, MD, USA 2006. III. D.
[15] Ibid. IV. D. 4.
[16] Ibid. IV. D. 5.

Chapter 6: Documentation

CHAPTER 6

Documentation

Abstract: Documentation is an essential GMP feature. If the PQS is something like a nervous system, then the documents are the nerves which carry information and which keep an organism alive and operational. This information has to be exact, clear and delivered safely where it is necessary. This is why the lifecycle of documents is critical. It is indispensable ensuring that they are well written and reviewed and approved by the right persons. Personnel using these documents have to receive copies and get well acquainted with them. This is vital, but not easy to ensure. Documents should reflect reality. This is why they have to be kept updated and superseded documents have to be returned to QA. Documents are crucial because they define how operations have to be performed, but also because they allow for traceability in the operations. The documents of a PQS are so numerous that document management requires hard work. Consequently there is always the risk of considering it something unworthy and boring, to be allotted to unlucky novice technicians. As a matter of fact documents reflect so trustworthy reality that is almost impossible doing wrong and showing good documentation or doing right and providing poor documentation, and this is why inspectors pay particular attention to documentation. Disorganized documentation is the hallmark of a disorganized company. Although documentation is usually associated to paper, this is not exact. Documentation is information on any support, ensuring traceability, safety and readability at any time. Tentative lists of the documents which are required in a manufacturing laboratory are given in this chapter.

Keywords: Accessibility, approval, BMR, code, controlled copy, data back-up, drawing, instruction, label, log (log-book), master document, master formula, master record, procedure, record, retention time, review, SOP, specification, version.

WHAT DOCUMENTATION IS

"Documentation" is the general term used to designate the documents of an organization (*i.e.* a group of people working together in a structured way for a shared purpose). Documents are pieces of information (*i.e.* data which has a meaning) on a support (traditionally paper but nowadays usually stored electronically or otherwise).

GMP acknowledges that documentation is an indispensable element of the Pharmaceutical Quality System (PQS). It fixes, preserves and diffuses company knowledge (*i.e.* what has to be done, why, by whom, when, *etc.*) and, besides, this diffusion is free from the misunderstandings linked to spoken communication. Documentation allows for the traceability of operations. As it was described in the previous chapter PQS requires process monitoring and evaluation and it is evident that this necessitates documentation, either on paper or electronic.

Jordi Botet

DOCUMENTATION LIFECYCLE

Although documents are simply instruments used to convey information on the processes of an organisation, their production and management constitute a process too. Thus, documentation requires a lifecycle approach (see chapter 2), as shown in Fig. (**1**).

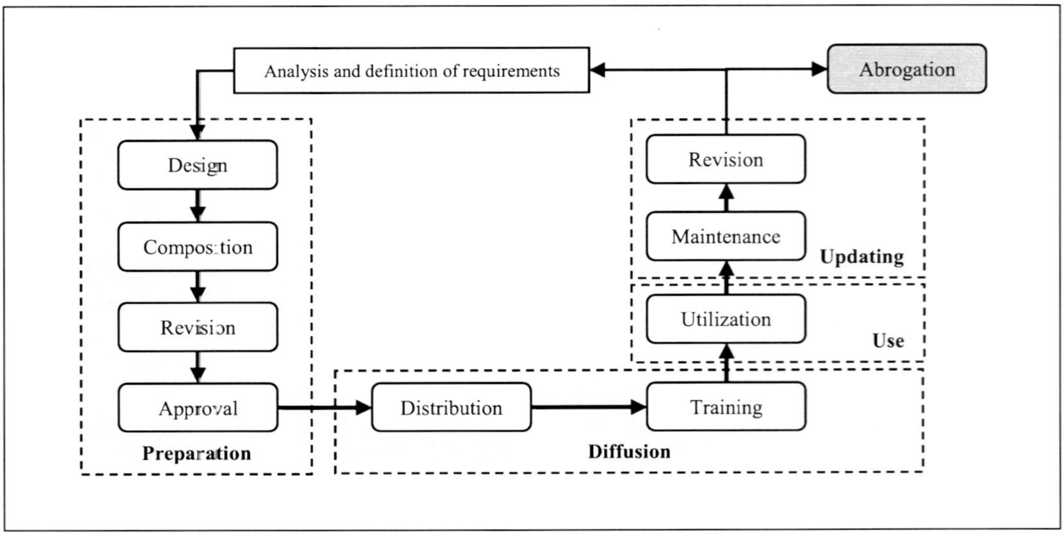

Fig. (1). Lifecycle of documents.

Design

Although it is evident that good presentation does not improve a bad document, an appropriate design enhances a suitable document.

Organizations design documentation according to their needs but also consider that documents are a kind of visiting card. This is why internal procedures often describe in detail how documents should be designed, even defining the font to be used, and they are developed on templates for ensuring homogeneity.

Each company has established its "own format" for the documents, which differentiate them from those of other organizations. Although there are not defined models, following is given general orientation on this matter.

Some people prefer documents with pages limited by margin lines, because this ensures to the lector the entirety of the text when printing or photocopying.

Cover Page

The cover page (or first page) is different from the other because it presents the document. A quite practical approach is using this front page for displaying all the general information about the document (identification, signatures, version control and distribution of copies), while the technical contents of the document start on the following page.

Thus, a first page could contain this information (Fig. **2**):

(A) Document identification

- The company logo and name;
- The related area of the document (project, plant, unit, department, process, system, *etc.*);
- A short and concise description (title);
- The type of document (see below);
- Code. It is a set of alphanumerical characters used as a reference for the document. Each organization uses its own system and all are equally acceptable, provided that they allow for the unambiguous identification of the document. They usually consist of three parts. The first one identifies the type of document. The second one the unit, division or department to which the document belongs. And, finally, the third one specifically identifies the document, which is often consecutive numbering. Thus, SOP-WAR-005, would mean: standard operating procedure of the warehouse number 5.
- Version of the document. There is no defined norm for the numbering of the versions of a document. Some prefer to consider that the first writing of a document is version 0 (zero), whereas other consider it version 1 and consequently do not have a version 0. Any option is correct, but it should be indicated in the appropriate procedure.

The version of a document can be included in the code (*e.g.* SOP-WAR-005-01), but then, when a new version is released (*e.g.* SOP-WAR-005-02), it is necessary to publish also new versions of all the documents which mentioned the old version. Instead, a code without version does not change when new versions are edited.

(B) Signatures of responsible persons

- A table with names, posts, dates and signatures for the responsible persons of the document (writing, revision and approval). Although the number of people participating depends on the particular structure of each organization, it is normally better to limit their number to prevent long delays.

Drug Pharm

Area

Type of document

Title of the document

Code

Version

Signatures

Name	**Responsibility**	**Post**	**Date**	**Signature**
	Writing			
	Review			
	Approval			

This document comes into force 10 days after its approval
This document is valid for 3 years.

Change control

Date	Version #	Reason for issuing a new version
dd/mm/yyyy	01	Original version

Distribution of copies

☐ Non controlled	☐ Controlled / No.	Assigned to:

Fig. (2). Sample of front page.

- Dates of coming into force and revision. Many organizations include a date in the heading of the document. Then, although each page is dated, it has to be decided whether this is the date of coming into force or the date of writing. As in large organizations an important delay often exists between the writing and approval of a document, it is then preferable not to include a date on the heading. In this case, the date of coming into force is the date of approval. A more elaborate option is to indicate, for instance, that the document is enforced ten days after its approval and that it should be reviewed after, say, three years.

(C) Change control

- Control of versions.

The history of the document is described by listing its versions, with the date of coming into force and the reason for the revision.

(D) Distribution of copies

- Space for controlling the distribution of copies.

The cover can have neither header nor footer (*i.e.* first page different from the others) or simply have the same header and footer than the other pages. If this latter solution is adopted, then, the above mentioned "(A) Document identification" information can be eliminated (or simplified) from the cover, not to repeat the same data.

Header

In general, it seems preferable to use the header to identify the document including all the information therein, whereas the footer is just reserved for pagination and special remarks (*i.e.* confidential, non authorized reproduction of this document is prohibited, *etc.*).

Experience also shows that to avoid editing errors it is better, whenever possible, to have a single header for the whole document (*i.e.* cover page either with a blank header or with the same header of all the other pages).

The header summarizes the essential information on the document identification before mentioned (Fig. **3**):

- Company logo and name;
- Related area (project, plant, department, process, system, equipment, *etc.*), as necessary;
- Type of document (see below);
- Title of the document;
- Code and the version of the document.

✱ **Drug Pharm**	Type of document		
	Title of the document		
	Area/Project/Unit/Department	Code	Version

Fig. (3). Sample of header.

Footer

Although it is possible to eliminate the footer and transfer the page number which is an essential element of information to the header, in general it can be said that a footer with a separation line as in the figure has the advantage of better enclosing the text of the document.

Often (Fig. **4**) it includes a reminder of the property of the document (*e.g.* this document cannot be reproduced without authorization) and the number of page and the total number of document pages (*e.g.* page 3/12 or page 3 from 12).

This document cannot be reproduced without authorization	Page 3/N

Fig. (4). Sample of footer.

In order to have homogeneous documentation each company chooses its own type of font and outline. The type of font of the company is indicated in the general procedure on documentation. The outline of the document is partly described in this same document (with examples of it either in the text or annexed). However, for practical reasons this is usually handled by the QA (Quality Assurance) department which keeps templates of the documents which can be handed to the persons who have to prepare a new document. When the QA department reviews a new document not only checks its contents but also its outline.

Composition

Before preparing a document it is necessary to think carefully about its intended purpose, the requirements to be met and to whom it is addressed. Nevertheless, as documents are necessary (and often compulsory) and usually there is little time to prepare them, this stage is sometimes overlooked and that has a direct influence on their quality level (*i.e.* vague purpose, unclear regulatory background, text not adapted to its readers, *etc.*).

Documents are designed following similar patterns everywhere. Every document has two well defined sections, the first one comprises general parts present in all documents, whereas the second one is variable and develops the particular contents of the document. Often there is a third section which is constituted by the annexes. See Fig. (**5**).

Documents should be above all useful and this means that they are required to be clear and understandable. This statement might be surprising (why to prepare a document not to be understood?), but unfortunately practice shows that not always documents are easy to understand. In fact, the rule of thumb of documentation is that a document should be understandable for a normal person with the training required for the post to which this document is linked.

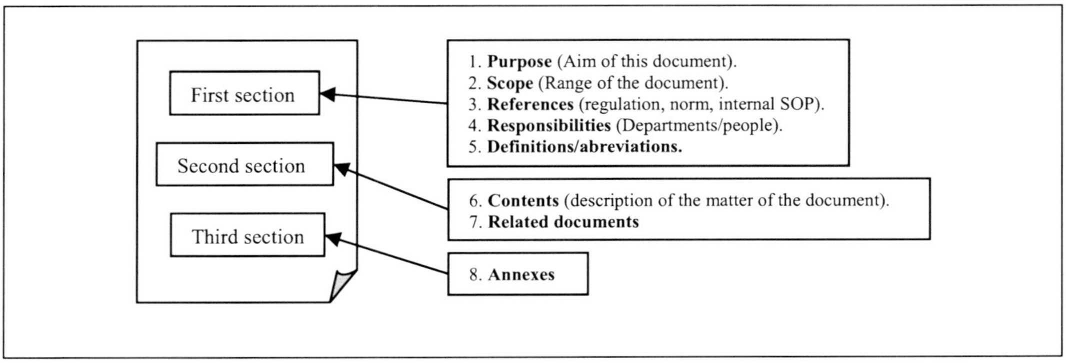

Fig. (5). Structure of a document.

Although some of the characteristics required to documents by GMP are rather vague, they can be summarized as follows:

- Their contents should be clear and unambiguous.
- Their title, kind of document and objective should be clearly and accurately presented.

- They should be logically structured in order to be easy to read and to understand.

- *They should comply with the relevant parts of the manufacturing and marketing authorizations* [1].

- If documents are reproduced (usually they are either a photocopy or a printing) than they should be easily readable (*i.e.* lack of toner may lead to a defective copy) and reproduce faithfully the approved original.

Usually documents are written by the person or persons who know better the matter, then they are revised with the objective of confirming that technically their contents are correct and that they comply with GMP, with authorizations and with internal procedures. And finally they are approved by a person possessing the company endorsement for empowering the documents. Thus, in a document should intervene at least three persons (writer, reviser and approver), who should sign and date. In some cases, because of the content of the document it is preferable that more people get involved. Each company has its own policy regarding who should intervene. In general, experience shows that the more people get involved the less brisk becomes the process.

In practice the draft document is normally reviewed by all the persons who will be later involved with its revision and approval in order to get consensus on it before being formally printed.

Documents, as said before, are allotted to a department which is identified in the code. Most of documents are clearly linked to a department (*e.g.* "Maintenance of vacuum pumps" – Maintenance; or "Study of the ongoing stability of products" – Quality Control), but sometimes this is not the case (*e.g.* "Initial and continuing training management" – Manpower or QA?). Fortunately this is not a real problem because what counts is not to which department a document belongs, but that the persons who have written and revised it possess the necessary knowledge. Here the chosen approach takes into account two points (Fig. **6**):

1st Documents are allotted to the department which is more involved with the practical handling;

2nd QA should contribute in the writing of many documents but should not be too involved in practical handling, because its main responsibility is supervision to ensure GMP compliance, not operation.

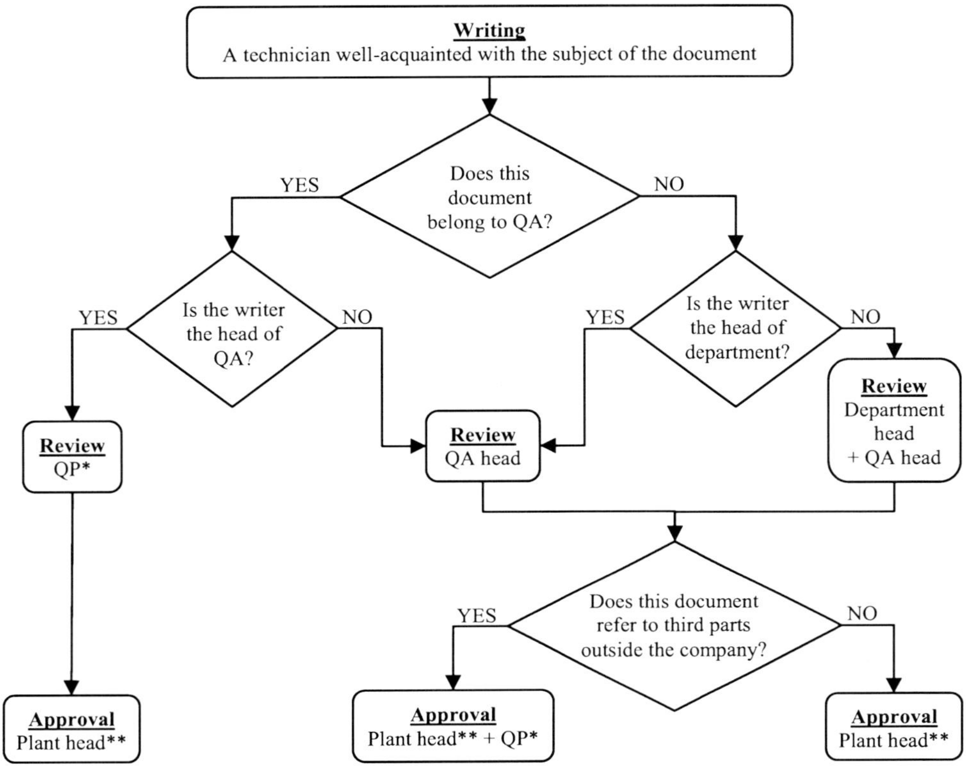

* If the qualified person (QP) is also the QA head, then the QC head might substitute her/him

** The Senior Director can also **approve** documents particularly those which don't have a pure technical contents

Fig. (6). Tentative flowchart for determining the approach to review and approval of documents.

As GMP indicates that documents have to be clear and not lead to interpretation errors, it is preferable to avoid using acronyms or specialized terms, unless they are described in the same document (the inclusion of a glossary is highly recommended). When document users participate in the creation of the documents or, at least, are consulted, the chances of getting clearer documents increase dramatically.

Revision

When a document is written by a specialist in the matter, revision is mainly understood as review by Quality Assurance in order to verify that the document is correct from the GMP point of view and that its outline and contents agree with the procedures of the company. But if a document is written by a technician of the team, then usually the head of the department (or a specialist) gets involved in the revision too.

Approval

GMP-related documents should be approved by officially designated persons, such as the key staff (head of production, head of quality control, qualified person). In high level documents or when it is preferable to have a "political" sanction documents are approved by the high direction.

Distribution

Documents are prepared to hand over copies of them to interested persons. These copies may be controlled or not:

- Controlled copies are given to persons or departments having the responsibility to enforce the document and who, therefore, should always be provided with its current version. In other words, controlled copies are "official" copies. The department responsible for the control and distribution of documents (usually QA) should keep a list of the controlled copies of any document, verifying that each registered user gets the new version while the old one is withdrawn (Fig. 7).

- Non-controlled copies are distributed, in principle, without any rule or limit.

The distribution of a document should take into account the following features:

- Quality Assurance is responsible for keeping the master copy of the document. Besides, in order to maintain a historical traceability, QA should preserve the master copies of all versions of a document;

- The controlled copies received by a department or person are numbered and the receiver (*i.e.* the person or the responsible of the department) should sign on the distribution list. QA should have a tally detailing for every document who should receive a controlled copy and these departments/persons should always possess the current version. This means careful distribution of a new version and retrieving of the previous one.

- When controlled copies are distributed to a department they should be easily accessible for any person of the department using them (*i.e.* when departments are scattered within the premises it might be advisable to provide more controlled copies; copies should be available to users for using them while working).

- Controlled copies are usually kept in a single box or folder to impede that they get dispersed and eventually lost. Then the question may arise: do I have all necessary documents? Or put differently, are here all the controlled copies that I should have? An answer to this question would be including in the box or folder a list of all the controlled documents. This, of course, means some more work for QA, because the distribution of a new document should be accompanied with a copy of the extended list of documents.

- It is also possible to hand over "uncontrolled copies". These, as the name shows, need not to be subjected to any control because they are considered as purely informative (*i.e.* without formal use).

Drug Pharm	Type of document: **Record**		
	Title: **Follow-up of controlled copies**		
	Area/Project/Unit/Department	Code	Version

Document	
Title:	
Code/Version:	

Copy #	**Handed to**	**Date**	**Signature (received)**	**Previous version withdrawn**	**Comments**
1				☐ **Yes**	
2				☐ **Yes**	
3				☐ **Yes**	
4				☐ **Yes**	
5				☐ **Yes**	
.				☐ **Yes**	

Fig. (7). Example of register for controlling the distribution of controlled copies of a document.

It has proven useful to use paper in other color to distinguish "master copies of the documents" (for instance, yellow paper) from their copies (common white paper). The master document, which can be numbered as copy #0 (zero), is kept by QA, whereas user controlled copies are numbered consecutively starting from #1. A specific table can be included for this purpose on the front page of the document.

Training

Before being applied, documents have to be known and understood by their users. A common procedure for ensuring this is organizing a training session when a new document or version is issued and distributed. Then, a record of this, including the signatures of people having taken part in it, is kept by the department to which the document belongs. See chapter 7.

In order to ensure that operators have really understood the document it is advisable to complement the training session with an exercise (written or practical testing). The key point is ensuring that people who are going to use it have enough understanding and knowledge for being capable of carrying out it correctly.

Use

Documents can provide information on how operating (*e.g.* procedures) or recording data regarding operations (*e.g.* records). These latter are forms which have free spaces for gathering data. Records should be documented when the action is performed. Thus, the traceability of all the significant activities pertaining to the manufacture of pharmaceutical products is ensured. Data concerning the operations should be clear, readable and indelible.

It is generally considered that ballpoint pens (biros) provide indelible writing, as required by GMP, whereas fountain pens or felt tip pens might be prone to blotting or be too thick for writing clearly. In any case the instrument should write clearly and indelibly. Pencils and the like are forbidden because they can be erased.

As reproduced documents are normally printed in black, in many organizations users are compelled to use blue ink ballpoint pens, to offer the best contrast. Blue ink also permits an easy differentiation of original documents with recorded data from photocopies.

Any alteration realized on a document because of errors or changes (*e.g.* in the document a measure was supposed to be done by using a certain instrument but in practice it was necessary to use another one) has to be done allowing the lecture of the existing information (without hiding the existing data). A simple line is drawn on the wrong data and the new information is written aside accompanied by the date and signature of the corrector. If necessary it is possible to indicate the reason for the change too. Erasing the data or covering them with correctors is not permitted.

Data (either register forms filled with data or electronic files) should be surely archived and safely preserved, because they provide evidence of the activities performed within the PQS.

When information is kept on paper, documents should be archived in a closed board or room in order to protect them for being taken away and lost by people. The most critical documents are usually kept in special fire-proof precincts. Written documents can also be scanned and kept as electronic or photographic data, but this method should offer the same level of safety than traditional paper.

When using computerized systems for recording data, they should offer the same reliability as handwritten entries in registering forms [2]. That is:

(a) Accessibility and safety of recorded data: The system has to provide recorded process data in a humanly understandable form. And this recorded data has to be safely protected (*i.e.* with a back-up system).

(b) Access control and identification of operators: Only authorized people can access the system and operators are identified by their electronic signatures (which provide the same identification security as a handwritten signature).

When electronic signatures are not based on biometric recognition, they should be composed of two different components: identification code and password. Electronic signatures based on biometrics should be conceived to ensure that can be used by a single person only. Non- biometric signatures should only be used by the designed owner.

A continuous session should be started by using both components, but afterwards just one component might suffice. Instead, in a non-continuous session it should always be required to use both components.

(c) Audit trail: The date and time of data entries/modifications should be recorded. Record changes should not prevent from reading previously recorded information.

(d) Validation: The computerized system has to be validated.

Maintenance

Documents should reflect the reality (*i.e.* they should describe how operations should be done; and operations should be realized as described in them). Consequently, documents must be regularly revised and updated, if necessary.

Changes in a process (*e.g.* updated requirements, modified operations, innovative equipment, *etc.*) require writing new versions of the documents related to this process, but even if there are not apparent modifications it is necessary to perform periodic revisions in order to confirm that documents still correspond to the reality.

The periodicity of revision is determined by each company in terms of compromise (too much time means great risk of deviation, whereas too short time may suppose too much revision work). Although there is no established term for the review of documents, many organisations institute a period of 3 or 5 years. Other set up a period of 2 years, after which they verify the document and if everything is correct than they fill an apposite form on the last page declaring that the life of the document is extended for a couple of years. Completed this new period of two years the document is considered out of date and a new version is prepared. Whichever be the term chosen it should be respected (*i.e.* there should not be outdated documents in the plant). In any case, changes in documents, like any other change within the PQS, have to be realized in a controlled manner (*i.e.* by the change management system). There should be a system in place for ensuring that copies of superseded versions of the documents are not unintentionally used (*e.g.* they can be destroyed or marked as obsolete).

Abrogation

Documents which are no longer necessary, either because the operations which they describe have ceased or because of a reorganization of the same documents (*i.e.* merging the contents of two or more documents), can be discontinued. In any case it should be taken into account what is said about the retention time for documents in order to ensure that as long as there are products on the market the related documentation will be kept. Abrogated documents, like obsolete ones, should not be inadvertently used.

RETENTION TIME FOR DOCUMENTS

The baseline objective is to ensure that no document will be thrown away while there is still some associated product on the market. Once this objective is satisfied, it has to be kept in mind that historical data are necessary for trend evaluation and also that older information might one day, who knows, give the clues for a problem. Unfortunately paper fills a lot of place and it is cumbersome to file and to retrieve. Thus, a composite approach could help. Highly significant protocols, reports, procedures or instructions could be archived as paper documents, whereas records and other less important documents might be scanned and archived by electronic systems (this would guarantee that data are preserved). The following rules should apply:

- Superseded documents (procedures and instructions): QA should keep the complete story of each document. Thus, if necessary, it will be always possible to know which procedure or instruction was used at a given date. In case of lack of space the older documents (*e.g.* more than 10 years after being out of date) can be scanned and then filed electronically.

- Records: *Records should be retained for at least one year after the expiry date of the finished product* [3]. *Any Quality Control documentation relating to a batch record should be retained for one year after the expiry date of the batch and at least 5 years after the certification* [4]. *Any production, control, or distribution record that is required to be maintained in compliance with this part and is specifically associated with a batch of a drug product shall be retained for at least 1 year after the expiration date of the batch or, in the case of certain OTC drug products lacking expiration dating..., 3 years after distribution of the batch* [5].

ELECTRONICALLY STORED DATA

As said before, they have to offer the same level of safety than traditionally written data. That means:

- That they have to be protected from loss by a periodic program of back-up transfer on storage media at a separate and secure location.

- That stored data have to be readily available and retrievable throughout the period of retention.

- That the retrieved data should be readable.

TYPES OF DOCUMENTS

As commented in chapter 5 the documents of the PQS can be distributed in four logical groups according to its level of importance. The documents of the two higher levels (Quality Manual and general procedures) have already been described there. Now it is the turn of the two lower levels constituted by documents directly linked to products or processes/operations.

Documents Directly Linked to Products

The documents directly linked to products belong to three categories:

- The "specifications" for starting and packaging materials, and for intermediate, bulk and finished products. A specification can be defined as *a list of detailed requirements with which the products or materials used or obtained during manufacture have to conform. They serve as a basis for quality evaluation* [6].

- The documents descriving the formula and the manufacturing process of a product. They are known collectively as "manufacturing formulae" or separately as "master formulae" plus "processing and packaging instructions" (Table **1**).

Thus, a "master formula" can be defined as *a document or set of documents specifying the starting materials with their quantities and the packaging materials, together with a description of the procedures and precautions required to produce a specified quantity of a finished product as well as the processing instructions, including the in-process controls* [7].

Formally authorized Manufacturing Formula and Processing Instructions should exist for each product and batch size to be manufactured. They are often combined in one document. There should be formally authorized Packaging Instructions for each product, pack size and type [8]. With this information it is possible to prepare a practical guide for the preparation of a lot of finished product. This guide contains blank spaces which are filled with data gathered during the process and is known as "master record", which can be defined as *a document or set of documents that serve as a basis for the batch documentation (blank batch record)* [9].

Table 1. Manufacturing formulae.

Document	Contents
Master formula	- Denomination and reference code of the product. - Description of the dosage form and of its presentation, potency and batch size. - List of starting materials with references and quantities (including substances which might disappear during production).

Table 1: contd...

	- Intermediate anticipated yields with acceptance ranges, as necessary. - Final anticipated yield with acceptance range.
Process instructions	- Description of the processing rooms and equipment. - Description or reference to a procedure/instruction regarding the preparation of critical equipment. - Detailed description of how to perform the operations, including verification, duration, temperature, *etc.*). - In process controls, including acceptance ranges; - Keeping of intermediate of bulk products (container, label, conditions, *etc.*). - Any other necessary information.
Packaging instructions	- Product denomination - Presentation, potency and batch size - Packaging size (number, weight, volume in the container) - List of packaging materials with code/reference number and quantity. - If adequate reproduction of printed materials and indication of places where to print batch numbers and expiry date. - Precautions (line clearance). - Description of equipment and operations. - In-process controls, sampling and acceptance ranges.

For each batch processed is prepared a "batch manufacturing record (BMR)", defined as *all documents associated with the manufacture of a batch of bulk product or finished product. They provide a history of each batch of product and of all circumstances pertinent to the quality of the final product* [10]. Each batch manufacturing record should be identified with the number of the batch being manufactured.

Documents Directly Linked to Operations/Processes

- "Procedures", known more precisely as "standard operating procedures" (SOP) describe processes or sets of operations. A SOP can be defined as *an authorized written procedure giving instructions for performing operations not necessarily specific to a given product or material (e.g. equipment operation, maintenance and cleaning; validation; cleaning of premises and environmental control; sampling and inspection). Certain SOPs may be used to supplement product-specific master and batch production documentation* [11]. They often have associated records, in which the data generated by the operations are written.

- "Instructions" describe how to perform operations. They often have associated records too. The distinction between procedures and instructions is purely conventional, as both types of documents have the same objective (*i.e.* to explain how things must be done). However, procedures are more general documents referring to processes or sets of activities or operations, whereas instructions refer to a given activity or operation (*i.e.* use of an instrument, cleaning a piece of equipment, control of an operation, *etc.*). There are organizations which do not distinguish procedures from instructions and both types of documents are simply known as procedures.

- "Records" or "registers" are forms used to gather data of the operations. They are associated to a procedure or instruction.

- "Plans" or "programs" schedule operations (maintenance, training, calibration, *etc.*). These documents, generally laid out in the form of tables, project and organize activities. They are often provided with spaces to gather data. They can be very varied. There are some very basic plans which exist in all laboratories (*e.g.* calibration of critical instruments, maintenance of systems and equipment, cleaning of premises, pest control, training, *etc.*).

- "Log books" or "logs" are note-books pertaining to equipment and where all operations of a given piece of equipment are registered. The more important or critical pieces of equipment and clean rooms should be accompanied by log-books where the different operations are chronologically registered indicating date, operation (*i.e.* production, validation, calibration, maintenance, cleaning, repair, inspection) and the identity of the person who performed it. In production operations it is necessary to register the hour, the product and the lot number.

- "Labels" are pieces of paper or other material which are applied to rooms, equipment, containers, *etc.*, for the sake of identification or description. The format and utilization of labels should be described in a document. In most organizations the wording on the labels is enhanced by colors which define the state (*e.g.* green means accepted/clean, yellow is quarantined, red shows rejected/dirty).

DOCUMENTATION OF A PLANT

A frequently asked question is how many procedures are necessary in a pharmaceutical organization to fulfill GMP requirements. This question does not have a straightforward answer, because each case is different and often diverse approaches are possible to attain the same objective.

This problem can be tackled by analyzing the processes of the organization and then establishing which procedures are necessary for each of them (Fig. **8**).

The representation of all the processes of an organisation is known as "process mapping" (see chapter 5 for the identification of the processes).

Folowing are provided lists of "topics/documents" that are in fact lists of matters which should be documented either as listed or brought together in different documents. What counts is the completeness of the information. The number or documents is irrelevant.

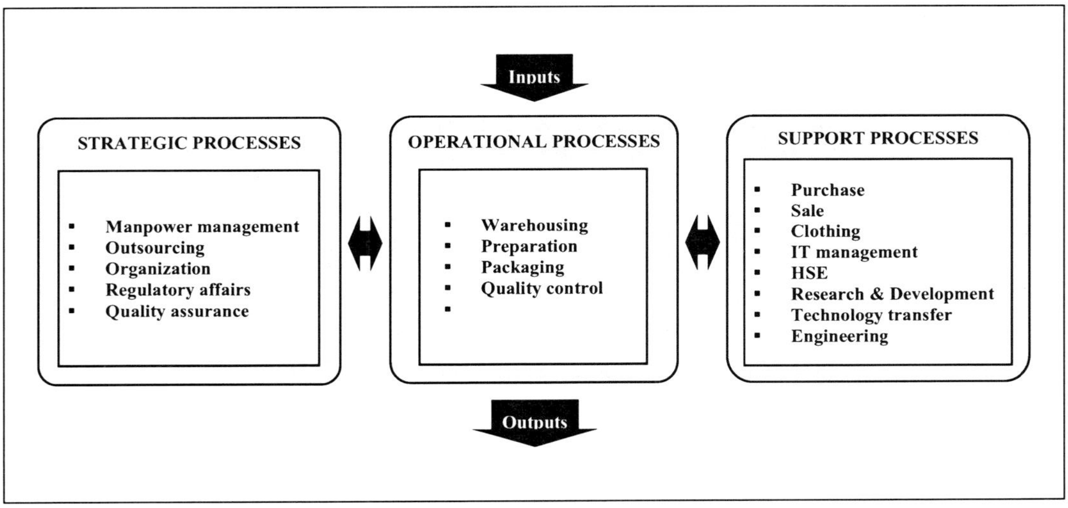

Fig. (8). Reminder of process map.

Moreover, for a more practical distribution of the documents some processes can be grouped (*e.g.* Organization and Outsourcing are grouped as ADM - from Administration; Purchase, Sale and Clothing are grouped as LOG - from Logistics). In the example which is here discussed, documents can belong to 14 groups, which are identified by a symbol composed of three letters.

Strategic Processes

These processes determine the approach of the organization to quality and as such they put into order not only the operations which are developed in the plant, but also those which are realized outside either regarding manufacturing activities (outsourcing) or ordered by the competent pharmaceutical authorities (regulatory affairs). Since operations are performed by people their appointment and training are very important and this is why it is spoken of Manpower management. And finally, QA is the overall company "watchdog" on the PQS. See Table **2**.

Table 2. Strategic processes and their groupings.

Process	Purpose	Symbol
Manpower management	Ensure that the plant has the necessary personnel and that they possess the adequate level of training and experience.	MAN
Organization	Arrange, plan, resource, control and guide the activities of the plant.	ADM
Outsourcing	Select and manage contract acceptors of production or analysis operations.	
Regulatory affairs	Prepare and present documentation to competent authorities in order to be authorised to manufacture pharmaceutical products.	RAF
Quality assurance	Develop, implement and manage a quality system to ensure that products meet their specifications.	QAS

Manpower Management

A high level general procedure "Personnel management" describes the approach of the company to manpower, including its training. Thus the following documents could be written in order to develop this general procedure. Some of them might be unnecessary if their contents were already included in the general procedure. See Table **3**.

Table 3. Tentative list of Manpower management documentation.

	Topic/Document	Contents
01	Job descriptions.	Account of duties and responsibilities associated with the organization posts.
02	Key personnel responsibilities.	
03	Personnel hiring.	Personnel employment and their arrangement to a system (selection, appointment, organization, *etc.*).
04	Personnel qualification for posts.	
05	Personnel organization.	
06	Rules for transfer of information during changes of shift.	
07	Rules for absence from work.	
08	Personnel education and training.	Personnel education and instruction (initial and continual).
09	Personnel professional CVs.	
10	Personnel training tallies.	
11	Training plans.	
12	Basic GMP norms for external personnel.	

Table 3: contd...

13	Personnel identification on documents.	Signature/initialization.
14	Access control of personnel to the premises	Supervision and handling of personnel health and sanitary conditions.
15	Personnel hygiene and clothing.	
16	Personnel health surveillance.	
17	Instructions for pregnant, puerperal or in lactation women.	
18	Sanitary surveillance.	
19	First aid management.	
20	Accident statement and analysis.	

Organization

Under this name is designed what could be called "administration and direction of the plant". It comprises both leadership and government. A high level general procedure, Management review, concerns directly the senior direction of the organization. Procedures might comprise the aspects shown in Table **4**.

Table 4. Tentative list of Organization documentation.

	Topic/Document	Contents
01	Material and product codification system.	Identification of materials and products.
02	Internal labeling system.	
03	Internal batch numbering system for materials	
04	Batch numbering system for products.	Place production orders.
05	Preparation and flow of documentation to produce a batch.	
06	Rules for the entry of data in records	Entry and correction of data and alteration of documents.
07	Systematization of communication flows of information in the company.	Methods used in the organization for ensuring the transmission of information (from top to bottom and bottom to top).
08	Rules on the flows of materials/products, waste and personnel in the premises.	General organization.
09	Rules for the use and handling of pallets	
10	Rules for the entrance of persons and vehicles in the premises of the organization.	
11	Management of emergencies.	
12	Restarting of the facility after stopping or after an emergency stop.	
13	Allocation of resources.	Resource management
14	Budget control.	

Table 4: contd...

15	Approach for improvement of performance (lean management and 6σ).	Improvement of performance

Outsourcing

As seen in chapter 5 any outsourced operation/process falling within the scope of the PQS should have the same guarantee of GMP compliance than in house operations/processes. A high level general procedure, Outsourcing, provides information on the formal agreement (contract) which should exist between both parts in order to ensure compliance (Table **5**).

Table 5. Tentative list of <u>Outsourcing</u> documentation.

Topic/Document		Contents
01	Contract production and analysis management.	Conditions and flows of information in case of work done by other organizations.
02	Documentation relevant to external services/working.	

The documents of Outsourcing and Organization processes are identified as "Administration".

Regulatory Affairs

Documents prepared by this department are directed to the competent regulatory authorities. Here are considered two topics. On one side the description of the organization of the department and the management of regulatory activities and on the other the management of pharmacovigilance (Table **6**).

Table 6. Tentative list of <u>regulatory affairs</u> documentation.

Topic/Document		Contents
01	Regulatory affairs organization and management.	Description of the department of regulatory affairs and its arrangements.
02	Responsibilities and organization of pharmacovigilance.	Description of how the company meets pharmacovigilance requirements.

Quality Assurance

As commented before, QA as guarantor of the PQS intervenes in all documents, but also there are documents which concern QA directly. Besides the high level general procedures already mentioned (Documentation management; Change management; Risk and knowledge management; Incident, deviation and OOS management; CAPA system; Process performance and product quality review;

Internal audits; Product quality review; Qualification/Validation policy) the following topics can be mentioned (Table **7**).

Table 7. Tentative list of QA documents.

Topic/Document		Contents
01	Review and evaluation of Master Batch records.	Revision, certification and release of product batches.
02	Certification and release of product batches.	
03	Supplier assessment and auditing.	Internal and external GMP-compliance auditing.
04	Self-inspection (internal quality audits).	
05	Cross contamination and mix-up prevention, control, and investigation.	Prevention of contamination, cross-contamination and mix-up.
06	Prevent objectionable microorganisms in drug products not required to be sterile.	
07	Prevent contamination of steriles.	
08	Handling of OOS.	Treatment of non-compliant batches.
09	Handling of complaints.	
10	Handling of recalls.	
11	Vigilance of changes regarding GMP and legal requirements.	Procedure for keeping information on requirement updated.

Operational Processes

These are the core processes that contribute in transforming materials into the products of the organization. See Table **8**.

Table 8. Operational processes and their groupings.

Process	Purpose	Symbol
Warehousing	Receive and store materials. Store intermediate, bulk and finished products. Dispatch and distribute finished products.	WAR
Production	Transform materials into intermediates and bulk products.	PRO
Packaging	Transform bulk products into finished products.	PAC
Quality control	Sampling and testing materials and products (intermediate, bulk and finished) and product. Environmental sampling and testing.	QCO

Warehousing

Under the name of warehousing are considered different, although closely connected processes: reception of materials, storage of materials under quarantine, storage of approved materials, storage of products under quarantine, storage of approved products, preparation of delivery orders, shipping, and distribution. And this requires a good amount of documents. See Table **9**.

Table 9. Tentative list of Warehousing documents.

	Topic/Document	Contents
01	Handling of returned and recalled products.	Handling of non conformities.
02	Handling of rejected materials and products.	
03	Handling of outdated materials and products	
04	Disposal of unsalable stock.	
05	Reception, identification, cleaning, labeling, quarantine and storage of starting materials.	Reception, identification, handling, quarantine and storage of the different types of items.
06	Storage of temperature sensitive materials.	
07	Storage of solvents in tanks.	
08	Storage of controlled, narcotic or habit forming starting materials.	
09	Handling and storage of hazardous materials (flammable substances, highly toxic substances, strongly smelling materials, pressurized gases).	
10	Reception, identification, quarantine and storage of printed and non printed packaging materials.	
11	Reception, identification, quarantine and storage of intermediates and finished products.	
12	Storage of intermediates and finished controlled narcotic and habit forming products.	
13	Reception, identification, quarantine and storage of product samples.	
14	Reception, identification and storage of promotional material.	
15	Reception, identification and storage of other types of wares.	
16	Handling of batches in stock (FIFO).	
17	Handling of rests of small quantities of single approved batches.	
18	Handling of spillages in the warehouse	
19	Cleaning of containers in/out of the warehouse.	
20	Inventories/revision of stocks.	
21	Temperature mapping, monitoring and recording. Handling of temperature excursions.	Control of storage temperature.
22	Preparation of sales orders.	Distribution of finished products.
23	Delivery of sales orders.	
24	Handling and transporting of shipped products.	
25	Monitoring of transport conditions.	

Table 9: contd...

26	Extending expiry date.	Recuperation of materials/products.
27	Repacking damaged stock.	
28	Cleaning of the warehouse.	Cleaning.
29	Cleaning/sanitization of the sampling area.	

Production

The documentation related to production is very rich (Table **10**). However, most of the operations/processes cannot be shown specifically on the list because they are very different and depend on the type of products manufactured.

A high-level procedure, "Qualification/Validation" policy, is developed here by a Validation Master Plan (VMP) and instructions for the validation of production processes and for the validation of cleaning methods.

Table 10. Tentative list of Production documents.

Topic/Document		Contents
01	Preparation of manufacturing master formulae, processing and packaging instructions and batch master records (BMRs).	Preparation of documentation and materials for production.
02	Instructions for the weighing of starting materials and their transfer to production.	
03	Assembly, utilization, verification/check, cleaning/sanitization, calibration/maintenance of...	Directions on handling and use for each piece of equipment/tool/instrument/(as necessary).
04	Entering and exiting of personnel into and out of clean rooms/aseptic areas. Instructions for the donning of clothing.	Rules for personnel in production areas, both in clean and conventional rooms.
05	Behavior in the production areas in general and in the clean rooms in particular.	
06	Instructions for the donning and use of gloves and masks in the production areas.	
07	Handling of spillages in the production areas.	
08	Realization of the operation/process...	Directions on the realization of each operation/process, as necessary (*e.g.* filtration, weighing, loading, *etc.*)
09	Entry/Exit of materials in clean areas.	Instructions for producing adequately.
10	Incidence and deviation handling during production.	
11	Reconciliation (balance of materials) and estimation of yields in production.	

Table 10: contd...

12	Recovery of materials/products in production.	
13	Reprocessing of materials/products in production.	
14	Instructions for the compilation of the batch master record (BMR) during production.	
15	Instructions for the use of water in production (cleaning and compounding)	
16	Instructions for sampling during production.	
17	Instructions for the recording of environmental parameters (T, RH, ΔP) during production.	
18	Instructions for the realization of in-process controls.	
19	Log-book management.	
20	Optical controlling of ampoules and vials filled with liquid.	
21	Handling of flexible pipes.	
22	Validation Master Plan.	Validation.
23	Instructions for the validation of production processes.	
24	Instructions for the validation of cleaning methods.	
25	Aseptic work evaluation by means of media fills.	
26	Preparation of materials/tools/instruments/equipment for sterilization/depyrogenation.	Directions on sterilization/depyrogenation.
27	Steam (humid) sterilization.	
28	Oven (dry) sterilization/depyrogenation.	
29	Ethylene oxide sterilization.	
30	Hydrogen peroxide/peracetic acid sterilization.	
31	Rules for the organization of washing rooms	Washing of equipment and utensils
32	Instructions for cleaning of clean rooms.	Cleaning/sanitization.
33	Instructions for sanitization of aseptic areas.	

Packaging

The documents here listed for secondary packaging are similar to those described for the preparation of bulk products, but they are considered apart because of the separation of both physical areas (*i.e.* bulk products are prepared in clean rooms, but final packaging is realized in non classified areas). See Table **11**.

Table 11. Tentative list of Packaging documents.

	Topic/Document	Contents
01	Instructions for the preparation and transfer of packaging materials to packaging.	Preparation of materials for packaging

Table 11: contd...

02	Assembly, utilization, verification/check, cleaning, calibration/maintenance of...	Directions on handling and use for each piece of equipment/tool/instrument/(as necessary).
03	Realization of the operation/process...	Directions on the realization of each operation/process, as necessary (*e.g.* weighing, labeling, marking, *etc.*).
04	Instructions for the validation of packaging processes.	Validation.
05	Behavior in the packaging areas.	Instructions for packaging adequately.
06	Incidence and deviation handling during packaging.	
07	Reconciliation (balance of materials) and estimation of yields in packaging.	
08	Instructions for the compilation of the batch master record (BMR) during packaging.	
09	Instructions for sampling during packaging.	
10	Instructions for the realization of in-process controls.	
11	Log-book management.	
12	Transfer of finished products to the warehouse.	
13	Instructions for cleaning of the packaging areas	Cleaning.

Quality Control

The quality control laboratory is a completely different world by itself. This is why it is separated and treated independently from the production areas. It is true that GMP provides some general orientation regarding the laboratory and this is logical because of its key role for ensuring quality. Anyway, it is GLP which offer specialized guidance on the organization of the laboratory. The quality control laboratory is normally composed of two autonomous, separated and very different parts: physico-chemistry (P) and microbiology (M). And sometimes it is possible to add other ones like biology or radioisotopes, which are not considered here.

Most of documents can apply to the QC department in its entirety, but its specialized sections require some specific documents. See Table **12**.

Table 12. Tentative list of Quality control documents.

	Topic/Document	Area	Contents
01	Behavior and clothing of personnel in the QC laboratory.	P/M	Rules for laboratory personnel

Table 12: contd...

02	Sampling, inspecting, and testing starting materials.	P/M	Sampling and testing. (Sampling plans, techniques and equipment. Precautions for preventing cross-contamination and for protecting unstable and/or sterile materials. Recording of the visual appearance of materials and of unexpected or unusual circumstances).
03	Sampling, inspecting, and testing packaging materials.	P/M	
04	Sampling and testing intermediate and bulk products.	P/M	
05	Sampling, inspecting, and testing finished products.	P/M	
06	Sampling and testing of clean rooms (environmental monitoring). Study of trends. Handling of deviations.	M	
07	Sampling and testing of personnel/clothing. Study of trends. Handling of deviations.	M	
08	Reception, storage and handling of samples in the QC laboratory.	P/M	
09	Control of well/mains water and drinkable water.	P/M	
10	Control of purified water.	P/M	
11	Control of water for injection/highly purified water.	P/M	
12	Control of pharmaceutical steam	P/M	
13	Control of pharmaceutical compressed air	P/M	
14	Handling of analytical raw data and calculations.	P/M	Data handling and organization.
15	Handling of laboratory log-books.	P/M	
16	Procedure for the emission of analytical certificates.	P/M	
17	Treatment of Out of Specification results and laboratory investigations.	P/M	
18	Vigilance of changes (pharmacopoeial and other) and updating of analytical specifications and procedures.	P/M	Procedure for keeping information on requirement updated.
19	Instructions for the assembly, utilization, verification/check/adjustment, cleaning/sanitization, calibration/maintenance of...	P/M	Directions on handling and use for each apparatus/instrument/piece of equipment/tool (as necessary).
20	Realization of the operation...	P/M	Directions on the realization of each operation, as necessary (*e.g.* weighing, filtration, thin layer chromatography, *etc.*).
21	Analytical method for the determination/identification of...	P/M	Description of the procedure for analyzing each material, intermediate, bulk, product (as necessary).
22	Rules for the preparation of specifications.	P/M	Description of the critical parameters and their acceptable ranges for each material, intermediate, bulk, product (as necessary).
23	Specifications for	P/M	

Table 12: contd...

24	Handling of reagents, solutions, and standards.	P/M	Preparation, control, labeling and storage.
25	Verification of analytical scales in the QC laboratory	P/M	Handling of analytical scales.
26	Rules for the reanalysis of starting materials	P/M	Handling of reanalysis.
27	Cleaning and sterilization of laboratory glass.	P/M	Cleaning/sanitization.
28	Cleaning of the physico-chemical department of the laboratory.	P	
29	Cleaning of the microbiological department of the laboratory.	M	
30	Laboratory waste treatment and disposal.	P/M	Waste handling.
31	Preparation, control and labeling of solutions for microbiology.	M	Practical work instructions.
32	Handling and control of culture media.	M	
33	Handling and control of reference microbiological strains.	M	
34	Handling of chromatographic columns.	P	
35	Preparation and sterilization of culture media.	M	
36	Verification of the fertility of culture media.	M	
37	Preparation and sterilization of containers and tools.	M	
38	Introduction and use of materials in the aseptic area.	M	
39	Identification of microorganisms.	M	
40	Control and use of biological indicators.	M	
41	Assay of endotoxin.	M	
42	Sample dispatch to external laboratories.	M	
43	Control of cleaning equipment.	P/M	Qualification/Validation.
44	Qualification of laboratory equipment.	P/M	
45	Instructions for the validation of analytical methods.	P/M	
46	Management of reference and retention samples.	P/M	Collection, storage and handling.
47	Stability studies.	P/M	Collection, storage and analysis.
48	Instructions for entrance and exit of personnel in the laboratory.	P/M	Control of access into the laboratory and use of clothing.
49	Safety measures and utilization of personnel protective equipment (PPE) in the QC laboratory.	P/M	Safety procedures.
50	Handling of spillages in the QC laboratory	P/M	
P = Physico-chemistry/M = Microbiology			

Support Processes

These are auxiliary processes that assist in the fulfillment of the strategic and manufacturing processes. See Table **13**.

Table 13. Processes and their groupings.

Process	Purpose	Symbol
Purchase	Buy the necessary items for the adequate operation of the organization.	LOG
Sale	Sell the products of the organization.	
Clothing	Provide adequate clothing for the manufacturing activities.	
Information technology management	Use of computers and other electronic equipment to store and retrieve information.	ITE
HSE (Hygiene, security and Environment)	Remove dirt and sanitize premises.	HSE
	Ensure clean and safe environment inside and outside of the plant.	
Research and development	Improve existing products and develop new ones.	RDE
Technology transfer	Control of the transference of a process with their related documentation and professional expertise between R&D and production or between two production sites.	TTR
Engineering	Provide adequate premises and equipment for the manufacturing processes.	ENG

Purchase

The purchase of materials is the first step of the supply chain and thus it influences its entirety (Table **14**).

Table 14. Tentative list of Purchase documents.

Topic/Document		Contents
01	Purchase management.	Preparation and handling of purchase orders.
02	Supplier management.	Supplier selection and qualification.
03	Delivery conditions for suppliers.	Packaging, quantities, documentation, *etc.* to be supplied.
04	Supply management of auxiliary materials and analytical reagents.	Rules for supplying auxiliary materials and analytical reagents.

Sales

The traceability of sales in order to have adequate information for a recall is very important (Table **15**).

Table 15. Tentative list of Sale documents.

Topic/Document		Contents
01	Management of selling orders.	Administration of sales.
02	Maintenance of logistic data on sales.	Only authorized organizations can buy pharmaceutical products.
03	Traceability of sales into the market.	Distribution of drug products (records of the distribution of each batch for recalls).
04	Measure of customer satisfaction.	Indicator for improvement.
05	Research of marketing targets and promotion.	Commercial organization.
06	Revision system for price lists.	
07	Handling of sample requests.	

Clothing

Clothing plays a twofold role in a pharmaceutical plant (Table **16**). On one hand it protects the products from the particles shed by personnel. On the other it identifies the operators of different areas. See chapters 4 and 8 for more details on clothing.

Table 16. Tentative list of Clothing documents.

Topic/Document		Contents
01	Instructions on clothing in the plant.	General organization of clothing
02	Washing and handling of clothing.	Clothing for non aseptic areas.
03	Washing, sterilizing and handling of clothing.	Clothing for aseptic areas.

Information Technology Management

These documents should ensure that electronic data, as it has been previously discussed, offer the same level of security that traditionally recordings of data on paper (Table **17**).

Table 17. Tentative list of Information technology documents.

Topic/Document		Contents
01	Data archive and retrieve.	Handling of the computer system.
02	Back-up and restoration of services.	
03	Description of computer network.	
04	Auditing to suppliers of computerized systems.	

Table 17: contd...

05	System & application security.	
06	System & application retirement.	
07	Validation of computerized systems.	Validation
08	Handling, filling and validation of excel spread-sheets.	
09	Instructions for the utilization of the ... system.	For the existing managing system/s (*e.g.* LIMS).
10	Instructions for the maintenance of the ... system.	
11	Instructions for back-up and restoration of the ... system.	
12	Emergency plan of the ... system.	
13	Organization and maintenance of the room of the server	Room of the server.

Hygiene, Security and Environment (HSE)

As the name shows, HSE documentation covers different situations. Although part of them fall outside of the scope of GMP it is evident that they are so closely related to manufacturing that all organizations treat them as any other GMP document. See Table **18**.

Table 18. Tentative list of HSE documents.

Topic/Document		Contents
01	General safety plan. Safety rules.	Safety based on hazard identification, evaluation. Preventive measures. Control measures in case of accident. There are MSDS (Material Safety Data Sheets).
02	Environmental impact of the industrial activities: study and handling.	
03	Instructions for the handling of dangerous materials.	
04	Instructions for the use of personal protective equipment (PPE).	
05	Fire prevention, protection and handling.	
06	Handling of outdated materials and products	Waste handling.
07	Waste handling: general criteria.	
08	Treatment and control of waste water.	
09	Decontamination and elimination of wastes.	
10	Cleaning of premises: general rules.	This is a general document which describes the general cleaning procedures for the premises outside from clean rooms (which are usually cleaned by the own personnel of the department, and which require specialized cleaning/sanitization described in other more specific documents of the departments).

Table 18: contd...

11	Insect and pest management.	Instructions for the use of suitable rodenticides, insecticides, fungicides and other agents in other to keep the premises free from vermin. It should include plans with the position of the traps and directions for the identification of the trapped species of vermin.

Research & Development

Here are given some essential documents which are directly related to the R&D activity, but as R & D is normally a completely separated unit, it requires many of the documents described above and, particularly, those listed for the operational processes. See Table **19**.

Table 19. Tentative list of R & D documents.

Topic/Document		Contents
01	Research and development management.	Description of the organization and handling of the R & D activities.
02	Handling of investigational products.	
03	Starting and planning of a R&D activity.	

Technology Transfer

Herewith are given documents required for the technological transfer (table **20**).

Table 20. Tentative list of Technology transfer documents.

Topic/Document		Contents
01	Technology transfer management.	Description of the organization of the research and development department.
02	Identification of product requirements.	Description of the requirements (regarding premises, facilities, personnel, materials, *etc.*) for the transfer of a new product from the R&D department to the manufacturing plant.
03	Instructions for the establishment of the Quality Target Product Profile (QTPP).	A practical description of how to establish the Quality Target Product Profile (QTPP) of a product.
04	Instructions for the identification of product and process critical attributes and variables.	A practical description of the application of HACCP (or any other equivalent approach in order to establish the critical attributes and variables of a manufacturing process.
05	Quality Target Product Profile (QTPP) of...	Description of the Quality Target Product Profile (for each product).
06	Identification of critical variables for the manufacturing of...	Identification of critical attributes and variables of the manufacturing process of (for each product).

Engineering

Engineering is a very specialized department in a pharmaceutical plant and it plays a paramount role for ensuring quality. Its documentation is grouped in a few concrete areas: codification/identification of items; maintenance/calibration; insurance of adequate environmental conditions; qualification of systems and equipment; and management of purchases/projects. See Table **21**.

Table 21. Tentative list of Engineering documents.

	Topic/Document	Contents
01	Instructions for the codification of rooms, instrumentation and equipment.	Codification/Identification.
03	Instructions for the identification, register and use of drawings.	
04	Preventive maintenance of premises, facilities and equipment.	Description of the general approach towards maintenance.
05	Repairing interventions on premises, facilities and equipment.	
06	Instructions for the maintenance of …	For each apparatus/instrument/tool/piece of equipment/system (as necessary).
07	Instructions for the calibration of …	
08	Maintenance plan of …	Usually for each calendar year.
09	Calibration plan …	
10	Instruction for the control of weighing equipment: verification and calibration.	Control of weighing equipment.
11	Instructions for the replacement of filters.	Change of filters: HEPA, air-filters, water-filers, *etc.*
12	Instructions for the monitoring of differential pressures (rooms, HEPA filters).	Description of the monitoring of ΔP. Pressure gauges should have indicated their acceptance ranges.
13	Instructions for the realization of T mappings.	Control of T/RH.
14	Instructions for the control of T/RH in the premises.	
15	Instructions for the T/RH control of refrigerators, freezers, ovens and climatic chambers.	
16	Qualification Master Plan.	Qualification.
17	Instructions for the qualification of equipment and systems.	
18	Instructions for the qualification of clean rooms.	
19	Instructions for the management of projects.	Handling of purchases and projects

Table 21: contd...

20	Instructions for the preparation of URS (User Requirements Specification).	
21	Instructions for the purchase of technical materials.	

CONCLUDING REMARKS

Documentation allows for the establishment, the preservation and the transmission of information and as such is a key element of the PQS. Thanks to good documentation personnel can be adequately trained and processes can be faithfully realized and monitored. But all this is only true if documents are correct and well written and this requires a careful lifecycle approach where all stages are well defined, understood and executed. A detailed analysis of the PQS processes permits determining which documents might be needed and this is important because if documents are written at random, without any systematic approach, there is a high risk of getting an entangled mass of documents which becomes very difficult to manage (*e.g.* if clothing needs are described in several different documents without clear interrelation, then training becomes difficult and if there are changes in clothing it is complicated to modify all the necessary documents).

CONFLICT OF INTEREST

The author confirms that this chapter contents have no conflict of interest.

ACKNOWLEDGEMENT

Declared None.

REFERENCES

[1] WHO (World Health Organization). WHO Good manufacturing practices for pharmaceutical products: main principles. In: WHO Expert Committee on Specifications for Pharmaceutical Preparations. Forty-eighth report (WHO Technical Report Series, No. 986). WHO, Geneva, Switzerland 2014. Annex 2. 15.2.

[2] European Commission. Health and Consumers Directorate General. Computerised Systems. In: EudraLex. The Rules Governing Medicinal Products in the European Union. Volume 4. Good Manufacturing Practice. Medicinal Products for Human and Veterinary Use. European Commission. Brussels, Belgium 2010. Annex 11. 10.

[3] WHO (World Health Organization). WHO Good manufacturing practices for pharmaceutical products: main principles. In: WHO Expert Committee on Specifications for Pharmaceutical Preparations. Forty-eighth report (WHO Technical Report Series, No. 986). WHO, Geneva, Switzerland 2014. Annex 2. 15.8.

[4] European Commission. Good manufacturing practices. Medicinal products for human and veterinary use. The rules governing medicinal products in the European Union. Volume 4. Brussels. Part I. 6.8.
[5] US National Archives & Records Administration. Federal Register. Code of Federal Regulations (CFR). Title 21 (Food & drugs). Part 211. Section 180.a.
[6] WHO (World Health Organization). WHO Good manufacturing practices for pharmaceutical products: main principles. In: WHO Expert Committee on Specifications for Pharmaceutical Preparations. Forty-eighth report (WHO Technical Report Series, No. 986). WHO, Geneva, Switzerland 2014. Annex 2: Glossary.
[7] Ibid.
[8] European Commission. Good manufacturing practices. Medicinal products for human and veterinary use. The rules governing medicinal products in the European Union. Volume 4. Brussels. Part I. 4.14/15/16.
[9] WHO (World Health Organization). WHO Good manufacturing practices for pharmaceutical products: main principles. In: WHO Expert Committee on Specifications for Pharmaceutical Preparations. Forty-eighth report (WHO Technical Report Series, No. 986). WHO, Geneva, Switzerland 2014. Annex 2: Glossary.
[10] Ibid.
[11] Ibid.

CHAPTER 7

Personnel and Training

Abstract: Personnel are certainly the weakest ring of the quality chain of the pharmaceutical industry. On one side, their adequate level of training is difficult both to reach and to monitor. On the other, they are the only known source of contamination and mix-up which is voluntarily allowed to enter a manufacturing unit. It is true that automation and computer-assisted monitoring systems have contributed in diminishing this problem. Nevertheless personnel still holds the center of the scene. Education and a good deal of training can provide an acceptable level of knowledge and skills, but keeping this "state of training" is not easy. Training programs are a must for any laboratory, but ensuring their efficiency requires a good deal of dedication, not to say of ingenuity. It is well known that when the root causes for a deviation are investigated often one of them is "lack of adequate training", then training is repeated and rather commonly this becomes a vicious circle because the problem was not lack of training but inadequate training. Hygiene is a must too, but can training change behavior? The answer should be yes, of course, but this requires convincing people of the real impact of hygienic practices on the quality of products. This chapter describes the GMP approach to personnel and training, analyses well-known problems and proposes solutions for them. The organization and documentation of training is studied in detail. Particular attention is drawn to the existing methods of training and to the measure of their effectiveness.

Keywords: Analysis of requirements, annual training program, appointment, confidentiality agreement, continuing training, evaluation of effectiveness, general admission training, job description, job specification, personnel lifecycle, personal training matrix, personal training tally, post profile, professional CV, selection, specific admission training, trainees, trainers, training methods, training records.

PERSONNEL: AN UNSOLVED PROBLEM

Personnel are at the same time the hero and the villain of pharmaceutical manufacturing. It is evident, at least for the time being, that in spite of the increasing automation persons still play a key role in production. They are educated and trained to possess the necessary competence for performing and supervising production. They are aided by specifically designed documentation and they work in GMP-compliant premises provided with purpose-build facilities and equipment. And in spite of that, personnel, as it was seen in previous chapters, keep always being a source of hazard because of their intrinsic capacity of microbiological contamination, not to mention how easily they may act as vectors of cross-contamination. Besides, human beings are prone to make errors and mix-

Jordi Botet

ups. In other words, personnel organize, supervise, perform and monitor production and they are intended to do this with the lowest possible quality risk but at the same time, for the simple reason of being there, they increase significantly the level of quality risk regarding contamination, cross-contamination and error/mix-up.

As we have already considered in chapter 4, this is a hazard which cannot be eliminated. Thus, only palliative solutions can be envisaged:

- Separation of personnel from products (clothing);
- Separation of products from personnel (isolators, RABS, closed systems);
- Education and training to avoid unhygienic practices and errors derived from lack of practice;
- Supervision by other personnel of the critical operations to detect errors/mix-ups.
- Use of automated systems as far as possible.

Automation of manufacturing processes is useful because it allows for an important degree of separation between products and operators, eliminates (at least in theory) mistakes and can be used as an independent supervisor of manual operations. Nevertheless, still many processes rely on critical operations performed by human workers.

PERSONNEL LIFECYCLE

As it was described in chapter 2 the lifecycle model can be usefully applied to the management of personnel, as shown in Fig. (**1**).

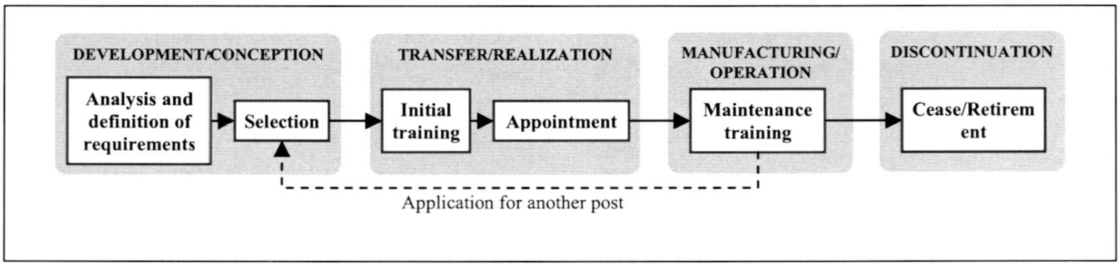

Fig. (1). Personnel lifecycle

Consistent with the important role played by personnel in pharmaceutical manufacturing a policy directed to their management is of paramount importance. The aims of this policy are:

- Determining the manpower needs in terms of quantity and quality (educational and training level).
- Selecting people meeting these specifications.
- Providing selected persons with the initial training to familiarize them with the company organization and the Pharmaceutical Quality System (PQS).
- Prepare them for the concrete tasks they should perform.
- Appointing selected and trained persons to the posts.
- Detecting training needs and providing people with adequate continual training.
- Promote people to different posts to meet new manpower needs or just to fill vacancies.

As it can be seen, these actions correspond to the steps of a lifecycle model which match closely that of the products or of the premises, equipment and utilities. See chapter 2 for more details on lifecycles.

The objective of the PQS is implementing the quality policy and ensuring that the quality objectives are attained and this can be obtained by adequately trained personnel provided with the adequate documentation working in well-designed pharmaceutical plants. As it was described in chapter 6, documentation (or better said, the information that it conveys) is the backbone of the PQS. And in this sense, documents are crucial for the adequate development and control of the personnel lifecycle.

Analysis and Definition of Requirements

The need of educated and trained personnel in sufficient amount is not only imperative for logistic reasons, but also because it is a GMP requirement: *The establishment and maintenance of a satisfactory system of QA and the correct manufacture and control of pharmaceutical products and active ingredients rely upon people. For this reason there must be sufficient qualified personnel to carry out all the tasks for which the manufacturer is responsible* [1].

The exact practical meaning of sufficient is not self-evident. It is clear however that an inspector finding that some tasks have not been performed might attribute it only to two causes: lack of knowledge/training or insufficient personnel (or even to both). Thus, it can be said that there should be enough personnel for carrying out the programmed manufacturing operations and all the tasks described in the PQS documentation.

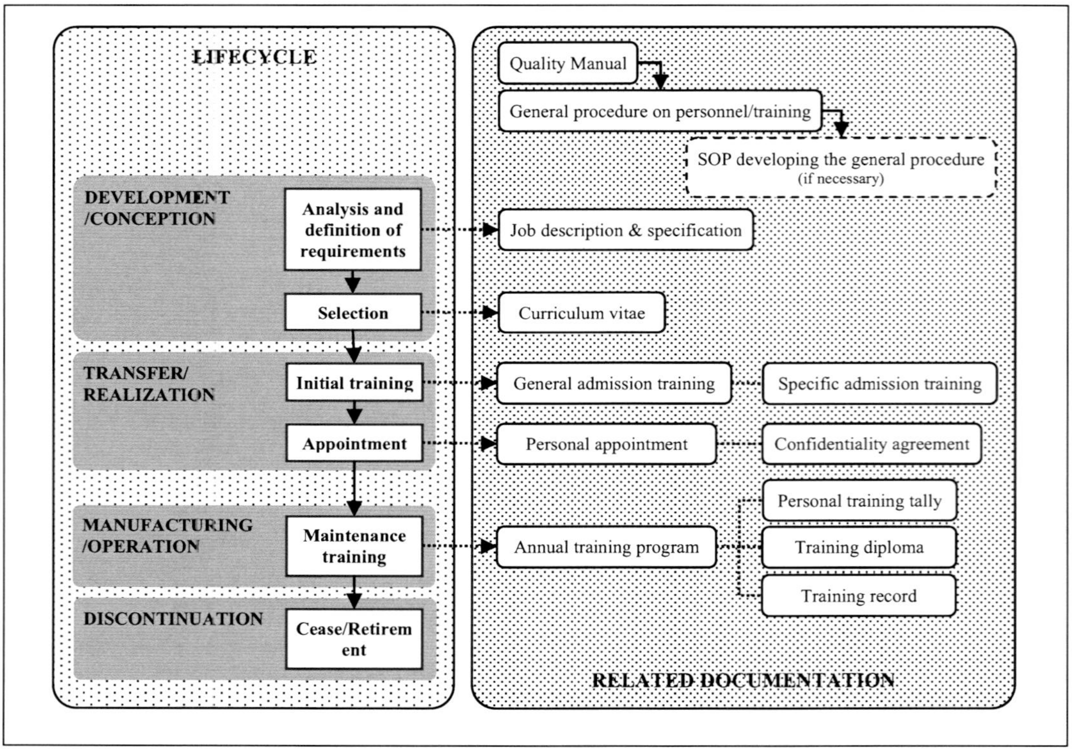

Fig. (2). Personnel lifecycle and related documentation.

There should be an organization chart showing the respective relations of all the posts in the organization and for each of them a job description and a job specification. The former is a written statement that defines the functions (purpose, responsibilities and duties) for a given job, whereas the latter is an analysis of the qualifications needed by the person who holds the post (degree of education, experience, skills, and training requirements). Both documents can be separated or form a unique job profile document (Fig. **2**).

As the first step regarding personnel management is determining which posts will be considered in the plant and which will be their organic relations it is necessary to start by filling job (or post) descriptions. As this paper usually also explains the organic relations with other posts and includes the education and experience requirements for the person holding the post it can be named job (or post) profile (Fig. **3**).

Usually this document is written by the department to which the post belongs. It is revised either by QA (particularly if there are GMP issues) or by the manpower department and it is approved by the head of the plant. Most of the contents of these post profiles are not dictated by GMP but by purely logistic reasons. Thus, it is only necessary to ensure respect to GMP and to the Quality Manual and the procedures which develop it regarding human resources. In key personnel posts it is necessary to take into account what states GMP, but outside from these requirements companies can organize posts as they wish. See chapter 1 for detailed information on the tasks which correspond to the key personnel according to GMP.

* **Drug Pharm**	Type of document: **Record**	
	Post profile (job description and specification)	
	Related to SOP-XXX-nnn (---)	Date:

Post name:	
Code/Reference:	

Item		**Description**
Functions	Purpose	
	Responsibilities	
	Duties	
Organic relations	Answering to	
	Answered by	
Qualification needed	Degree of education	
	Experience	
	Skills and abilities	
	Training requirements	
Special requirements		

Written by:	Signature:	Date:	**Revised by:**	Signature:	Date:	**Approved by:**	Signature:	Date:

Fig. (3). Post profile (job description & specification).

Job descriptions and specifications may be defined in a general way for the whole organization or be considered subdivided by departments, areas or specific projects.

Selection

Personnel applying for the post send a letter explaining why they are interested in this post and why they consider that they deserve holding it. To this letter should be annexed a professional CV (curriculum vitae) in order to show that education and experience match the post requirements.

Then, the manpower department, accompanied by representatives of the departments directly affected by the post, as necessary, evaluates if the CV of the person shows him adequately prepared for the post and, if this is the case, she/he is selected for an interview to get a better knowledge of her/him. Sometimes the candidate must fill a questionnaire and/or a test.

In fact, in order to reduce the amount of work and the selection time, normally the candidates are subjected to different levels of filtering. Thus, only those who pass one filter are submitted to the next one. Often a first general interview is performed by the manpower department and only those candidates who are filtered are interviewed in a more specialized way by the involved departments.

Risk ranking and filtering (RRF), the comparing tool described in chapter 3 is very appropriate for the selection of personnel. It is only necessary to establish which elements are going to be taken into account (education, experience in general, experience in a similar post, place of residence, income, *etc.*) and their respective values.

Sometimes it is difficult to decide among several candidates, but this is good news. Whereas at times it is impossible to find a candidate meeting the basic requirements and this is, evidently, bad news. This latter situation would constrain the company to choose a not very good candidate and then provide her/him with the necessary complementary training to meet minimal post requirements.

The selection of applicants for a job is not an easy undertaking and requires a good amount of time. This is why many organizations outsource this task (or at least the first and more general stages) to specialized companies. This latter approach permits reducing the workload of the organization and at the same time taking advantage of the experience of the manpower consultancy firms on this matter.

It is important to underline that the objective of the manpower department: attracting endowed people into the organization depends not only on the intrinsic value of their activities. People are attracted by the image of the organization, namely its prestige in the world of pharmaceutical manufacturing, and by the possibilities of promotion. Money of course is important but if it is not accompanied by other qualities it is doubtful that really talented personnel will stay longtime in an organization.

In any case the front line document for any person in the organization is an updated professional CV. It is convenient to keep this CV, both in paper and in electronic form. A paper with a handwritten signature is filed in the personnel archive, whereas an electronic copy can be sent to other organizations to show, on demand and after authorization by the person, the education and experience level of a given employee. The annexed document (Fig. **4**) shows an example of CV form which is filled by the employee once it joins the organization. This CV contains the spaces to answer the questions which are interesting for the organization, whereas the CV which is sent to get a post may contain much irrelevant information.

✱ **Drug Pharm**	Type of document: **Record**	
	Professional curriculum vitae (CV)	
	Related to SOP-XXX-nnn (---)	Date:

Full name:	
Personal data	
ID/Passport nº:	
Date of incorporation into the organization:	
(1) **Education:**	
(2) **Specialized training**	
(3) **Professional experience:**	
(4) **Other:**	
Annexed CV supplied by the employee?	☐ **Yes**/☐ **No**

Head of manpower:	Signature:	Date:	**Reference:**

Fig. (4). CV (curriculum vitae).

Initial Training

Training is the process of learning the skills that personnel need to do a particular job or activity. The aim of training in the pharmaceutical industry is ensuring that personnel involved in the manufacturing processes will always have the appropriate technical competence (very important the adverb "always" because it implies the need of continual training).

There should be a training program for all people entering the production and quality control areas, this includes both people involved in production directly and indirectly (technical, maintenance and cleaning). The basis on which all the training activities of an organization relies is job specification, which defines the respective training requirements. These needs should be specified in writing (see Fig. **3**).

Initial training on admittance into the organization should be of two kinds:

- Wide-ranging admission training for everybody

  and

- Specialized admission training to provide additional knowledge for specific tasks.

Both training activities should be recorded and their effectiveness tested.

Untrained people in principle should not enter the manufacturing areas. In particular cases, visitors and technicians may be allowed to enter the above mentioned areas without the basic training provided in the organization, but only after receiving the minimal guidance regarding clothing and behavior within the premises and they should always be supervised and accompanied by trained personnel. It is not necessary to insist on the fact that these untrained people should not intervene in any of the manufacturing processes.

Temporary personnel pose a particularly difficult problem because logic says that in order not to jeopardize quality (or increase the quality risk level) their preparation level should be equivalent to the training level of permanent personnel. Thus, they should either be given training similar to that of permanent personnel or receive a limited specific training for the tasks they are going to undertake, while reserving the more complex tasks for permanent personnel. This latter option means increased supervision because they cannot be considered operators like the others. Many organizations provide "cross-training" in order to have people prepared to perform different tasks in the department. This reduces the impact of absentees.

Besides basic training on the theory and practice of GMP, newly recruited personnel should receive training appropriate to the duties assigned to them [2].

The concept of quality assurance and all the measures which aid its understanding and implementation should be fully discussed during the training sessions [3].

General Admission Training

All employees should receive minimal general training on admission as defined in a procedure (SOP). See Fig. (**5**).

Drug Pharm	Type of document: **Record**		
	General admission training		
	Related to SOP-XXX-nnn (---)	Date:	
Full name:			
ID/Passport nº:			
Purpose:	Obtain a minimal general "admittance" training,		
Training:	As detailed in SOP:		
Comments:			
We, the undersigned, confirm that this person has been trained as planned and consequently is considered to be ready for admission into the organization.			
Manpower head ***Signature:*** ***Date:***		***Quality Assurance*** ***Signature:*** ***Date:***	

Fig. (5). General admission training activities.

This initial general training should be independent from whichever specific task they undertake, and should at least cover:

- Presentation of the organization: origin, history, idiosyncrasy (values), objectives, structure, *etc.*
- Quality policy and organization (PQS).
- Internal norms and procedures, as necessary.
- Basic GMP.
- Behavior and clothing norms in manufacturing areas.
- Information on environmental protection, security, and hygiene measures.

Specific Admission Training

First of all every operator should know and understand the documents related to her/his work. Ideally this should be done not only by reading and commenting the documents, but also by performing practically the operations which they describe (Fig. **6**).

Outside from this, GMP consider necessary some complementary training:

- Risks for the patients: it is of the outmost importance that personnel involved in the manufacture of pharmaceutical products understand that these are very special products and that if they do not possess the intended quality (because of contamination, cross-contamination, degradation or mix-up) they might put the life of patients at stake.

- Specific requirements to the type of product: Personnel should comprehend that each type of product has its own requirements (*i.e.* the production of oral solid products supposes an important risk of cross-contamination and of operator contamination because of the release of dust, whereas the production of oral liquid products is always threaten by the microbiological contamination of water or solutions).

- Personnel working in clean areas: they should understand that contamination is a hazard and how products and tools are contaminated. This means that they should be aware of hygienic measures and have a minimal knowledge on microbiology.

- Personnel working in areas where hazardous materials or infectious microorganisms are handled: they should understand the risks linked to the manipulation of highly active, sensitizing, and toxic starting materials and the existing protecting measures. Operators should know the different levels of biohazard and how to protect themselves from infectious microorganisms.

- Personnel working in areas where radioactive products are manufactured: They should understand the risks linked to these products and the protection measures available.

- Personnel involved with computerized systems: They should receive training on how to operate them adequately and they should understand the restricted access measures to ensure the security of data.

- Specific training on validation: Personnel involved in qualification/validation should receive specialized training on these matters.

✱ **Drug Pharm**	Type of document: **Record**	
	Specific admission training	
	Related to SOP-XXX-nnn (---)	Date:
Full name:		
ID/Passport n°:		
Purpose:		
Proposed training:	**Theoretical:**	
	Practical:	
Comments:		
We, the undersigned, confirm that this person has been trained as planned and consequently is considered to be ready to develop the activities for his job.		
Department head Signature: Date:	**Quality Assurance** Signature: Date:	

Fig. (6). Specific admission training activities.

The objective of these two levels of admission training is ensuring that operators have adequate training for performing the entrusted operations. In practice the result should be obtaining a training matrix similar to the one given in Fig. (7).

✱ **Drug Pharm**	Type of document: **Record**	
	Personnel training matrix	
	Department: **Oral solid prod**	Period of validity: **xxx - zzz**
	Related to SOP-XXX-nnn (---)	Date:

Task	Operator						
	JH	AO	BS	GH	PG	AS	KH
Weighing	✓					✓	
Compounding	✓		✓	✓			
Milling and sieving			✓	✓			
Tableting (compression)		✓				✓	
Coating		✓			✓		
Room cleaning	✓						✓
Equipment cleaning					✓		✓

Fig. (7). Schematic example of personnel training matrix.

Besides possessing a personnel training matrix table like the one given here and which helps the supervisors in their task, in some companies the operators possess personnel identification cards where this information is loaded.

In any case the personal training matrix should include trained substitute operators able to perform the task when there is some absence.

Appointment

Appointed people are inscribed in the organization file (Fig. **8**). This is a document to assign a job to an employee or declare him competent to perform specific tasks. The original document is kept by the organization, normally in the human resources archives, while the concerned person receives an authenticated copy, stamped and signed by the appointed head of department.

This is the formal procedure; in practice this can be substituted by personal ID cards (*i.e.* provided with bar codes or magnetic bands). Then, when the employee has to identify himself before an operation, the system detects if he has been appointed to use a determinate room or instrument or piece of equipment.

Drug Pharm	Type of document: **Record**	
	Personal appointment	
	Related to SOP-XXX-nnn (---)	Date:

According to paragraph. of the Manual of Quality/SOP:., this is to confirm the appointment of:

. [indicate the person's name]

As. [indicate the job profile]
Since she/he fulfils the training and experience requirements and is acquainted with the functions below:

.

., Date.

We, the undersigned, confirm that this person has been trained as planned and consequently is considered to be ready to develop the activities for his job.

Manpower responsible	Area manager:	QA manager

Fig. (8). Personal appointment.

A particular case, which was already shown in Fig. (**1**) by a discontinuous line, appears when an employee is transferred to another post in the same organization. In principle the process requirements are similar to those followed for the admission of new employees in the organization, but taking into account that she/he is well-known. Generally speaking, it is possible to say that normally an employee of the company does not need any general admission training. However, specific admission training would usually be necessary to make her/him acquainted with the particularities of a new post.

Another document is a confidentiality agreement to be signed when a person is appointed (Fig. **9**). With this document an employee commits herself/himself to keep any information regarding his job confidential. It may or may not be deemed necessary by an organization. Although usually there are no problems regarding confidentiality, experience shows that an agreement regarding this subject is often very useful since it clarifies matters.

Drug Pharm		Type of document: **Record**
		Confidentiality Agreement
	Related to SOP-XXX-nnn (---)	Date:
According to paragraph. of the Quality Manual/SOP:. The undersigned employee,. [indicate the person's name] As. [indicate the person's job] Swears not to divulge information on., nor publicize nor broadcast. . (date).		
Employee:	Area manager:	Manpower head

Fig. (9). Agreement on confidentiality.

Continuing Training

It is evident that training should be a permanent activity, both because there are always changes in the existing situation (new or modified operations/processes requiring new or modified documentation, GMP updating, regulatory changes, *etc.*) and also because human beings tend to forget things unless there are periodic reminders.

Continuing training should also be given, and its practical effectiveness periodically assessed. Approved training programs should be available. Training records should be kept [4].

Training in current good manufacturing practice shall be conducted by qualified individuals on a continuing basis and with sufficient frequency to assure that employees remain familiar with CGMP requirements applicable to them [5].

Thus, during the last quarter of the year (or the first quarter of the year under consideration, depending on the organization and its time-limits for processing the year reviews), a general training program for the following year should be established and approved. These training activities may be performed by personnel from the organization or be outsourced.

The annual training program (Fig. **10**) is established taking into account two points of view:

1st The evaluation of what has happened during the year:

- Incidents/Deviations/Non-conformities (OOS) and their corrective and preventive actions.
- Observations of audits or inspections
- Insufficiencies detected by area managers or supervisors.
- Needs detected by personnel (surveys, suggestions, inquires, *etc.*).
- New processes or modification of the existing ones.
- New legal requirements.
- New internal requirements.
- Monitoring of products and processes.

2nd The need to keep a proficient GMP knowledge and an adequate internal organizational level:

- Sufficient GMP awareness.
- Thorough knowledge of the instructions for entering and exiting clean rooms, of the established cleaning and hygiene practices and of the adequate behavior in clean rooms.

Drug Pharm	Type of document: **Plan**		
	Annual Training Program for .... (yyyy)		
	Area/Project/Unit/Department	Code	Version

Quarter	*Training activities*	*Duration (hours)*	*Purpose*	*Assisting personnel*	*internal/external*
1					
2					
3					
4					

Head of human resources	Date:	Signature:	**Head of production**	Date:	Signature:
Head of QA	Date:	Signature:	**Head of QC**	Date:	Signature:

Fig. (10). Annual training program.

Besides, these training activities formally included in the annual program might be complemented with additional unforeseen training activities which appear as a result of particular needs. If these new training requirements concern several persons of the organization there is no problem in preparing a modified version of the annual training program incorporating new training activities. But if they just affect some isolated persons, then the training activity must be considered a complementary training activity provided for a particular technician of the organization and it is not necessary to include it in the annual training program.

Thus training activities deemed "general" are included in the annual training program, whereas "particular" ones need not be included. In any case, both types of training activities should be recorded and their effectiveness tested.

Cease/Retirement

Personnel leaving the organization should be withdrawn from the "dynamic" file. Documentation related to them should be kept for the length of time specified in the procedures. In fact the approach should be the same that has been described for the products; while there is product on the market, information regarding all the elements which have intervened in its manufacturing, and this includes personnel, have to be kept.

TRAINING: ANOTHER (OFTEN) UNSOLVED PROBLEM

Training should be considered a process, where "inputs" are transformed into "outputs" (Fig. **11**). The former are constituted by the manpower hired by the department of Human Resources. The latter consist of a workforce possessing the adequate knowledge and skills. It is true that this process is particular because outputs are continually becoming inputs again, because of the requirement of continuing training.

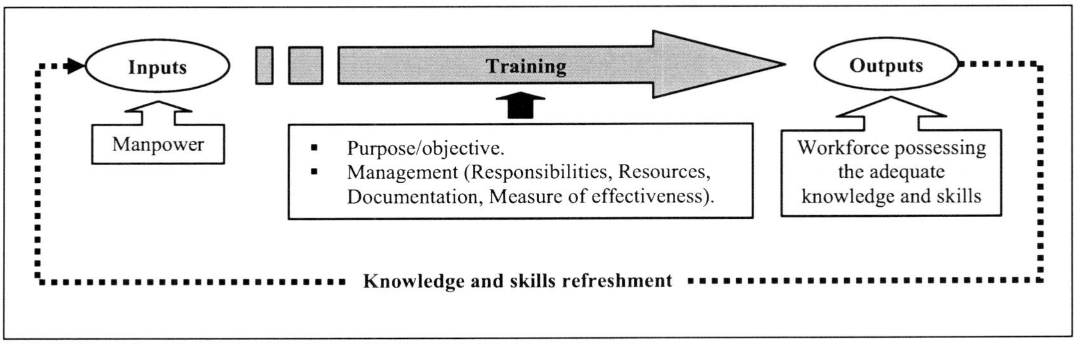

Fig. (11). The process of training.

Purpose/Objective of Training

Above all it is important to bear in mind that training, in a GMP context, means meeting all the following points:

- There are written job descriptions (detailing the duties and responsibilities of the post, its hierarchical relations and the requirements in terms of education and experience for the employee).
- There are procedures describing the policy and management of training in the organization.
- There are periodic training plans or programs describing the training activities for a given period of time (usually one year).
- Everybody knows his/her duties and responsibilities.
- Personnel have the appropriate education, knowledge and skills to hold the posts.
- Personnel know GMP and, if necessary, the related regulations, guidelines, *etc.* The level of knowledge which is necessary depends logically on the type of post held.
- Personnel know and understand the documentation (procedures, instructions, registers, *etc.*) associated to their posts.
- Personnel receive initial and continuing training to ensure that they are prepared to perform adequately the assigned functions.
- The effectiveness of training is verified.
- Only personnel with the appropriate education, knowledge and skills undertake a specific task.
- Information on personnel education, qualification, experience and training is kept updated by the department of manpower (human resources).
- Follow-up of the PQS shows that there are not significant problems derived from inadequate personnel training.

Responsibilities

Although the exact distribution of responsibilities may vary in each organization, the department of Human Resources is usually the manager of the training activities. See Fig. (**12**).

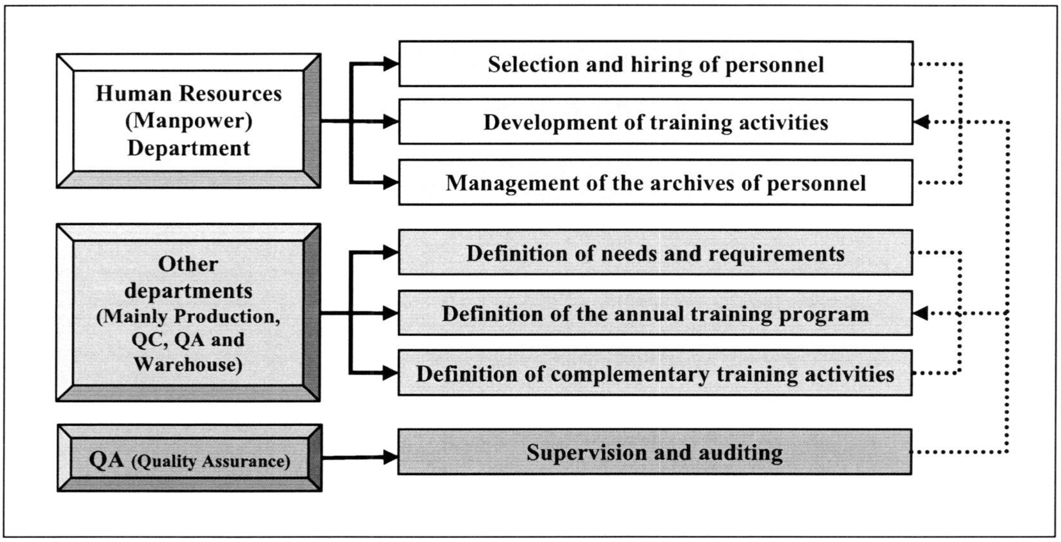

Fig. (12). Organization of the training activities.

The other departments define their training needs (both general and particular), whereas Quality Assurance supervises the implementation of the programs and attests the effectiveness of training (by audits and general follow-up of the performance of the PQS).

In any case, training activities have to be carefully planned, listening to all the actors not to affect negatively the manufacturing operations.

Documental Frame

There should be written procedures and the associated records of actions taken or conclusions reached, where appropriate, for. personnel matters including training [6].

Documents regarding personnel in general and training in particular can be organized in different ways. Here we follow the approach described in chapters 5 and 6:

1st. The policy of the organization is described in the Quality Manual.

2nd. Detailed guidelines of this policy are given in the general operational procedure (GOP) "Personnel management" which might include, like this chapter, both personnel and their training".

3rd. Other documents of lower level are usually necessary to describe practically how to carry through the previously mentioned guidelines. The number of necessary documents depends on each particular case.

Whatever the number and organization of the documents the following points should be considered:

- Organization chart.
- Job descriptions and specifications.
- Personnel recruitment: conduct and responsibilities.
- Admittance training requirements.
- Training activities and responsibilities.
- Training evaluation: conduct and responsibilities.
- Training maintenance: plan/program, development and evaluation.
- Personnel resignation/retirement: conduct and responsibilities.

Definition of Requirements

Training requirements are determined as the result of different activities, from which we may emphasize the following:

- Quality risk Management;
- Process Performance and Product Quality Monitoring System
- Product quality reviews
- Corrective Action/Preventive Action (CAPA) System
- Change Management System

- Management review
- Audits (both internal and external)

Quality Risk Management

Below is given a general example (Table **1**), which might be adapted to the particular case of each organization. In it are analyzed the hazards which may hamper the effectiveness of a training program.

Table 1. Sample of PHA for training.

Hazard	Cause	Preventive measure
Persons who need training are not offered training	Persons not included in the training program.	All new employees receive the admission training. All employees are included in the annual training program.
Persons do not receive the type of training they need	Error in the distribution of trainees in the training groups.	Employees hold a post and training is linked to the post.
Training is not adequately provided	Trainer does not know enough the subject.	Trainers have to provide a CV showing their knowledge and experience.
	Trainer has not enough training experience	
	Training material is poor.	Training material has to be prepared carefully.
Trainees do not pay attention to the trainer	Trainees are not interested/motivated.	Effectiveness of the training is tested.
		Trainees with good results in training get a diploma and some advantages in the organization.
	Training time-table is not adequate.	Training courses should not last for too long with too many sessions and be programed very late in the day.
	Training sessions are too long.	A session should not last more than 90 minuts (and preferably 60).Tea/Coffee breaks are very important.
	Trainer does not attract the attention of trainees.	Trainer has to create an agreable atmosphere.
Trainees do not understand the trainer	Trainees are in the wrong training group.	Employees held a post and training is linked to the post.
	The trainer is not adequate.	Trainers have to provide a CV showing their knowledge and experience.
Trainees forget what they have learned	They are not included in the program of continuing training.	All employees are included in the annual training program.

Risk analysis can be used for determining which are the most important hazards linked to the personnel in the manufacturing processes (Table **2**). This example can be developed for the operations which are realized in each organization.

Table 2. Sample of PHA for manufacturing operations taking into account the operators.

Type of hazard	Hazard description	Hazard cause
(Outer) Contamination	Entrance of particles (dust, pollen, *etc.*) and vermin from outside	Doors are left open.
		Dirty incoming containers are not cleaned.
	Build-up of dust/dirt in the premises and equipment	Inadequate cleaning.
	Product contamination	Persons are carriers of contamination because of poor hygiene.
		Persons do not wear appropriate clothing.
		Tools/pipes are dirty and carry contamination.
Cross-contamination	Diffusion of particles	Doors are left open.
		Operators pass from an area to the other with the same clothing covered with dust
	Cross-contamination during sampling/weighing and production	Liberation of dust during operations.
		Inadequate separation of products and poor cleaning.
		Equipment dirty.
		Direct passage of contamination by hand contact.
Environmental contamination	Unawareness of danger	Lack of information on the hazards
	Diffusion/liberation of hazardous organisms/products	Lack of separation
		Liberation of drops/dust.
		Lack of decontamination
		Contaminated hands
		Doors left open
		Lack of primary containment/Leakage/Spillage
		Staff unaware of HVAC failure
		Operator moves around with contaminated suit
		Organisms are not kept in closed systems even if they have not been inactivated.

Table 2: contd...

		Inadequate handling of waste and effluents
		Same equipment used for different processes in different areas
	Loss of system control	Accident or emergency
Error/mix-up	Mix-up of operations or materials/products	Flows and separations are not respected
		Unclear identification and status
	Confusion on the state of quarantine/approved and of rejected/recalled/returned materials/products	Unclear identification and status
		Unsure segregation
	Mix-up of printed materials	Unsafe storage
	Error during operations	Poor practice and lack of verification
	Confusion of fluids	Lack of identification
		Interchange of connections/adaptors
	Use of defective equipment	Presence of non identified faulty equipment
	Misuse of the facilities	Inadequate knowledge of the facilities
	Inappropriate donning of cloths	Poor practice and lack of verification
Degradation	Degradation of materials/products during reception and dispatch.	Materials/products exposed to weather.
	Degradation of materials/products during production and storage	Materials/products exposed to inadequate T/RH
		Materials/products sensitive to light.
		Product kept at inadequate conditions because of lack of information

The hazards that are pointed out here are typically present in all pharmaceutical plants. They are raised by GMP and have to be present in all the basic training programs, not to mention continuing training programs. Some are general and require providing complementary information to the operators, while most of them (*e.g.* leave doors open in order to facilitate passage during operations or leave moist tools or pipes) are specific and require permanent insistence on them.

Process Performance and Product Quality Monitoring System and Product Quality Reviews

Although they are not primarily intended for evaluating personnel performance, in case of lack of performance and detection of deviations, it is evident that this might indicate that personnel is not adequately trained.

Product Quality Reviews

Neither product quality reviews are thought for detecting training needs, but as they assess all the topics related to the quality of products, they may provide some hints on lack of proficiency as far as personnel is concerned.

Corrective Action/Preventive Action (CAPA) System

CAPA system is directly linked to personnel performance, as many of the actions consist in improvement of the level of training of the personnel. Here, however it is necessary to make an important comment. Speaking in a rough general way, it can be said that deviations are the outcome of an operation that was not performed as intended and the cause of this is that a machine didn't work as programmed or that an operator didn't realize an action as foreseen. Then, further analysis on the failure of the machine might lead to breakdown, to wrong adjustment or to inadequate programming. In all these cases the cause could be the same, namely operator deficiency. And this might be seen as a problem of training. Thus, a preventive action would be "train again the operators". However, it is likely that here there was not really a problem of lack of training but of lack of the adequate training. Repeated training on the same subject without substantial improvement might show that training is not adequate (or that operators are not appropriate…).

Management Reviews

The objective of these reviews is evaluating the performance of the PQS and, eventually, redistributing the allocation of resources. One of the elements of the system which is analyzed is the effectiveness of training (Fig. **13**).

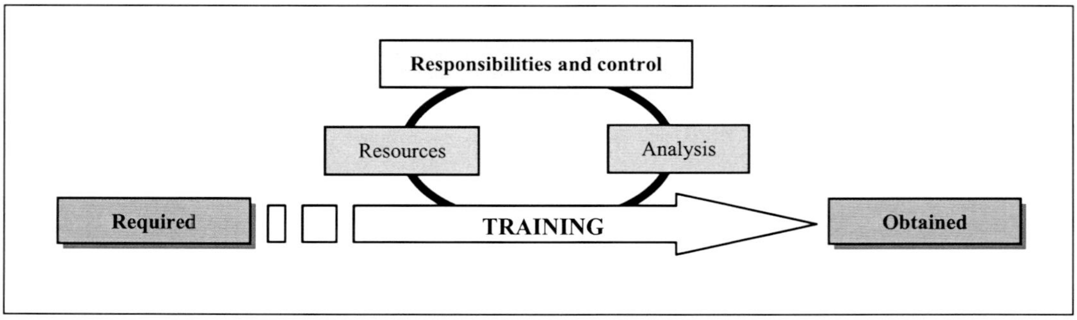

Fig. (13). Continuous improvement in training.

Audits

Audits, both these internals and those realized by third parts, are very significant as a tool for discovering deficiencies regarding personnel and their level of training. Each deficiency launches a corrective/preventive action which may be translated into modifications of the admission training and/or of the annual training program, (*i.e.* new activities or changes in the program).

Resources

The resources which are necessary for training in terms of equipment are normally irrelevant (*i.e.* they consist in not much more than photocopies for the training notes, a projector for the slides or videos, a video camera...). They focus mainly on economical terms and here have to be taken into account both the direct costs of the activity and the indirect costs (the working hours used for training). The directs costs are very different if the employees are sent outside to training events or if they are trained on-site (in house training)

Outside Training

The advantages of this type of training are evident. Employees of the organization are sent to an event where well-known trainers can provide specialized training. There they can get some knowledge and also meet other people with whom to exchange experiences. The drawbacks are clear too. It is expensive to send people outside from the plant, both in terms of direct expenses (event, board and lodging, travel) and indirect costs (lost hours during training and travel). Expenditures can be reduced by sending only a person (or at most two) and then when she/he comes back from the event she/he prepares a presentation on the event for other technicians of the organization. This is a much cheaper way of providing external specialized training to the whole group of interested personnel.

In-House Training

Employees are trained in the plant and thus they do not lose time traveling and costs are reduced. Trainers can either be competent technicians of the organization or external consultants. Both approaches are correct and have their pros and cons.

In house trainers know better people and their needs, but often it is difficult for some trainees to see people with whom they speak every day and share lunch as trainers.

External trainers can be taken more seriously but do not know trainees and their needs are only indirectly known (*i.e.* when they are hired the organization explains them which are their needs).

Summarizing, it can be said that probably the best option is to combine internal and external trainers. Internal trainers can perform the training linked to internal documentation and some basic training (*e.g.* admission training), whereas external trainers can offer more specialized training and also complement internal trainers by providing a different vision. Generally speaking, it can be said that changes in persons and approaches can help in making training more attractive for trainees.

External trainers should attest an adequate level of qualification and experience by providing their CV.

Consultants advising on the manufacture, processing, packing, or holding of drug products shall have sufficient education, training, and experience, or any combination thereof, to advise on the subject for which they are retained. Records shall be maintained stating the name, address, and qualifications of any consultants and the type of service they provide [7].

Training Records

Approved training programs should be available. Training records should be kept. [8].

Each training activity has to be adequately reported and filed. The department of human resources should open a portfolio (this information can be kept on paper or digitally, by scanning the registers; often a combination of both systems is adequate) for each training activity, containing the following,

- Information on the contents of the activity: A copy of the approved program and of the training notes;
- Information on the duration of the training activity: Hours (this is clearly stated in the training records);
- Information on the qualifications of the trainer/s: A professional CV is normally sufficient.
- Information on the attendees: The training records should be signed both by the trainer and the trainees. Thus assisting people are controlled.
- Evaluation of the training: Trainees should pass an evaluation test which is kept in the training file.
- Attestation of the training: Trainees having shown a good understanding of the training are given a diploma or an equivalent document showing that they have received satisfactorily this training.

The training records are intended to control any training activity. Attendees and trainers sign as an acknowledgement of their participation (Fig. **14**).

Training records should be maintained and periodic assessments of the effectiveness of training programs should be made [9].

Drug Pharm	Type of document: **Record**	
	Training Record	
	Related to SOP-XXX-nnn (---)	Date:

Record for the recording of courses/training activities (A sheet will be completed for each daily session of a course or training activity)	
Name of the course/activity	
Organization/Person Responsible	
Location	
Date	
Reference (as appropriate)	

Trainees

Name	**Signature**	**Remarks** (as appropriate)

Trainer/s

Name	**Signature**	**Remarks** (as appropriate)

Fig. (14). Training record.

Although there is no formal requirement to issue diplomas to the trainees of a training activity, this document tends to enhance the prestige of the training and can contribute to some increase in the motivation of trainees. It is therefore advisable to issue a diploma for personnel taking part in training activities and having shown their competency in the evaluation tests (Fig. **15**).

✱ **Drug Pharm**
Training Diploma
Related to SOP-XXX-nnn (---)
Ms./Mr. has been trained in: . . (place), (date) Her/His practical competency has been assessed by means of a test. Contents of the training activity: . . Duration of the training activity:. hours
Signature by the trainer: Signature by Manpower or QA head

Fig. (15). Training diploma.

Outside from controlling people assisting to the training activities by filling a training record form, each employee has a personal training tally (Fig. **16**) where all the training activities that she/he has attended as a trainee are registered. In the archive of human resources CVs inform about the education and experience of the person before entering the organization, whereas personal training tallies gather the training she/he has received while being in the organization and, thus, it completes CVs.

✱ **Drug Pharm**	Type of document: **Record**				
	Personal Training Tally				
	Related to SOP-XXX-nnn (---)			Date:	
Full name:				**Page:** ____	
ID/Passport nº:					
Date of incorporation into the organization:					
Name of the course/training activity	**Date**	**Duration (hours)**	**Trainer**	**Test past?**	**Remarks**
				□ Yes/□ No	
				□ Yes/□ No	
				□ Yes/□ No	
				□ Yes/□ No	
				□ Yes/□ No	
				□ Yes/□ No	
				□ Yes/□ No	

Fig. (16). Personal training tally.

Conduct

The annexed Fig. (**17**) describes an approach towards training organization which considers methods, testing and evaluation of effectiveness.

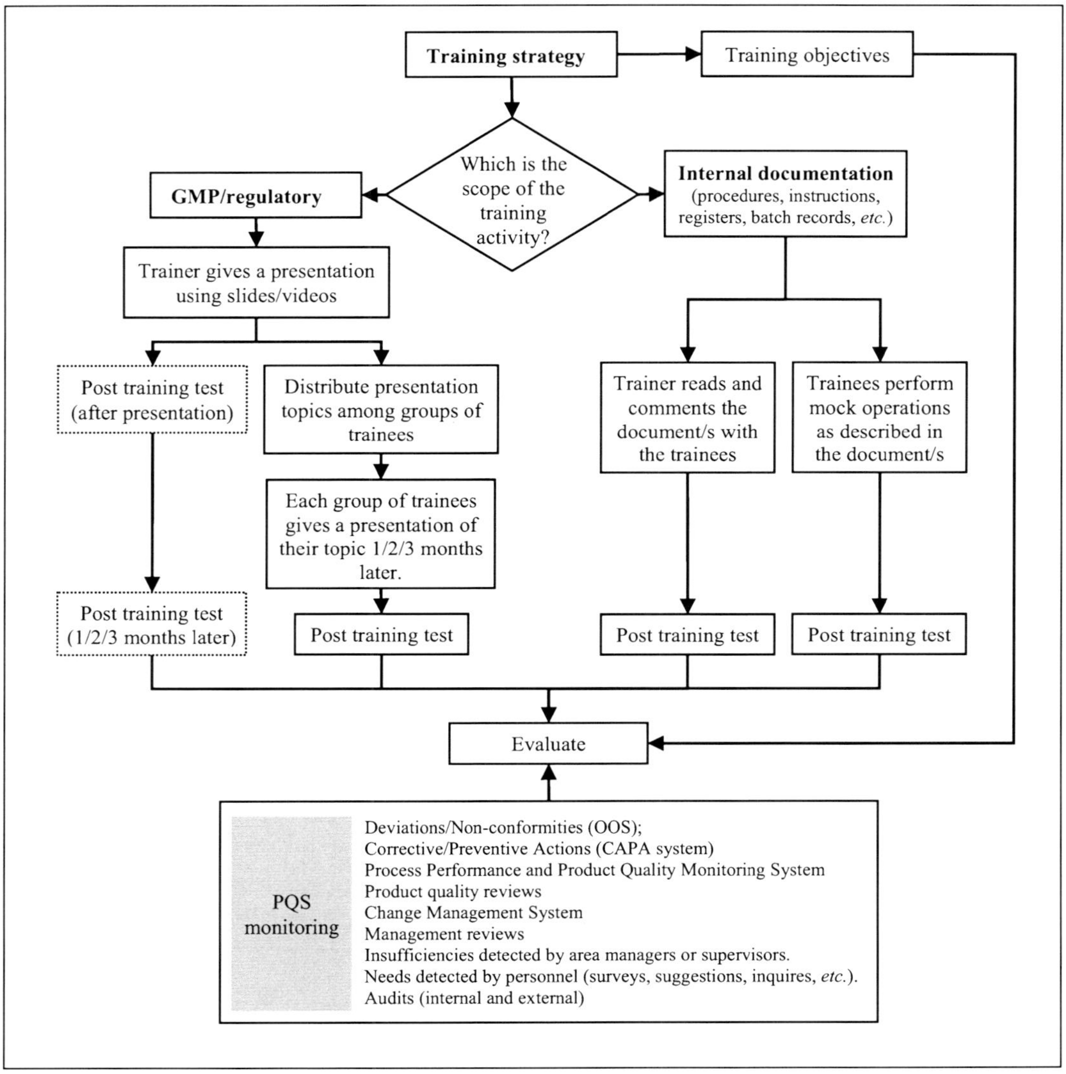

Fig. (17). Organization of training.

GMP/Regulatory Training

As we have seen, pharmaceutical training is focused on GMP. Although the contents of GMP are very good, they are far from being easy to "digest" and to remember. Although at first sight GMP might seem relatively simple, in reality they are quite complex because they involve many different aspects. Let us see two examples:

Access to production premises should be restricted to authorized personnel [10].

This is a simple and clear rule, even if in fact contains two requirements. On one hand it is necessary to define who is allowed and how she/he is authorized and on the other it has to be defined how this control of access is performed.

Electrical supply, lighting, temperature, humidity and ventilation should be appropriate and such that they do not adversely affect, directly or indirectly, either the pharmaceutical products during their manufacture and storage, or the accurate functioning of equipment [11].

Instead, here many different elements are put together. Although it is a logical sentence and its meaning is easy to understand, it has a very complex meaning. Just to mention a few: utilities (electricity, lighting and HVAC), processes (manufacturing and warehousing), equipment, and products. Besides, it is necessary to clarify what is meant by "appropriate" and what is an "adverse effect".

GMP training requires decomposing its text and reordering it in a systematic way (*e.g.* in the second example: utilities, operations and equipment) in order to better understand and remember it. And, evidently, always bearing in mind who are the trainees and which level of information they need.

Training on Internal Documentation

The simplest way for delivering training regarding internal documents is providing the employees with a copy of the document and after reading it signing a document declaring that they have read and understood it. This is evidently not a very satisfactory approach. An improvement would be organizing a session where a trainer reads and comments the text. It is also possible to include practical training. The operations are performed as indicated in the document, first by the trainer and then by the trainees.

Training Methods

Slides

Probably the best and simplest way of training on GMP is preparing good slides which can be used by the trainer to expose the matter in a systematic way, well adapted to the knowledge and needs of the trainees. But, attention! Slides are not intended for crushing the trainees under an avalanche of data, but just for helping the trainer to expose concrete and organized information. Moreover, slides should be clear, readable and connected in a logical sequence. Unfortunately slides are often inadequate. To be useful they have to meet some simple requirements:

- Avoid introducing too much information in one slide
- Do not use small letter sizes (*e.g.* minimum font size 18).
- Do not write more than 12 lines in a slide.
- Provide clear orientation on the subject of the slide and its position in the presentation (chapter, part, *etc.*) and write its number.
- Present the logo of the organization, the reference of the author and a date or year.

Fig. (**18**) shows an example of acceptable slide. Notice that it has a clear title (PROTECTION OF PRODUCTS), that the font sizes allow for an easy reading, that the number of the slide is written (#34) and that the subject (Introduction to GMP) and the chapter (5 – HVAC system) are given. Besides, it identifies the organization ("Drug Pharm"), the author (JBF) and the year of preparation.

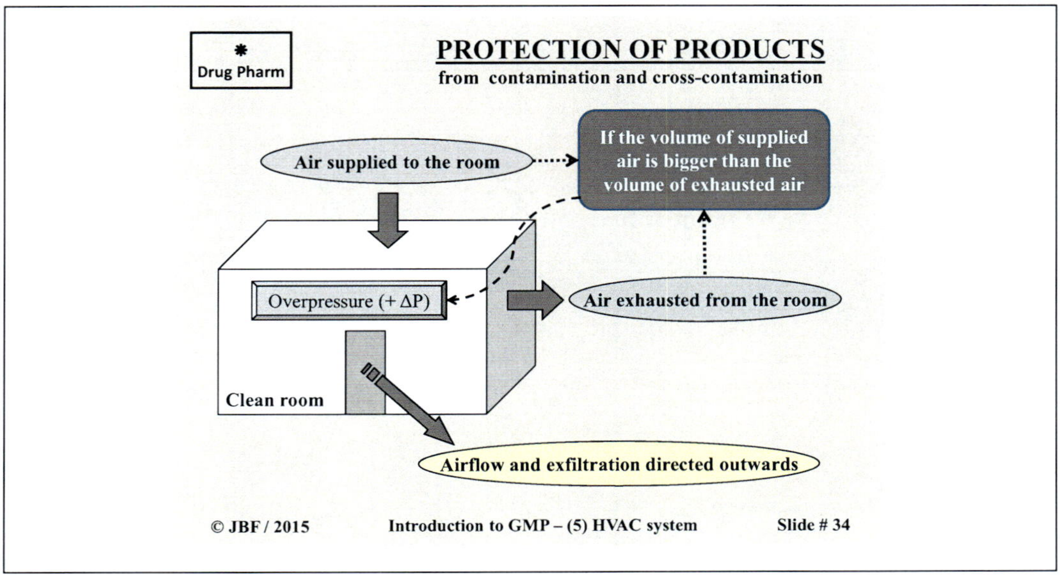

Fig. (18). First example of slide: A good designed slide.

Instead, Fig. (**19**) represents a slide which cannot be accepted. It has an identification of the organization, and this is good, but there is not any other reference. It contains a table too big to be given in a single slide. Consequently, it is very difficult to read, and probably trainees will not pay attention to it. Big tables pose always a problem in presentations. Although this supposes an important amount of work it is necessary either simplify the table or divide it in smaller tables which might be given in readable form in a slide.

Drug Pharm

Concerned sphere	Hazard description	Hazard cause	Preventive measures
Premises / Plant areas	Entrance of particles (dust, polen, mist, etc.) from outside	Outside air can get in	(#1.1) Separation from outside
			(#1.2) Separation inside the plant (GMP/non GMP areas)
		Dirty air moves between different areas	(#1.3) Separation inside the plant (QC/Production)
		Untidy plant surroundings	(#1.4) Plant location
		Dirty incoming containers	(#1.5) Receiving areas
	Entrance of vermine	No control of vermine	(#1.6) Vermine control
	Build-up of dust/dirt	Existence of points for the build-up of dirt	(#1.7) Design of premises
		Surfaces shedding particles and difficult to keep clean	(#1.8) Sanitary room construction
		Inadequate cleaning	(#1.9) Room cleaning
Utilities / HVAC	Entrance of particles and inadequate air system	Air is not adequately treated and does not meet requirements	(#1.10) Air supply to classified areas (clean rooms)
			(#1.11) Air supply to non-classified areas
Utilities / Dust exhaust	Entrance of outside particles (dust, polen, etc.)	Outside air can get into the rooms by the exhausting ducts	(#1.12) Protection against air flow inversion
	Diffussion of particles	Disruption of the pressure cascade	(#1.13) Protection against modification of ΔP
Utilities / Water for pharmaceutical use	Water not meeting requirements	Entrance of contamination into the system	(#1.14) System design
		Inadequate treatment system	(#1.15) Water treatment
		Stored water is contaminated	(#1.16) Protection of the water
Utilities / Steam for pharmaceutical use	Steam not meeting requirements	Build-up of contamination	(#1.17) System design
		Passage of water contaminants to steam	(#1.18) Source of water
Utilities / Compressed air	Compressed air not meeting requirements	Source air contaminated	(#1.19) Source of air
		Air contaminated by the compressor	(#1.20) Compressor type
		Condensation of water	(#1.21) System configuration
Utilities / Compressed gases	Compressed gas not meeting requirements	Gas is not of pharmaceutical quality	(#1.22) Gas quality
Operations / equipment	Equipment contamination	Inadequate installation	(#1.23) Installation
		Inadequate cleaning	(#1.24) Cleaning
	Product contamination	Inadequate surfaces	(#1.25) Surfaces in contact with materials and products
		Acces of contamination	(#1.26) Design
			(#1.27) Separation
Operations / Personnel	Product contamination	Persons act as carriers of contamination	(#1.28) Hygienic measures
			(#1.29) Wear appropiate clothing
		Tools and pipes act as carriers of contamination	(#1.30) Beware of tools and transfer pipes

Fig. (19). Second example of slide: A poorly designed slide.

In any case, it is important to bear in mind that in order to introduce difficult concepts it is better to place them in a context where they are combined with lighter concepts than to produce a bare group of difficult concepts. You can easily swallow a pill or two with a good cup of tea/coffee, but it will be difficult to ingest a whole group of bitter pills.

Thus, placing difficult concepts within general descriptions helps in understanding and remembering them.

Video

An even better method is using video. It is possible to film both examples of good procedures (*i.e.* what should be done) and bad procedures (*i.e.* what should not be done). This approach is evidently very good for GMP training but it is even better for training on internal procedures or instructions. Unfortunately, this approach requires more time and the participation of many of the trainees themselves.

Group Training

A frequently encountered problem of training is that it is too passive. Trainees just listened to the trainers. A possible way for overcoming this problem is, once that the exposition of the trainer/s is finished, distributing the trainees in small groups which shall explain the training topics by themselves.

Practical Training

Of course the most effective training is practical training on-site. Trainees realize or see practically the problems related to the subject.

It has to be emphasized the great importance of providing practical training on hygienic practices to operators unfamiliar with microbiology. This can be done, for example, by taking samples of the hands of the operators before washing, after a poor washing and after a good washing performed according to the internal procedures. Culture media are inoculated with these samples and after incubation they are shown to the trainees. This way, they will understand the importance of hygienic practices.

Efficacy Assessment

A key point for the efficacy of a training activity is that people who attend it are interested and have the adequate preparation for understanding and benefiting from it. Although there will often be some exceptions, in general these problems can be overcome by the adequate assessment of CVs and of history training by the department of human resources.

Usually technicians are highly motivated and interested in increasing their knowledge (training is related with the specialty they themselves have chosen), even if passing successfully training tests is not linked with internal advancements. But this is often not the case with non specialized operators. They might be working in the pharmaceutical industry just because there was not another choice or just because it was the most advantageous job in terms of wages, location, *etc.* Thus, how to motivate them? This is not easy and there are not many alternatives left, but we can name the following three. First of all, the organization can devise some type of reward for the more competent trainees. Secondly, trainers should attract the attention of the trainees. And lastly, as they are submitted to a final training evaluation, if they want to pass it they are obliged to pay a minimal level of attention.

The key question for the organization is: Has the training been effective? This leads to another question: Which were the expectations of the organization?

Efficacious training means that it meets the objectives. And the objectives of training are self-evident: trainees should acquire knowledge and skill for performing the operations described in the documents and adequate knowledge on GMP guidelines. Or said differently, they should integrate training into their work.

The expectations of the organization were, consequently, that the resources allocated and the methods used for training would lead to meeting the above mentioned objectives. These expectations were formulated when programming the training activity. If personnel perform correctly the operation, which constituted the training topic, it is evident that training was correct, but showing the efficacy of GMP training, which is more general, is more difficult. However, audits and incidents and deviations show clearly the way.

In order to be successful training has to fulfill several conditions:

- Trainees should identify with its purpose;
- It has to be understood by the trainees;
- It has to be connected to their work and applicable (at least to a certain measure);
- It has to meet their expectations.

However, experience shows that these conditions are hard to meet, because they cannot be controlled by the trainer alone.

If training shows itself as not effective it is necessary to change the approach in order to get a real improvement.

When analyzing in the laboratory a non-compliant result it is unacceptable to repeat simply the essay and if it is then compliant consider it right. This would only be acceptable if it had been discovered a clear failure in the first testing. This approach must be used in training too. A corrective action should not be simply retraining, because probably even accepting that the training is necessary the problem lays in the inadequate form it was delivered. The failure was not being able to ensure that personnel were adequately trained.

Understanding

A simplest way for verifying if the trainees have understood the training is having a test. It can be done after completing the training activity or, better, after a few days or weeks. And alternative, even if cumbersome, approach might be performing both tests. This latter dealing would provide a hint on what happens with the knowledge as time goes by.

A more sophisticated method which might be applied when the training refers to practical operations is showing by the trainees that they can realize adequately these operations.

Satisfaction

This is usually performed by trainees who fill a form with questions regarding the training (*e.g.* trainer appraisal, interest for them of the subject, did they consider that it was useful for them, can apply it to their work).

CONCLUDING REMARKS

In spite of the impressive advances in automation and in computerized systems personnel continues to play a key role in pharmaceutical manufacturing. And this means that the difference between success and failure may be the quality of persons in terms of education and training.

Training procedures, generally speaking, are well-known and, in principle, there is not much to add, but selection of trainees, preparation of training programs, motivation of trainees, and realization and evaluation of the effectiveness of the training activities are always difficult to manage. And these latter are the key points which determine the success of training.

Supervision and auditing activities are oriented towards detecting problems in the PQS and, once they are found, towards discovering the root causes for these problems. Often the "human factor" is deemed guilty (*i.e.* is it not true that persons design, build and use machines and computerized systems?) and training is the tool used for redeeming people. Often, however, redemption is not obtained simply by repeated training, but by providing adequate training.

CONFLICT OF INTEREST

The author confirms that this chapter contents have no conflict of interest.

ACKNOWLEDGEMENT

Declared None.

REFERENCES

[1] WHO (World Health Organization). WHO Good manufacturing practices for pharmaceutical products: main principles. In: WHO Expert Committee on Specifications for Pharmaceutical Preparations. Forty-eighth report (WHO Technical Report Series, No. 986). WHO, Geneva, Switzerland 2014. Annex 2. 9.1.

[2] Ibid. 10.2.

[3] Ibid. 10.4.

[4] Ibid. 10.2.

[5] US National Archives & Records Administration. Federal Register. Code of Federal Regulations (CFR). Title 21 (Food & drugs). Part 211. Section 211.25.a.

[6] European Commission. Good manufacturing practices. Medicinal products for human and veterinary use. The rules governing medicinal products in the European Union. Volume 4. Brussels. Part I: 4.26.

[7] US National Archives & Records Administration. Federal Register. Code of Federal Regulations (CFR). Title 21 (Food & drugs). Part 211. Section 211.34.

[8] WHO (World Health Organization). WHO Good manufacturing practices for pharmaceutical products: main principles. In: WHO Expert Committee on Specifications for Pharmaceutical Preparations. Forty-eighth report (WHO Technical Report Series, No. 986). WHO, Geneva, Switzerland 2014. Annex 2. 10.2.

[9] WHO (World Health Organisation). WHO Good manufacturing practices for biological products. In: WHO Expert Committee on Specifications for Pharmaceutical Preparations. Thirty-third report (WHO Technical Report Series, No. 834). WHO, Geneva, Switzerland 1993. Annex 3. 3.8.

[10] WHO (World Health Organization). WHO Good manufacturing practices for pharmaceutical products: main principles. In: WHO Expert Committee on Specifications for Pharmaceutical Preparations. Forty-eighth report (WHO Technical Report Series, No. 986). WHO, Geneva, Switzerland 2014. Annex 2. 16.7.

[11] Ibid. 12.8.

CHAPTER 8

Premises/Clean Rooms

Abstract: Pharmaceutical premises determine the manufacturing flows and provide the setting for manufacturing equipment and for the complementary utilities. Clean rooms, where production operations can be performed within a controlled environment, are the result of combining sanitary internal architecture and HVAC systems. Premises have to be well designed in order to impede the entrance of outside contamination and the diffusion of internal cross-contamination. Moreover, personnel, because of their inherent contamination, put at risk the quality of the internal environment of the premises and therefore their access has to be controlled and performed through changing rooms, where operators put on appropriate clothing for the operations to be performed. When products happen to be potentially harmful, it is necessary to protect operators and outside environment too. This requires specially designed premises where the above-mentioned protection of products is coupled with the protection of operators and environment. This latter requirement is fulfilled by means of two steps of contention, primary within closed devices and secondary within the rooms by a combination of differential pressure and air filtration. Qualification allows for the demonstration that premises perform as intended.

Keywords: Action limits, airborne particles, air changes, airflow, airlock, internal architecture, clean area, clean room classification requirements, clean room conditions, clean room monitoring, clean room qualification, clothing, containment, design, differential pressure, material flow, personnel flow, sanitary construction, turbulent airflow, UDAF.

PREMISES FROM THE GMP POINT OF VIEW

Pharmaceutical premises are not just a physical space where equipment and personnel perform the manufacturing operations. Their layout determines flows and separations. Besides, the internal architecture complemented with the HVAC system allows for the creation of a controlled environment where manufacturing takes place.

A pharmaceutical manufacturing plant is defined by the operations which are or can be performed:

- Scope of operations: Although traditionally in the same premises were prepared many different products with varied dosage forms (multiproduct plants), nowadays the tendency is often towards specialized plants for given dosage forms or for reduced number of

Jordi Botet

products or production stages. In some cases logistic and economical reasons can even lead to plants dedicated to a single product (single product plants). In other cases plant specialization is a GMP requirement to impede cross-contamination (*e.g.* penicillanic antibiotics).

- Dosage forms: The characteristics of the premises depend on the dosage form, because of its physical characteristics (solid, semi-solid or liquid) and environmental requirements (aseptic production or not).

- Technology: It is evident that equipment is chosen in function of the type of operations which are needed and that this equipment, then, determines the lay-out of the facility (utilities which are required, space filled by equipment, material and personnel flows, *etc.*). The separation of the dirty parts of equipment outside the clean production zones in order to allow maintenance and repair without affecting the products is a GMP requirement. This means that production areas have to be complemented with technical zones.

- Other considerations: Adaptability to changes in product and batch size, packaging materials (containers, closures) ready for use or cleaned/sterilized *in situ*, production and storage requirements. HVAC equipment is bulky and heavy and requires a good amount of space. It is installed above the production rooms in a specially designed technical zone or outside.

The production rooms can be distributed in a single floor or in different floors. In the first case movement is easy because of the even surface. Whereas in the second, starting materials are taken upstairs by elevators and then the operations take advantage of gravity for the displacement of materials and products until attaining the lowest level.

The partitions and false-ceilings of the premises, known as "internal architecture" play a purely passive role, but a very important one. They contribute in controlling and limiting access to the different areas. They allow for the separation of areas within the premises and determine the flows. And they provide a sanitary setup.

The adjective sanitary is applied to the design based on the know-how of engineers and architects in order to control the risk of contamination during operations:

- Smooth surfaces not shedding particles. This is why brick-build walls with plaster or wood coverings are not accepted. The best-suited material for partitions and false-ceilings are sandwich panels with external coating of enameled metal or phenolic resin. Floors are covered either with PVC sheets or coated with resins.
- No cracks or open joints. Paneling joints have to be filled with silicon.
- Limitation of shelves. They accumulate dust and therefore they should be absent in the most critical areas.
- Utilities (pipes, sockets, luminaries, *etc.*) should not have recesses difficult to clean. Whenever possible utilities should be installed outside from the production rooms or fitted in the partitions and embedded.
- Corners with rounded union profiles.
- Flush surfaces (window panes, doors, *etc.*) to avoid ledges.
- Avoid uncleanable recesses where dust can gather. This is why sliding doors are not recommended. In low risk areas they are often substituted by rolling doors.
- Control of sinks, drains and floor channels. They should be installed in low risk areas (grade C and D) but not in grade A and B areas and be provided with easily cleanable traps and with air breaks to avert backflow. Floor channels should be open, shallow and easily cleanable and be linked to drains outside the area in a way that prevents the access of microbial contamination.

CLEAN AREA/CLEAN ROOM CONCEPT

During manufacturing operations materials and products should only be exposed to the environment in clean areas, which can be described as areas *with defined environmental control of particulate and microbial contamination, constructed and used in such a way as to reduce the introduction, generation, and retention of contaminants within the area* [1]. The rooms composing a clean area are clean rooms (or cleanrooms).

As it can be inferred from the definition, the clean area notion mixes different concepts:

Control of the airborne particulate contamination

- Dusting by filtration.
- Pressure differentials in order to ensure that airborne particulate contamination does not pass from one room to another.

Control of the introduction of airborne particulate contamination

- Airlocks for materials and equipment.
- Changing rooms for personnel.
- Special ad hoc clothing.

Sanitary construction

- Use of materials that do not liberate particles.
- Use of materials which can be cleaned and disinfected.
- No recesses.

Appropriate procedures

- Behavior of personnel.
- Cleaning and maintenance.

Monitoring

- Of particles.
- Of microorganisms.
- Of ΔP.
- Of T and, sometimes, RH.

CLEAN AREA/CLEAN ROOM CLASSIFICATION

Clean areas are classified according to airborne particulate limits. Particulate materials may have any form and composition. They can also act as "carriers" of bacteria. This is why **non-viable** (or inert) **particles** and **viable particles** are recognized. This distinction is made in relation to the possibility of development of colonies when particles are cultured. If particles carry microorganisms they will develop colonies when put on culture medium.

Usually the terms "particles" and "particulate contamination" refer to both types of particles, viable and non-viable (*i.e.* to any particle which can be numbered by a particle-counter), whereas viable particles are explicitly denoted as such or as "microbiological contamination".

Airborne particles are counted by m^3 (or cubic feet) and, logically, when contamination diminishes, the level of cleanliness increases and rooms have a higher classification.

In pharmaceutical plants this classification is done for a determined condition, according to the maximum permitted number of particles per m^3 of a size equal or larger than 0.5 and 5 µm (according to WHO and European GMP) or to particles larger than 0.5 µm (according to US CGMP). Currently two different classification systems are used.

Clean Room Conditions

Clean rooms can be considered in three conditions or occupancy states (Fig. **1**):

As-built (after construction): This situation exists when the construction of the clean area is finished and the HVAC system is already functioning, but manufacturing equipment, not to mention materials and personnel, are not present.

At rest: This situation exists when the clean area is complete and equipment has been installed and is ready for operation (but turned off). Neither materials nor operating personnel are present.

In operation (operational) or dynamic: This situation exists when the clean area works under conditions of normal production (*i.e.* with working equipment, materials and personnel).

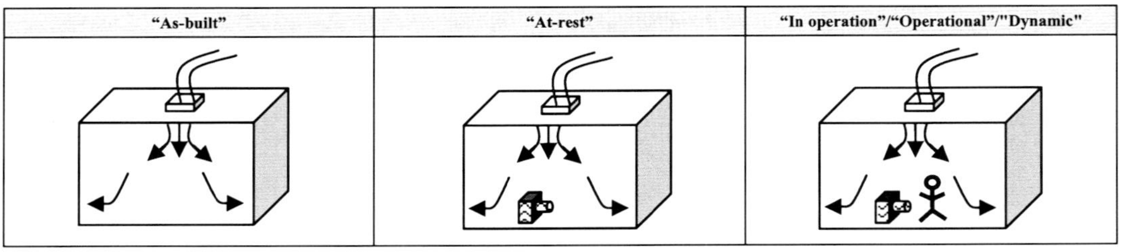

Fig. (1). Conditions (occupancy states) under which the classification of a clean room can be defined

The as-built condition exists only when a new or modified installation is started. Afterwards there are only at-rest or in operation/operational/dynamic installations.

Classification Approaches

This is one of the few aspects which now show significant differences between US CGMP and GMP (WHO and Europe).

US Approach to Clean Area Classification

Federal Standard 209

Americans were the first to establish a system for the classification of zones with a controlled environment according to the required airborne particulate characteristics. Federal Standard 209 appeared in 1963. Until its abrogation in 2001, this standard had had 6 versions (original, A, B, C, D and E) [2].

The system of classification set up by Federal Standard 209 in its E version was never readily accepted, whereas its D version (1988) was so successful that today, although obsolete, it is still quoted. In Federal Standard 209 D the denomination of a class coincides with the maximum permitted number of particles per cubic foot of a size equal to or above 0.5 µm, which makes it very practical (Table **1**).

In 2001 American authorities decided not to publish any new versions of Federal Standard 209 and substitute it by the international norm ISO 14644. This standard has the advantage of proposing both a system of classification, published in 1999, and test methods to determine this classification.

Table 1. Classification of clean areas: USA – Federal standard 209 D (1988). Obsolete.

Class	Maximal permitted number of particles of a size equal to or above (≥)			
	0.5 µm/cubic foot	0.5 µm/cubic meter	5 µm/cubic foot	5 µm/cubic meter
1	1	35	not defined	not defined
10	10	350	not defined	not defined
100	100	3,500	not defined	not defined
1,000	1,000	35,000	7	245
10,000	10,000	350,000	70	2,450
100,000	100,000	3,500,000	700	24,500

ISO 14644

Standard ISO 14644 is a wide-scope norm, not just limited to pharmacy, that establishes 9 classes of particulate cleanliness, which are defined by "N" (number of classification) [3]. See Table **2**.

Table 2. Calculation of the maximal permitted concentration of particles according to norm ISO 14644.

The maximal permitted concentration for each defined particle size (**C_n**), for a given ISO class, is determined by means of the following equation, where N is the number of ISO class and D the considered particle size in µm:	$\mathbf{C_n = 10^{N} \cdot (0.1/D)^{2.08}}$

Six particle sizes are taken into account (0.1 µm, 0.2 µm, 0.3 µm, 0.5 µm, 1 µm and 5 µm). See Table **3**.

Table 3. Classification of clean areas according to norm ISO 14644.

"N" Number of classification	**Maximum permitted number of particles of a size equal to or above (particles per m^3 of air):**					
	0.1 µm	**0.2 µm**	**0.3 µm**	**0.5 µm**	**1 µm**	**5 µm**
Class ISO 1	10	2				
Class ISO 2	100	24	10	4		
Class ISO 3	1,000	237	102	35	8	
Class ISO 4	10,000	2,370	1,020	352	83	
Class ISO 5	100,000	23,700	10,200	3,520	832	29
Class ISO 6	1,000,000	237,000	102,000	35,200	8,320	293
Class ISO 7				352,000	83,200	2,930
Class ISO 8				3,520,000	832,000	29,300
Class ISO 9				35,200,000	8,320,000	293,000
Note: The norm considers the possibility of using intermediate numbers of class ISO (for instance: 4.8)						

It has to be pointed out that US FDA applies this classification but with the following criteria:

- Although this norm does not indicate occupancy states (this is a point which has to be agreed), FDA considers that particles should always be counted in dynamic conditions;

- Only particles of a size equal or above 0.5 µm are taken into account.

This has relevant consequences which are considered further on.

GMP (WHO and Europe) Approach to Clean Area Classification

WHO [4] and Europe [5] GMP have established 4 grades of clean areas (A, B, C and D) and distinguish two conditions, "at rest" and "in operation" (Table **4**).

Table 4. WHO and Europe GMP classification of clean areas.

GRADE	At rest		In operation	
	Maximum permitted number of particles per m^3		Maximum permitted number of particles per m^3	
	≥ 0.5 µm	≥ 5.0 µm	≥ 0.5 µm	≥ 5.0 µm
A	3,520	20	3,520	20
B	3,520	29	352,000	2,900
C	352,000	2,900	3,520,000	29,000
D	3,520,000	29,000	Not defined	Not defined

Comparison Between ISO and WHO/Europe Clean Area Classification

First of all, it is necessary to point out that whereas the airborne particle limits for particles of 0.5 µm are the same in both classification systems (Table **5**). The values for 5.0 µm particles are slightly different (*e.g.*, 2,930 and 2,900). Well, not always "slightly" different because 29 (ISO 5 class) represents a 45% of increase with reference to 20 (GMP grade A). In fact grade A corresponds to class ISO 4.8.

Table 5. Comparison of ISO 14644 and WHO/Europe GMP classifications.

	Class	Maximum permitted number of particles of a size equal to or above (particles per m^3 of air)]:			
		Condition: "at rest" or "dynamic" as defined			
		0.5 µm		5.0 µm	
ISO	ISO 5	3,520		29	
	ISO 6	35,200		293	
	ISO 7	352,000		2,930	
	ISO 8	3,520,000		29,300	
	Grade	Maximum permitted number of particles of a size equal to or above (particles per m^3 of air):			
		Condition: "at rest"		Condition: "dynamic"	
		0.5 µm	5.0 µm	0.5 µm	5.0 µm
GMP	A	3,520	20	3,520	20
	B	3,520	29	352,000	2,900
	C	352,000	2,900	3,520,000	29,000
	D	3,520,000	29,000	Not defined	Not defined

Aside from that:

- Class ISO 5 and grade A show an acceptable equivalence (with the above mentioned reservations).
- Class ISO 6 has no equivalence in GMP.
- Class ISO 7 corresponds to grade B dynamic and to grade C at rest.
- Class ISO 8 corresponds to grade C dynamic and to grade D at rest.

This means that the equivalence between both systems is mostly determined by the defined state or condition (at rest or dynamic). See Table **6**.

Table 6. Summarized equivalences between WHO/Europe GMP and ISO 14644.

GMP (WHO/Europe)	ISO 14644
Grade A	Class ISO 5 (for particles ≥ 0.5 μm)/ISO 4,8 (for particles ≥ 5.0 μm)
Grade B (at rest)	Class ISO 5 (for particles ≥ 0.5 and ≥ 5.0 μm)
Grade C (at rest)	Class ISO 7 (for particles ≥ 0.5 and ≥ 5.0 μm)
Grade C (dynamic)	Class ISO 8 (for particles ≥ 0.5 and ≥ 5.0 μm)
Grade D (at rest)	Class ISO 8 (for particles ≥ 0.5 and ≥ 5.0 μm)

Comparison Between USA and WHO/Europe Clean Area Classification

This comparison has to take into account that US FDA Guideline on Sterile drug products produced by aseptic processing indicates that measures should be performed in activity and that only particles ≥ 0.5 μm are considered [6].

Table 7. Comparison of US FDA and WHO/Europe.

	Class	Maximum permitted number of particles of a size equal to or above (particles per m^3 of air):
		Condition: "dynamic"
		0.5 μm
USA	ISO 5	3,520
	ISO 6	35,200
	ISO 7	352,000
	ISO 8	3,520,000

Table 7: contd...

	Grade	Maximum permitted number of particles of a size equal to or above (particles per m^3 of air):			
		Condition: "at rest"		Condition: "dynamic"	
		0.5 µm	5.0 µm	0.5 µm	5.0 µm
GMP (WHO/Europe)	A	3,520	20	3,520	20
	B	3,520	29	352,000	2,900
	C	352,000	2,900	3,520,000	29,000
	D	3,520,000	29,000	Not defined	Not defined

Thus (Tables **7** and **8**), ISO 6 has no equivalence in GMP and, generally speaking, it can be said that USA and WHO/Europe classifications match imperfectly.

Table 8. Summarized equivalences between US FDA and WHO/Europe classifications.

Classification US FDA (dynamic)		Equivalence GMP (WHO/Europe)
ISO	≥0.5 µm/m^3	
Class 5	3,520	Grade A (at rest and dynamic)/B (at rest)
Class 6	35,200	Without equivalence
Class 7	352,000	Grade C (at rest)
Class 8	3,520,000	Grade C (dynamic)/D (at rest)

CLEAN ROOM DESIGN

The cleanliness of a clean room is the consequence of a series of strategies involving different aspects [7]: design and construction, extent of filtration of air, number of air changes, type of airflow, separation between room environments and the operations performed within them. In general, in order to reduce costs, it is convenient to minimize the size of clean rooms. Equally, the limitation of the number of people within a clean room contrives to limit contamination. Critical areas of a clean room where operations at risk are carried out should be separated from doors and pathways (in order to avoid disturbing air-flows).

The adequate level of air filtration is obtained combining prefilters, filters and absolute filters (HEPA). See chapter 9. In order to obtain lower levels of airborne particles the HEPA filters have to be sited in the same false ceiling of the clean room (terminal) [8]. See Table **9**.

Table 9. Types of filtration used to attain the different cleanliness levels.

Type of zone		Classification		Required filtration level
		ISO 14644	WHO/European GMP	
Non pharmaceutical		---	---	G4
Pharmaceutical	Non controlled	---/Class 9	---	G4 and F8
	Controlled	Class 8	Grade D	G4, F8 and H13
	Protected	Class 7	Grade C	G4, F8 and H13*
	Critical	Class 5	Grade A/B	G4, F9 and H14*

* Terminal filters

Airflow Rates and Air Changes

The supply of filtered air into a room, by simple "dilution", diminishes the airborne particulate concentration. Thus, by increasing the number of air changes it is possible to diminish the concentration of particles in air.

In general it is considered that to reach grade D, the number of air changes should be at least 20 (although often a grade D is obtained with less air changes). For other grades, the number of air changes should be higher [9].

Types of Airflow

The flow of supplied air can either be turbulent, turbulent airflow, (*i.e.* non laminar) or unidirectional (*i.e.* laminar). In the former case airborne particles are diluted, whereas in the latter case airborne particles are displaced (Fig. **2**).

Turbulent (Non Unidirectional/Non Laminar) Airflow

The supply of air into a room (logically complemented with extraction) allows for a diminution in the number of airborne particles simply by dilution. Extracted air contains more particles than supplied air until a steady state is reached. Then, airborne particulate concentration would allow for the classification of the room. Air-flows within the room do not show any regularity. Supplied air (through terminal filters or diffusers) flows in all directions, until it reaches the air exhaust grilles.

A turbulent airflow requires a certain time to eliminate particulate contamination produced within the room and there is also a risk of displacing particles towards the critical areas where products are handled. Consequently, non-laminar air-flow does not allow attaining the cleanliness levels required for aseptic manipulation.

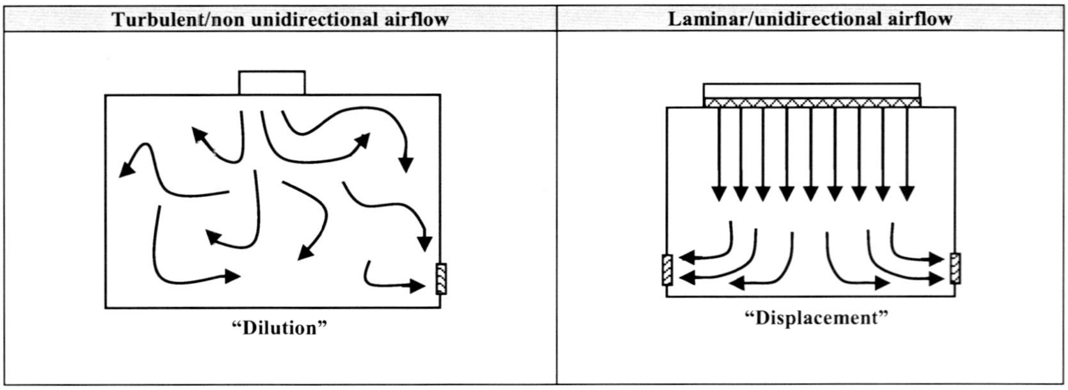

Fig. (2). Types of airflow in clean rooms.

Unidirectional (Laminar) Airflow

"Laminar flow" is an airflow moving in a single direction and in parallel layers at constant velocity from the beginning to the end of a straight line vector.

"Unidirectional flow" is an airflow moving in a single direction, in a robust and uniform manner, and at sufficient speed to reproducibly sweep particles away from the critical processing or testing area [10].

The customary denomination of "laminar flow" is being substituted by "unidirectional flow" because it reflects more accurately what really happens in practice (*i.e.* air really moves in a single direction but attaining true parallelism and speed uniformity is not so common). Nowadays laminar flow and unidirectional flow are used as synonyms, although the latter is considered more correct. Often it is spoken of UDAF, that is, "unidirectional airflow".

A "plenum", a cavity, placed before the HEPA filter allows for a homogeneous distribution of the airflow. The regular flow of air permits a rapid elimination of airborne contamination. Airborne particles are simply "pushed", displaced. Consequently, with this type of airflow it is possible to attain the high level of cleanliness required by aseptic manipulation.

According to the direction of the airflow with relation to the working plan, it is possible to distinguish between vertical and horizontal UDAF. Both kinds can ensure work place cleanliness, provided that air is allowed to flow freely. Any obstacle in the flow of air disrupts its unidirectionality creating whirls and this means a loss in the degree of protection provided by the UDAF. Thus, the kind of UDAF chosen depends on the type of equipment and on the operations.

However, it should be taken into account that by using a horizontal UDAF, operators are exposed to the product. Consequently it should not be used for the manipulation of products susceptible of being harmful to operators.

Normally UDAF provides a controlled environment with an airborne particulate concentration corresponding to grade A (WHO and European GMP) or class 5 (ISO 14644). Air has to attain a determined speed to be able to sweep the work place adequately.

Laminar airflow systems should provide a homogenous air speed in a range of 0.36 – 0.54 m/s (guidance value) at the working position in open clean room applications. The maintenance of laminarity should be demonstrated and validated [11].

A velocity of 0.45 meters/second (90 feet per minute) has generally been established, with a range of plus or minus 20 percent around the set point. Higher velocities may be appropriate in operations generating high levels of particulates [12].

Separation by Differential Pressure

It is possible to impede the displacement of airborne contamination between two adjacent rooms by regulating the amounts of air supplied and extracted. This establishes a pressure differential which allows for the control of the airflow. Pressure differentials (ΔP) should suffice to ensure that air will flow in a single direction, without flow inversion. The pressure differential between adjacent rooms is usually established between 10 and 15 Pa., with a tolerance of $\pm$ 3 Pa [13]. The differential pressures of the diverse clean rooms of a pharmaceutical plant create pressure gradients (also known as pressure cascades). These pressure differentials (or at least those deemed critical) should be monitored with pressure gauges and have appropriate alarm systems. Operating procedures require that personnel verify pressure differentials before starting any critical task.

It has to be kept in mind that pressure differentials are very small and thus exist only when doors are closed. This is why the maintenance of pressure gradients relies on a good design of the system and on personnel training.

When the HVAC system is turned off or fails the pressure differentials disappear and consequently there is no control on the airborne contamination. This is why:

- An alarm should complement the pressure gauges and alert personnel that the protection afforded by differential pressure does not exist any longer. Production should stop and products should not be exposed to the environment.

- In premises where sterile products are manufactured environmental requirements are critical and consequently the HVAC system cannot stop, because it would allow entrance of microbiological contamination. In order to save energy HVAC systems are designed so that they can operate in a stand-by mode when manufacturing operations are not taking place.

- The qualification of clean rooms includes the "recovery test" (see further on) which determines the time needed to reach its cleanliness level.

Control of Environmental Contamination

Maintaining positive pressure within the clean rooms protects them from the entrance of external contamination, not only through doors, but also through partition joints or false-ceiling cracks.

However, this general rule has an exception when harmful products are manipulated. Then, it is necessary to protect the outside environment from contamination and, following the same rationale previously acknowledged, maintaining a negative pressure within the critical rooms impedes the diffusion of these harmful products towards the outside. Besides, it is necessary to protect the products from the entry of external contamination and this requires adjoining them a protective "buffer" of positive pressure rooms (for example changing rooms and airlocks).

Control of Cross-Contamination

In clean areas where solid forms are produced, keeping a positive pressure in the corridor in relation to rooms impedes the displacement of dust outside the rooms. Whereas in zones where liquid or semi-solid forms are prepared, keeping a positive pressure in the rooms hinders the entrance of airborne contamination.

Airlocks

Maintaining the separation of clean room environments by means of pressure differentials is greatly facilitated by placing airlocks between rooms with different level of risk and, thus, provided with different pressure differentials and, maybe, different classification levels.

Characteristics of the Airlocks

- The doors (usually two, but certain lay-outs may require several doors) of an airlock are interlocked so as to impede simultaneous opening, avoiding thus the direct flow of air between adjacent rooms.

- The cleanliness classification level of an airlock should normally equal that of the cleaner adjacent room.

- With regard to pressure differentials, airlocks can be in gradient (cascade), in depression (sink) or hyperpressure (bubble) [14].

- As it has been said, the strategy of environmental separation by means of differential pressure is only effective if doors remain closed. It is critical not to leave them inadvertently open by personnel during manufacturing operations. This can be impeded by providing them with a system of automatic closure.

- Whenever possible, it is preferable that airlock doors open towards the positive pressure side (thus, air pressure assists in keeping them closed).

- Airlocks also constitute an element for physical separation of rooms having different temperature and/or humidity conditions. See Fig. (**3**).

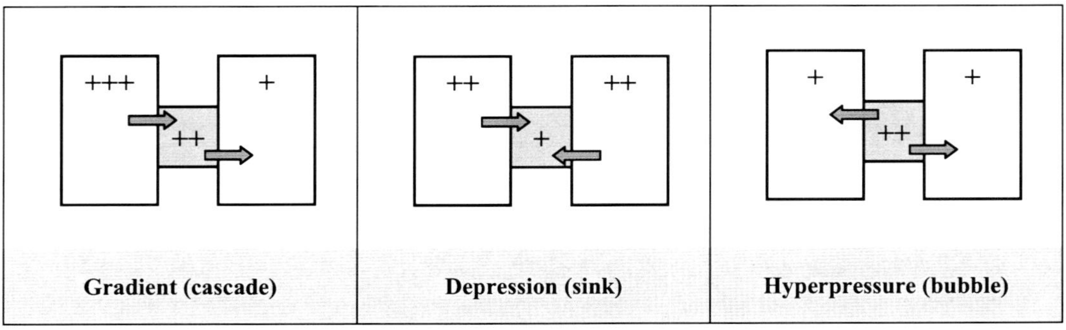

Fig. (3). Types of pressure differentials in an airlock (arrows show airflow direction).

CLEAN ROOM FUNCTIONAL PARAMETERS

Clean rooms are designed and built to meet previously specified requirements [15]. These depend on the operations performed and on the characteristics of the products manipulated therein.

Functional requirements comprise the following parameters:

- Airborne particulate cleanliness
- Ambient parameters
- Pressure differentials

Airborne Particulate Cleanliness

This is a basic point to establish. In practice, it is necessary to determine

- ✓ Which norm will be used for its classification: WHO/Europe GMP, US CGMP or ISO 14644.
- ✓ Which condition will be chosen for its classification (at rest or in operation).
- ✓ Which class will be required (or classes, because, for instance, in a grade B room, there can be a part of it provided with UDAF and, thus, grade A.

Area classes or grades are selected according to the operations performed there.

Changing Rooms

The last part of a changing room should have, in the at-rest state, the same classification as the area into which it leads.

Sampling and Weighing Areas

GMP does not establish any requirement for the classification of these areas. However, logic dictates that their cleanliness level should be the same that is established for the production stages where these same products are exposed to the environment. In practice, sampling and weighing are performed inside booths provided with UDAF (above the working surface) and with air exhaust (below the working surface for extracting any dust liberated during the manipulation of the materials). For non-sterile products, an airborne particulate classification of grade C, equivalent to class ISO 7 (ISO), is usually considered sufficient.

Production Areas for Non Sterile Medicinal Products

Regarding these areas GMP indicates that the rooms, where materials, products or clean, open containers are exposed to the environment should be ventilated with filtered air [16].

In practice, these areas are classified as grade D/class ISO 8. The intent is providing a reasonably clean controlled environment.

Production Areas for Sterile Medicinal Products

The requirements for environmental classification are linked to the level of risk which supposes for the product the contamination with particulate material and microbes. This is why in plants where sterile drug products are manufactured there are clean rooms with different cleanliness levels. Their classification depends on the type of operation and on the nature of the product (*i.e.* its proneness to develop microbes).

Table **10** shows the general GMP approach, exposed in WHO GMP [17], Europe GMP [18] and US CGMP [19].

Table 10. Clean room classification. General requirements.

Grade/Class	Operation
A/ISO 5	Aseptic processing line with high risk operations (aseptic filling, plates with closures, opened ampoules and vials, aseptic connections of equipment)
B/ISO 7 (at least)	Area surrounding class A for high risk operations. *FDA recommends that the area immediately adjacent to the aseptic processing line meet, at a minimum, Class 10,000 (ISO 7) under dynamic conditions. Manufacturers can also classify this area as Class 1,000 (ISO 6) or maintain the entire aseptic filling room at Class 100 (ISO 5). An area classified at a Class 10,000 (ISO 8) air cleanliness level is appropriate for less critical activities (e.g., equipment cleaning)* [20].
C or D/ISO 7 or 8	Less critical phases in the preparation of sterile products. *An area classified at a Class 10,000 (ISO 8) air cleanliness level is appropriate for less critical activities (e.g. equipment cleaning)* [21].

Attention! It is necessary to bear in mind that, as it has been discussed in previous sections of this chapter, the equivalence between WHO/Europe GMP and US CGMP environmental classes is imperfect. And this is particularly relevant for the area surrounding the aseptic line of high risk (see following table).

Besides, WHO GMP in some cases accepts grade C for the area surrounding the high risk zone. Here for simplification reasons and to provide a global advice, this is not taken into account and it is considered that the surrounding area for grade A should be grade B.

The environmental cleanliness required for the manufacturing operations of sterile products is basically determined by the process, which can be conducted aseptically or not (Tables **11** and **12**).

In the first case, the process can be either entirely aseptic in all its steps or just in a part of them. It is evident that aseptic operations require a very high-quality environment.

In the second case, although non aseptic processes require less strict environments, products should be protected from contamination too, because a very high bioburden puts at risk the terminal sterilization and also because there is a risk of particulate contamination. "Terminal sterilization" is defined as - *the application of a lethal agent to sealed, finished drug products for the purpose of achieving a predetermined sterility assurance level (SAL) of usually less than 10^{-6} (i.e., a probability of a non sterile unit of greater than one in a million)* [22].

Terminally Sterilized Products

Table 11. Environment requirements for terminally sterilized products.

<table>
<tr><th colspan="2">Type of operation</th><th>Minimal required environment grade/class</th></tr>
<tr><td colspan="2">In general, preparation of materials and products to obtain low levels of particles and microbes.</td><td rowspan="2">D/ISO 8</td></tr>
<tr><td colspan="2">Environment surrounding the blow/fill/seal (BFS) equipment used for the preparation of products.</td></tr>
<tr><td>In particular, preparation of materials and products in case of high risk of contamination:</td><td>- High susceptibility to microbial growth.
- Product is kept long time before sterilization.
- Product is processed in open recipients.</td><td rowspan="3">C/ISO 7</td></tr>
<tr><td colspan="2">In general, filling of products to obtain low levels of particles and microbes.</td></tr>
<tr><td colspan="2">In general, preparation and filling of sterile ointments, creams, suspensions and emulsions before sterilization.</td></tr>
<tr><td>In particular, filling of products in case of high risk of contamination:</td><td>- Filling process is slow.
- Containers with a wide opening.
- Exposition of the containers during filling for more than a few seconds during closing.</td><td>A/ISO 5 surrounded by B/ISO 7 (at least)</td></tr>
</table>

Aseptically Prepared Products

Table 12. Environmental requirements for aseptically prepared products.

<table>
<tr><th>Type of operation</th><th>Minimal required environment grade/class</th></tr>
<tr><td>Handling of starting materials and of packaging materials (after washing)</td><td rowspan="3">D/ISO 8</td></tr>
<tr><td>Background environment of an isolator for aseptic processing</td></tr>
<tr><td>Manufacture of pressurized metered dose aerosol preparations for inhalation</td></tr>
</table>

Table 12: contd...

Preparation of solutions that are to be sterilized by filtration.	**C/ISO 7**
Installation of a blow/fill/seal (BFS) unit provided with an effective grade A/ISO 5 air shower	**C/ISO 7** On condition that **A/B/ISO 5** clothing is used
Preparation of materials and products if solutions are not sterilized by filtration.	**A/ISO 5** surrounded by **B/ISO 7** (at least)
Handling and filling of products prepared aseptically.	
Handling of pieces of equipment previously sterilized.	
The transfer of partially closed containers (*e.g.* lyophilization).	
Preparation and filling of sterile ointments, creams, suspensions and emulsions, when the product is exposed without subsequent filtration.	
Before complete stoppering, as used in freeze drying, transfer in sealed transfer trays.	**B/ISO 5**

Ambient Parameters

It is necessary to establish set points and acceptable ranges for the ambient parameters: temperature, humidity, lighting and noise (depending on the products and on the operations). It is necessary taking into account personnel comfort too.

CLEAN ROOM QUALIFICATION

Once the construction of a clean room has been completed, it is necessary to perform trials to verify that it meets predetermined operational requirements.

Usually qualification is performed for all the rooms which make up a clean area and it includes not only testing within the rooms but also the associated external HVAC equipment. The start up of a clean area on completion is preceded by "as built" testing by the supplier as part of the commissioning testing. The aim of this testing is verifying that clean rooms meet their design requirements. Afterwards, when equipment is installed and the rooms are ready for starting production, the company (either by itself or by external technicians) performs "at rest" OQ testing. If tests pass the clean area can be used for production. Then it is possible to perform "dynamic" PQ testing and if everything is correct, the clean area can be deemed qualified. For OQ and PQ testing reference should be made to the methods described in standard ISO 14644 [23, 24]. See Fig. (**4**).

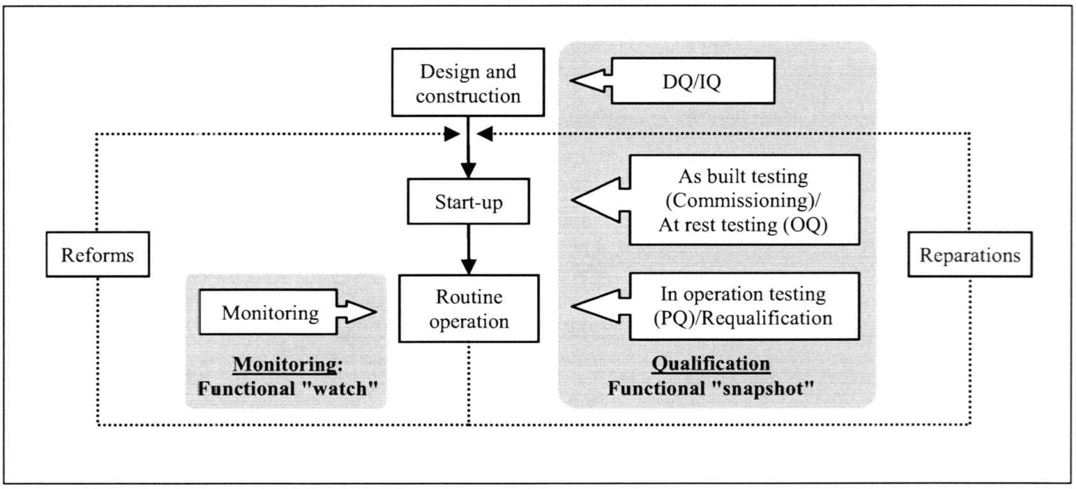

Fig. (4). Cleanroom qualification and monitoring.

Clean Room Qualification Tests

A clean room, from the construction point of view, is the combination of internal architecture and HVAC system (this system is dealt with in chapter 9).

Tests that are described here concern only the clean rooms and are performed within them.

(a) Design Qualification (DQ)

These tests are performed before starting the construction of the clean rooms:

- Verify that the proposed design agrees with the user requirement specification.

- Verify that the proposed design conforms to GMP/GEP.

(b) Installation Qualification (IQ)

- Check each room to its current tally (where its characteristics and fittings are described): size, elements (doors, windows, luminaries, wash basins, *etc.*), points of use of utilities (diffusers, terminal filters, grilles, sockets, water, compressed air, *etc.*).

  The purpose is showing that the finished clean rooms possess all the foreseen elements and fittings (in quality and quantity).

(c) Operational Qualification (OQ)

- Count airborne particles for classification.
- Measure airflow (airflow velocity, supply airflow rate and exchange rate).
- Measure air pressure difference (pressure differentials between rooms and between rooms and outside).
- Verify airflow direction (turbulent airflow)/Visualize airflow (UDAF).
- Verify installed filter leakage.
- Realize recovery test.
- Realize containment leakage test (as appropriate).
- Measure temperature.
- Measure relative humidity (as appropriate).
- Measure lighting.
- Measure noise.

(c) Performance Qualification (PQ)

- Count airborne particles for classification.
- Visualize airflow patterns.
- Measure temperature.
- Measure relative humidity (as appropriate)

Clean room Qualification Methods

Airborne Particle Count

The concentration of airborne particles is used for the classification of clean areas or rooms (Table **13**).

Table 13. Airborne particle count for the classification of clean areas or rooms.

Device/s used	Airborne particle counter by light diffusion. ➢ The probe of the particle counter should be adjusted in a direction that has been shown to obtain representative samples. ➢ *Portable particle counters with a short length of sample tubing should be used for classification purposes because of the relatively higher rate of precipitation of particles ≥5.0 µm in remote sampling systems with long lengths of tubing. Isokinetic sample heads shall be used in unidirectional airflow systems* [25].
Sampling points	The equation gives the minimal number of sampling points (N_L): ➢ For clean rooms with turbulent airflow, A is the total surface (m^2). ➢ For UDAF, A is the area (m^2) of the filter/s. $\mathbf{N_L} = \sqrt{A}$
	➢ As a result of risk analysis an increased number of sampling points may be justified.
Sampling volume	The equation gives the elementary sampling volume in each sampling point (V_s): $\mathbf{V_s} = (20/C_{n,m}) \times 1{,}000$
	$C_{n,m}$ is the number of particles per m^3 for the concerned class.
	➢ If according to the N_L equation there is only one sampling point, it is necessary to sample three times at this point (V_s). ➢ *For classification purposes in Grade A zones, a minimum sample volume of 1m³ should be taken per sample location. For Grade A the airborne particle classification is ISO 4.8 dictated by the limit for particles ≥5.0 µm. For Grade B (at rest) the airborne particle classification is ISO 5 for both considered particle sizes. For Grade C (at rest & in operation) the airborne particle classification is ISO 7 and ISO 8 respectively. For Grade D (at rest) the airborne particle classification is ISO 8. For classification purposes ISO 14644-1 methodology defines both the minimum number of sample locations and the sample size based on the class limit of the largest considered particle size and the method of evaluation of the data collected* [26].

Thus, a clean area or room has its specified airborne particulate classification when mean counts for each sampling point do not exceed the particulate concentration limits established by a given norm (GMP or ISO).

When performing an OQ the sampling points are distributed regularly on the surface of the room (or UDAF), but when realizing a PQ what counts is confirming the particle count in critical areas. Thus, samples should be taken at sites where the potential risk of contamination for the exposed product, for the containers and for the closures is higher.

"In operation" classification may be demonstrated during normal operations, simulated operations or during media fills as worst-case simulation is required for this [27].

Airflow Measurement (Airflow Speed, Supply Airflow Rate and Exchange Rate)

Variations in airflow velocity can cause turbulence and this means that the possibility of contamination is higher.

Periodic monitoring of the airflow speed is important to confirm that the conditions in the critical aseptic processing area are adequate (Tables **14** and **15**).

Table 14. Airflow measurement I (devices and points of measure).

Device/s used	The airflow speed can be measured with anemometers, which can be thermal or valve-type, or with flowhoods. ➢ Thermal anemometers have an electrically heated sensor which, when exposed to the air-flow, enables the determination of the air velocity by measuring the variation in heat transfer. ➢ Valve-type anemometers have a valve that turns when exposed to an air-flow; the revolution rate of the valve determines the air-flow velocity. ➢ Flowhoods collect the air-flow and concentrate it on the flowmeter, which measures an average velocity of the total section. ➢ Anemometers are habitually used for filters and air ducts and flowhoods with flowmeters for diffusers (but can also be used for filters).
Points of measure	The number of points of measure is the square root of ten times the air-flow area, expressed in m^2, but not less than four. $N_L = \sqrt{10 \times S}$ ➢ The air-flow velocity is measured at each measuring point. ➢ The measurement points have to be evenly distributed on the air-flow area. ➢ For each filtering outlet there should be at least one measuring point. ➢ Measures are performed at a distance of 15-30 cm from the surface of the filter. ➢ The speed of unidirectional air in the critical area should be measured at a distance of 15 cm from the HEPA-filter face and at a defined distance close to the work surface ➢ The duration of the measure should be sufficient to ensure a reliable reading. In practical terms, it can be said that the measuring time at each point should be at least 10 seconds, recording its maximum, minimum and average values.

The measurements should correlate to the velocity range established at the time of *in situ* air pattern analysis studies.

The measured speed should be within the speed range determined while performing the air pattern analysis studies.

HEPA filters should be replaced when the air speed across the filter area lacks uniformity or when airflow patterns may be negatively affected.

Table 15. Airflow measurement II (clean rooms, terminal filters/ducts, diffusers).

Measure of clean rooms supply	The measure of the air-flow speed in a clean room enables the determination of its supply air-flow rate and, consequently, its exchange rate (number of air changes per hour). The reports of this test usually indicate average air-flow by point of supply (filter/diffuser, duct), total air-flow (of the room) and the exchange rate (air changes per hour) of the room. The total supply air-flow of the room is obtained by adding the supply air-flows from each existing filter, duct and diffuser in the room. The number of air changes per hour is calculated dividing the total supply air-flow (m^3/hour) by the volume of the room (m^3).
Measure of air supply across terminal filters or ducts	The plane of the flow area (filter) is divided into grid cells of equal area. The centre of each one is a measuring point. The number of grids can be calculated either as the square root of the air-flow area, expressed in m^2, rounded up to a whole number, but no less than four points, or bigger than the square root of the flow area (filter surface), expressed in m^2, the number of measuring points never being less than three. Airflow speed is measured at the centre of each grid cell. The duration of the measure should be sufficient to ensure a reliable reading. In practical terms, it can be said that the measuring time at each point should be of at least 10 seconds, recording its maximum, minimum and average values.
	The equation gives the total supply air-flow rate (**Q**): $\mathbf{V_c}$ = Airflow speed at the centre of each grid cell $\mathbf{Q = \sum (V_c \times A_c)}$ $\mathbf{A_c}$ = Grid cell area
Measure of air supply across diffusers	As turbulences and currents make it very difficult to obtain precise measures with an anemometer, the air-flow velocity and the supply air-flow rate (**Q**) are preferably determined by means of a flowhood with flowmeter. The hood opening has to be placed completely covering the supply opening, to prevent any air bypass.

Air Pressure Difference Measurement

The maintenance of cascades of pressures in clean areas is a vital element for protection against contamination (Table **16**). This is why it is essential to verify that they are as per design and monitor them when production is going on. See chapter 4 for more information on the role of differential pressure.

Table 16. Air pressure difference measurement.

Device used	Differential pressure gauge (manometer).
Procedure	➢ It is advisable to start by measuring the central clean rooms (verifying differences between adjacent rooms) and then move outwards (determining differences in relation to the external environment). ➢ If rooms are provided with *ad hoc* connections it is possible to measure the pressure difference between each room and the external environment (for instance, in relation to the technical zone above the false ceiling).

Airflow Direction Verification (Turbulent Airflow)/Airflow Visualization (Laminar Airflow)

The airflow patterns should not distribute particles from areas of lower classification or from generating points (equipment, persons or processes) towards critical zones of high risk for the products. Even if clean room design is correct, operators and equipment can modify airflows and create stagnant air and turbulences. This is why this is a critical PQ test when particles can affect the quality of the product (e. g. aseptic processing). In case of UDAF this tests allows for showing the direction and regularity of the air-flow. See Table **17**.

Table 17. Airflow patterns visualization.

Device used	Tracer (smoke generator).
Procedure	The generation of an aerosol of droplets enables the visualization of airflows, which can be recorded (video).

Installed Filter Leakage Verification

This test is performed with an oil aerosol and allows verifying that the filter system is properly installed (*i.e.* there are no leaks, neither in the filter media nor in the frame sealant) and that the filter is well fitted (there is no air bypass between the filter and its gasket or the grid system). See Table **18**.

Leak tests are performed for E12 and H13 – H14 filters.

It is important not confusing the above described filter leak verification with efficiency testing, since an efficiency test is a general test used to determine the rating of the filter. An intact HEPA filter should be capable of retaining at least 99.97 percent of particulates greater than 0.3 µm in diameter [28].

This test is not only applied to HEPA filters of clean areas, but also to other HEPA filters (*e.g.* dry heat depyrogenation tunnels and ovens).

Table 18. Air pressure difference measurement.

Devices used	Aerosol generator and photometer.
Procedure	➢ The test is performed by introducing an aerosol challenge upstream of the filters and scanning with the photometer immediately downstream of the filters and support frames. Differences in upstream and downstream aerosol concentrations enable determination of leaks. Aerosol upstream concentration should be at least 10 mg/m^3. The photometer probe should be held at a distance of less than 5 cm from the downstream filter face

Table 18: contd...

	(approximately 3 cm). The filter face scanning is performed over the entire surface (filter, filter perimeter, filter frame and grid structure) by moving the probe slowly sideways (at a scan rate of less than 5 cm/s) and using slightly overlapping strokes. ➢ A single probe measure equivalent to 0.01% (10^{-4}) of the upstream aerosol concentration should be considered as indicative of a significant leak and then a replacement of the HEPA filter is required. When appropriate, repair in a limited area may be acceptable. Afterwards, retesting should show that corrective measures have been adequate. ➢ The aerosol is obtained with DOP (dioctylphthalate), DEHS (di-2-ethyl hexyl sebacate), PAO (poly-alpha olefin) or other equivalent materials (but they should meet specifications for critical physico-chemical attributes such as viscosity and they should not support microbial growth). The polydispersed aerosol is composed of particles with a light-scattering mean droplet diameter in the submicron size range including a sufficient number of particles of about 0.3 µm of diameter.

Recovery Test

The purpose of this test is verifying the capacity of a clean room to eliminate airborne particulates generated during the manufacturing operations. It is realized by determining the time necessary to recover the specified level of airborne particle concentration of the clean room after a short exposure to "dirtiness" (a test aerosol). See Table **19**.

This test is suitable for clean rooms having a turbulent (non laminar) airflow, in order to verify their capacity to recover its cleanliness level by air dilution (supply of clean filtered air and exhaust of dirty air).

Table 19. Recovery test.

Devices used	Aerosol generator and particle discrete-particle counter.
Procedure	➢ The capacity of recovery is determined by establishing the time needed for a reduction in the airborne particulate concentration from 100 to 1 (time needed to decrease the initial level of particle concentration by a factor of 0.01). ➢ It is preferable to determine this time by direct measure of the airborne particulate concentration, but when this is not possible, the evolution rate of the airborne particle concentration is estimated.

European GMP states that *the particle limits given for the "at rest" state should be achieved after a short "clean up" period of 15-20 minutes (guidance value) in an unmanned state after completion of operations* [29].

WHO GMP writes that the *airborne particle conditions for the "at rest" state should be achieved in the absence of the operating personnel after a short "clean-up" or "recovery" period of about 15–20 minutes (guidance value), after completion of the operations* [30].

Containment Leakage Test

The purpose of this test is to determine if there is an invasion of contaminated air (non-filtered air) across joints, junctions, seams, *etc.* See Table **20**.

Table 20. Containment leakage test.

Device used	Aerosol generator and particle discrete-particle counter.
Procedure	➢ The airborne particulate concentration is measured outside the clean room on a site close to the surface or doorway to be evaluated. The outer particle concentration should be greater than the clean room particle concentration by a factor of 10^4. If the concentration is less, then it is increased by generating aerosol. ➢ The concentration of particles inside the clean room is measured at a distance of not more than 5 cm from the enclosure, with a scan rate of less than 5 cm/s. ➢ To check the entrance of contamination at an open doorway, measures are performed at a distance of 0.3 to 1 m from the open door. ➢ The measuring points within the clean room are chosen according to the characteristics of the clean room. All readings greater than 10^{-2} times the measured external aerosol particle concentration are registered.

Temperature Measurement

The purpose of this test is to determine the capacity of the HVAC system to maintain the air temperature within pre-established limits. This test is performed as an OQ test and also as PQ test in order to show that under real production conditions temperature is maintained within its required range (Table **21**).

Table 21. Temperature measurement.

Device used	Thermometer.
Procedure	➢ This test is performed when the HVAC system has reached a state where temperature is stabilized. ➢ It is necessary to measure at least one point per room (when temperature control is a product requirement, there should be at least 3 measuring points). ➢ The temperature probe should be placed at work-level height for at least 5 minutes, with readings and recordings at least every minute.

Relative Humidity Measurement

The purpose of this test is to determine the capacity of the HVAC system to maintain the air humidity within pre-established limits, usually below a certain relative humidity (RH) value (Table **22**).

Table 22. Relative humidity measurement.

Device used	Hygrometer.
Procedure	➢ This test is performed when the HVAC system reaches a state where humidity is stabilized. ➢ It is necessary to measure at least one point per room (when humidity control is a product requirement, there should be at least 3 measuring points). ➢ The hygrometer probe should be placed at work-level height for at least 5 minutes, with readings and recordings taken at least every minute.

Lighting Measurement

Adequate lighting is a GMP requirement (Table **23**).

Table 23. Lighting measurement.

Device used	Luxmeter.
Procedure	➢ It is convenient to measure one point for about each 9 m^2. ➢ At each point it is necessary to take 3 measures ➢ Measures are taken at working level

Noise Measurement

The protection against noise is a HSE requirement (Table **24**).

Table 24. Noise measurement.

Device used	Sonometer.
Procedure	➢ It is convenient to measure one point for about each 9 m^2. ➢ At each point it is necessary to carry out 3 measures. ➢ Measures are carried out at working level.

Clean Room Qualification Report

According to ISO 14644 the report should contain these concepts:

- Information on the person/s who performed the tests (if they were performed by an external organization, besides the names, the address is necessary).
- Date of the test.
- Identification of the premises with diagrams showing the location of the measurement points.

- Performance criteria (acceptance limits), indicating under which condition (occupancy state).
- Test method used (mentioning any special condition or departure from the test method, *etc.*).
- Identification of the test equipment and their current calibration certificate.
- Raw measurement data.
- Test result and a compliance statement.
- Any other relevant information.

CLEAN ROOM REQUALIFICATION

When clean rooms are routinely operated, it is necessary to perform requalifications to prove continued compliance. See Table **25**.

Table 25. Clean room requalification: Tests to prove continued compliance.

Test	Maximum time interval between tests	
Airborne particle count	For class ISO 5/Grade A and B	6 months = average interval not exceeding 183 consecutive operation days (no interval exceeding 190 days)*
	For classes ISO 6 through 8/Grade C and D	12 months = average interval not exceeding 366 consecutive operation days (no interval exceeding 400 days)
Airflow measurement)	For all ISO classes/GMP grades	
Air pressure difference measurement		
Installed filter leakage verification		
Air-flow visualization		
Recovery test		
Containment leakage test		

* When in the clean room is performed continuous or frequent monitoring of airborne particle count and air pressure difference, this interval of time may be extended, but only if the monitoring results meet specified ranges.

Requalifications can be either programmed (when there are neither changes nor problems) or not (after performing changes and before resuming operations, and when problems have been detected). Although standard ISO 14644 provides this information on admissible requalification periodicity, in practice it is advisable to follow a risk assessment approach to establish a requalification program [31].

Standard ISO 14644 also suggests some events which should cause the requalification of a clean room:

- After a remedial action derived from an OOS condition.
- After a significant specification change.
- After a significant operational interruption which may affect its performance.
- After a maintenance operation which may affect its performance (*i.e.* change of terminal filters).

When test results meet requirements the clean room is considered in state of continued compliance.

CLEAN ROOM MONITORING

While qualification spans a very short period of time, monitoring is a long run exercise intending to show that the facilities are kept in state of continued compliance (*i.e.* in state of qualification). Clean room monitoring includes airborne particulate contamination, ambient parameters and microbiology [32].

Airborne Particulate Contamination

On-line particle counters provide information on the environmental cleanliness of a controlled environment while in operation. Standard counters provide information on particle concentration, but cannot differentiate between viable and non-viable particles (there exist, however, counters which are able to count viable particles but are not widely used yet). Experience shows that, roughly speaking, it is possible to say that the less particles (in general) there are, the less microbes (in particular) there are. However, it is not possible to correlate particle counts with microbial counts performed by standard particle counters.

GMP requires continuous particle counting during operation by means of dedicated on-line counters to control the particulate cleanliness in grade A areas and recommends it in other grades. Regular non-viable particle monitoring should be performed during each production shift by means of a remote counting system, which is normally less invasive than portable particle counters.

Physical Parameters

Different parameters like temperature, hygrometry, and pressure can be monitored by installing the appropriate on-line instrumentation. Column or gauge manometers are used both to watch the differential pressure between the rooms and the blocking of absolute filters.

Probes connected to a central system (*i.e.* SCADA) allow an automated control.

FDA recommends that pressure differentials between clean rooms be monitored continuously throughout each shift and frequently recorded. All alarms should be documented and deviations from established limits should be investigated [33].

Microbial Contamination

The estimation of the bioburden on air, equipment, surfaces, floor, walls, clothing and gloves and its trends throughout the time provides direct information on the quality of the manufacturing environment. The regular monitoring of clean areas allows for the detection of strains of resistant microorganisms.

Environmental Monitoring Program

The monitoring of controlled environments is carried out with an environmental monitoring program (Fig. **5**). The purpose of this program is to verify the quality of the air in the process areas (in relation to processed batches) and to detect shifting trends, in order to prevent contamination. This program has to include all the shifts and relevant aspects of work (operators, air, floors, walls, clothing, surfaces in general and particularly the surfaces of equipment which come into contact with the product or its containers and closures).

It is essential that the program should be able to detect changes timely, in order to be able to adopt appropriate preventive measures, before reaching a hazardous threshold. A monitoring program might be composed of the following 6 stages:

(1) Selection of the Sampling Points

A risk analysis allows the establishment of the sampling points. Critical points are selected on the basis of distance to the work site or of surfaces that may come in contact with the product or its containers and closures. These critical areas will require a closer monitoring than those far away from the exposed product, containers or closures, or not coming in contact with them. The procedure should have a list of sampling locations, sampling time (when and how long), sample size (surface, air volume), sampling procedure, alert and action levels, and actions in case of deviation from these levels. In aseptic production it is necessary to prove that critical locations remain sterile. It should be ensured that sampling methods do not contaminate the zones. After critical operations surfaces and personnel should be monitored. Samples of critical surfaces should be taken only after finishing the aseptic operations. Otherwise direct sampling of sterile surfaces could lead to contamination. The results of monitoring should be taken into account when reviewing the batch documentation for release of the finished product.

- Personnel monitoring: Surface samples of the gloves of each operator should be taken every day or in association with every lot manufactured. Surface samples of the gown should also be taken (frequency and location to be determined by risk analysis).

- Environmental monitoring (surfaces): The microbiological contamination of surfaces (floors, walls, equipment and, above all, those coming into contact with the products) should be determined by means of swabs and contact plates. The frequency of sampling is determined by risk analysis.

- Environmental monitoring (air): The microbial quality of air can be assessed by means of active and passive sampling devices. The amount of microorganisms per volume of air can be determined by means of active sampling devices. Instead, passive sampling devices only detect those microorganisms which settle onto the surface of settling plates which are exposed to the environment. These plates, which are Petri dishes containing growth medium, allow only for a qualitative or semi-quantitative air monitoring.

  Risk analysis is essential for obtaining significant results. It is necessary to determine the locations with highest risk for the product and the most appropriate media to detect low levels of microorganisms.

  The length of the exposition of the plates is another critical factor. It has to last enough to allow for the settling of organisms but it should prevent desiccation. The results acquired by passive air sampling should be analyzed in combination with data obtained by other types of sampling.

(2) Establishment of the Sampling Methods

Samples can be obtained by the following three types of procedures,

- Sedimentation: Uncovered Petri plates with growth medium are placed on the sampling points. It is important to ensure that they do not dry while they are exposed. Micro-organisms just "fall" on them (passive sampling).

- Contact: Regular, flat surfaces can be sampled directly by pressing contact plates onto them, known as Rodac (Replicate Organism Detection and Counting) plates. Irregular, uneven surfaces can be sampled by rubbing them with moistened swabs (swabbing). The counting of colonies obtained can be referred to the plate surface or to the swabbed surface (usually it is around 20-30 cm^2).

- Aspiration: Air can be actively sampled by using specialized equipment. Different types of equipment exist. They differ on the way air is absorbed and sent onto the culture medium,

- Air is aspirated through a slit (*i.e.* slit-to-agar sampler);

- Air is aspirated through a perforated plate (*i.e.* sieve impactor, sterilizable microbiological atrium);

- Air is aspirated by a turbine and sent onto a plate or strip (*i.e.* centrifugal sampler);

- Air is aspirated and sent to a plate surface (*i.e.* surface air system sampler);

- Air is aspirated through a gelatin filter and the trapped microbes can be subsequently liberated by dissolution of the gelatin and be counted.

(3) Definition of the Sampling Program

Sampling programs for a given controlled environment should be established with a two-stage rationale. As a start-up, risk assessment and qualification provide information on sampling points and methods. Then, subsequent experience will dictate the need for adjustments.

Monitoring is performed in order to ensure the quality of the operating environment. Thus, monitoring should be associated to manufacturing by providing, for each manufactured batch, information on the environment. A batch cannot be liberated without assessing the environmental quality during production (results from monitoring should be taken into account during the review of batch documentation which precedes the release of a finished product and this includes surfaces and personnel after critical operations). In other words, for grade A and B zones sampling has to be permanent during production, whereas for the other less critical grades (C and D) it can range from twice to once a week, depending on the criticality level.

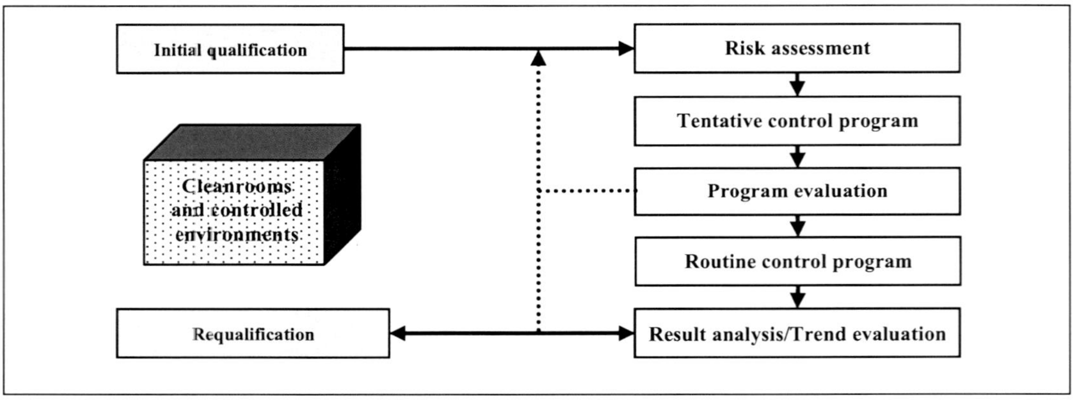

Fig. (5). Rationale of an environmental control program.

(4) Designation of Action Limits

Taking into account GMP and pharmacopoeial recommendations, results obtained during monitoring and risk analysis it is possible to set adequate limits (alert and action) for the routine monitoring of particles and microorganisms. Procedures should also define the corrective actions to be taken in case of excursion.

"Alert limit" can be defined as *an established microbial or airborne particle level giving early warning of potential drift from normal operating conditions and triggers appropriate scrutiny and follow-up to address the potential problem. Alert levels are always lower than action levels. Whereas "action limit" is an established microbial or airborne particle level that, when exceeded, should trigger appropriate investigation and corrective action based on the investigation* [34].

Changes in the quality of the environment are quickly detected by an adequate monitoring system and this allows for the implementation of corrective measures before reaching inadequate environmental conditions for the operations.

The limits for microbial monitoring should be related to the operations because they intend maintaining an adequate environmental control in the manufacturing premises. It is evident that sampling points closer to the work points should have more restrictive limits and those close to points where critical operations are performed should have the strictest limits. As said before, historical data (*e.g.* routine monitoring, qualification, media fills, sanitization studies, historical data from similar operations, *etc.*) should be taken into account when establishing monitoring limits. See Table **26**.

Table 26. Sample incubation [35].

Total count	Incubation (temperature/time)
Total aerobic bacterial count	30-35°C/48-72 h
Total combined yeast and mould count	20-25°C/5-7 days

Different recommended limits, expressed in "colony forming units", for the microbiological contamination in clean areas during operation have been proposed.

A "colony forming unit" or "cfu" is a microbiological term that describes the formation of a single macroscopic colony after the introduction of one or more microorganisms to microbiological growth media. One colony forming unit is expressed as 1 CFU [36].

WHO/Europe GMP recommend the following limits for microbial contamination (Table **27**):

Table 27. Monitoring of microbiological contamination in clean rooms (in operation/operational.

Recommended limits for microbial contamination (average values) (WHO GMP [37]/European GMP [38])				
Class	**Active air sampling (cfu/m³)**	**Settle plates/Ø 90 mm (cfu/4 hours) ***	**Contact plates/Ø 55 mm (cfu/plate)**	**Glove print/5 fingers (cfu/glove)**
A	< 1	< 1	< 1	< 1
B	10	5	5	5
C	100	50	25	---
D	200	100	50	---
* Individual settle plates may be exposed for less than 4 hours				

Whereas US CGMP recommends the following action levels for microbiological contamination (Table **28**):

Table 28. Monitoring of microbiological contamination in clean rooms (in operation/operational).

<table>
<tr><th colspan="7">Recommended action levels for microbiological contamination
(US FDA Guidance for Industry – Sterile drug products produced by aseptic processing) [39]</th></tr>
<tr><th rowspan="2">Class</th><th colspan="2">Particles ≥ 0,5 µm</th><th rowspan="2">Active air sampling (ufc/m^3)</th><th rowspan="2">Settle plates/ Ø 90 mm (cfu/4 hours)</th><th rowspan="2">Contact plates/"swabs"</th><th rowspan="2">Glove print/5 fingers</th></tr>
<tr><th>/foot</th><th>/m^3</th></tr>
<tr><td>ISO 5</td><td>100</td><td>3,520</td><td>1*</td><td>1*</td><td rowspan="4">Product contact surfaces, floors, walls, and equipment should be tested on a regular basis.</td><td rowspan="4">Monitoring should be accomplished by obtaining surface samples of each operator's gloves on a daily basis, or in association with each lot. This sampling should be accompanied by an appropriate sampling frequency for other strategically selected locations of the gown.</td></tr>
<tr><td>ISO 6</td><td>1,000</td><td>35,200</td><td>7</td><td>3</td></tr>
<tr><td>ISO 7</td><td>10,000</td><td>352,000</td><td>10</td><td>5</td></tr>
<tr><td>ISO 8</td><td>100,000</td><td>3,520,000</td><td>100</td><td>50</td></tr>
<tr><td colspan="7">* Samples from Class 100 (ISO 5) environments should normally yield no microbiological contaminants.</td></tr>
</table>

(5) Establishment of an OOS Plan

In case of non-conformity during monitoring, the procedure that should be followed is the same that is applied during qualification. The installation should be considered as non-compliant and a corrective action has to be implemented followed by requalification. Written procedures should prescribe which actions should be taken when limits (alert and action) are surpassed. They should detail the data review frequency and the corrective and preventive actions to be applied.

(6) Implementation of the Program

Procedures should also describe how the responsible managers will be regularly informed about the trends of monitoring and the results of the investigation in case of excursions.

It is well known that there are operations which produce great amounts of particles. Then during monitoring it is difficult to distinguish these particles from air contaminants. In these cases typical sampling close to the point of operation (30 cm) can be substituted by sampling at a position that detects environmental contamination instead of product powder. It is also useful to take as baseline data the results of the initial qualification of the line under operational conditions but without the product which generates the particles.

Table 29. Relations between clothing and the type of zone in a pharmaceutical plant.

<table>
<tr><th colspan="2" rowspan="2">Type of zone</th><th colspan="2">Classification</th><th rowspan="2">Clothing</th></tr>
<tr><th>ISO 14644</th><th>WHO/Europe GMP</th></tr>
<tr><td colspan="2">Non pharmaceutical</td><td>Non classified</td><td>Non classified</td><td>Normal outdoor clothing</td></tr>
<tr><td rowspan="4">Pharmaceutical</td><td>Non controlled</td><td>Non classified</td><td>Non classified</td><td>Undefined. Protective clothing used for identification and fit for operations (e.g. overall). Shoes should be covered with overshoes or appropriate internal shoes should be worn.</td></tr>
<tr><td>Controlled</td><td>8</td><td>D</td><td>Protective clothing (e.g. overall) should be worn. Street shoes should be covered with overshoes or use appropriate internal shoes.
The hair and beard and moustache, as necessary, should be covered. It is necessary to take appropriate measures to impede the ingress of contamination from outside the clean area.</td></tr>
<tr><td>Protected</td><td>7</td><td>C</td><td>A one-piece garment of trousers and top gathered at the wrists and provided with a high neck should be worn. Street shoes should be covered with overshoes or use appropriate internal shoes.
The hair and beard and moustache, as necessary, should be covered.
The clothing should shed neither fibers nor particulate matter.</td></tr>
<tr><td>Critical</td><td>5</td><td>A/B</td><td>Headgear should totally enclose the hair and, where relevant, beard and moustache. A one-piece jumpsuit, gathered at the wrists and with a high neck, should be worn. The headgear should be tucked into the neck of the suit. A facemask should be worn to prevent the shedding of droplets. Sterilized, non-powdered gloves of appropriate material and sterilized or disinfected footwear should be worn. Trouser-bottoms should be tucked inside the footwear and garment sleeves into the gloves. The protective clothing should shed virtually no fibers or particulate matter and should retain particles shed by the body [40].</td></tr>
</table>

CLEAN ROOM CLOTHING

It has already been indicated that human body is a very important source of contamination by particles. Brisk movements should be avoided as far as it is possible because they increase particle shedding. Clothing retains particles set free by the body and impedes their liberation to the environment. This is why the type of clothing is related to the cleanliness requirements of the process (Table **29**).

Gloves should be frequently disinfected during the operations. Both gloves and masks should be changed every working session.

Personal clothing should not be introduced in clean areas or changing rooms leading to clean areas of grade A/B or C (they should remain in the changing rooms before grade D). The processes of change of clothing and sanitization should follow written procedures with the aim of reducing the contamination of the clean areas.

Neither jewels nor wrist watches should be worn in clean areas. Cosmetics shedding particles should not be used by people working in clean areas.

Operators working in clean areas of class A or B/ISO 5 should receive clean and sterilized clothing every working session.

CONCLUDING REMARKS

Premises provide physical support to the facilities where pharmaceutical products are manufactured, but also isolate and determine the flows of personnel, materials, products and waste. Within the premises clean rooms are devised to protect products from contamination when they are exposed to the environment. This is possible because of different concurrent strategies. Firstly, clean rooms are built in a "sanitary manner" regarding partitions and floors with the object of not shedding particles and of being able to be thoroughly cleaned and, if necessary, sanitized. Secondly, clean rooms are ventilated with filtered air and this allows the control of its environment in terms of particles, airflows and ambient parameters. And thirdly, personnel wear protective clothing with the aim of limiting as much as possible the shedding of particles and the transfer of contamination.

The characteristics of the materials, the products and the operations which are realized within these clean rooms determine the particular environmental characteristics of the clean rooms and of the type of clothing to be worn by personnel.

Qualification and permanent monitoring of the clean rooms ensure that they work as purported.

CONFLICT OF INTEREST

The author confirms that this chapter contents have no conflict of interest.

ACKNOWLEDGEMENT

Declared None.

REFERENCES

[1] WHO (World Health Organization). WHO Good manufacturing practices for pharmaceutical products: main principles. In: WHO Expert Committee on Specifications for Pharmaceutical Preparations. Forty-eighth report (WHO Technical Report Series, No. 986). WHO, Geneva, Switzerland 2014. Annex 2. Glossary.

[2] IES (Institute of Environmental Sciences). U.S. General Services Administration. Federal Standard 209E. Airborne Particulate Cleanliness Classes in Cleanrooms and Clean Zones. IES, Mount Prospect, Illinois, USA 1992.

[3] ISO (International Organization for Standardization). Cleanrooms and associated controlled environments. Part 1: Classification of air cleanliness. International standard ISO 14644-1:1999(en). ISO, Geneva, Switzerland 1999.

[4] WHO (World Health Organisation). Good manufacturing practices for sterile pharmaceutical products. In: WHO Expert Committee on Specifications for Pharmaceutical Preparations. Forty-fifth report (WHO Technical Report Series, No. 961). WHO, Geneva, Switzerland 2011. 4.6.1.

[5] European Commission. Enterprise and Industry Directorate. Manufacture of Sterile Medicinal Products. In: EudraLex. The Rules Governing Medicinal Products in the European Union. Volume 4. EU Guidelines to Good Manufacturing Practice. Medicinal Products for Human and Veterinary Use. European Commission, Brussels, Belgium 2008. Annex 1. 4.

[6] U.S. Department of Health and Human Services. Food and Drug Administration. Center for Drug Evaluation and Research (CDER). Center for Biologics Evaluation and Research (CBER). Office of Regulatory Affairs (ORA). Sterile drug products produced by aseptic processing – Current Good Manufacturing Practice. Guidance for Industry. FDA, Rockville, MD, USA 2004. IV.

[7] ISO (International Organization for Standardization). Cleanrooms and associated controlled environments. Part 4: Design, construction and start-up. International standard ISO 14644-4:2001(en). ISO, Geneva, Switzerland 2001.

[8] WHO (World Health Organisation). WHO guidelines on good manufacturing practices for heating, ventilation and air-conditioning systems for non-sterile pharmaceutical dosage forms. In: WHO Expert Committee on Specifications for Pharmaceutical Preparations. Forty-fiftieth report (WHO Technical Report Series, No. 961). WHO, Geneva, Switzerland 2011. Annex 5. 4.2.

[9] Ibid. 4.1.6.

[10] U.S. Department of Health and Human Services. Food and Drug Administration. Center for Drug Evaluation and Research (CDER). Center for Biologics Evaluation and Research (CBER). Office of Regulatory Affairs (ORA). Sterile drug products produced by aseptic processing – Current Good Manufacturing Practice. Guidance for Industry. FDA, Rockville, MD, USA 2004. IV. B.

[11] European Commission. Enterprise and Industry Directorate. Manufacture of Sterile Medicinal Products. In: EudraLex. The Rules Governing Medicinal Products in the European Union. Volume 4. EU Guidelines to Good Manufacturing Practice. Medicinal Products for Human and Veterinary Use. European Commission, Brussels, Belgium 2008. Annex 1. 3.

[12] U.S. Department of Health and Human Services. Food and Drug Administration. Center for Drug Evaluation and Research (CDER). Center for Biologics Evaluation and Research (CBER). Office of Regulatory Affairs (ORA). Sterile drug products produced by aseptic processing – Current Good Manufacturing Practice. Guidance for Industry. FDA, Rockville, MD, USA 2004. IV. A.

[13] European Commission. Enterprise and Industry Directorate. Manufacture of Sterile Medicinal Products. In: EudraLex. The Rules Governing Medicinal Products in the European Union. Volume 4. EU Guidelines to Good Manufacturing Practice. Medicinal Products for Human and Veterinary Use. European Commission, Brussels, Belgium 2008. Annex 1. 53.

[14] WHO (World Health Organisation). WHO guidelines on good manufacturing practices for heating, ventilation and air-conditioning systems for non-sterile pharmaceutical dosage forms. In: WHO

Expert Committee on Specifications for Pharmaceutical Preparations. Forty-fiftieth report (WHO Technical Report Series, No. 961). WHO, Geneva, Switzerland 2011. Annex 5. 4. 7. 11.

[15] ISO (International Organization for Standardization). Cleanrooms and associated controlled environments. Part 5: Operations. International standard ISO 14644-5:2004(en). ISO, Geneva, Switzerland 2004.

[16] WHO (World Health Organisation). WHO guidelines on good manufacturing practices for heating, ventilation and air-conditioning systems for non-sterile pharmaceutical dosage forms. In: WHO Expert Committee on Specifications for Pharmaceutical Preparations. Forty-fiftieth report (WHO Technical Report Series, No. 961). WHO, Geneva, Switzerland 2011. Annex 5.

[17] WHO (World Health Organisation). Good manufacturing practices for sterile pharmaceutical products. In: WHO Expert Committee on Specifications for Pharmaceutical Preparations. Forty-fiftieth report (WHO Technical Report Series, No. 961). WHO, Geneva, Switzerland 2011. Annex 6.

[18] European Commission. Enterprise and Industry Directorate. Manufacture of Sterile Medicinal Products. In: EudraLex. The Rules Governing Medicinal Products in the European Union. Volume 4. EU Guidelines to Good Manufacturing Practice. Medicinal Products for Human and Veterinary Use. European Commission, Brussels, Belgium 2008. Annex 1.

[19] U.S. Department of Health and Human Services. Food and Drug Administration. Center for Drug Evaluation and Research (CDER). Center for Biologics Evaluation and Research (CBER). Office of Regulatory Affairs (ORA). Sterile drug products produced by aseptic processing – Current Good Manufacturing Practice. Guidance for Industry. FDA, Rockville, MD, USA 2004.

[20] Ibid. IV. B.

[21] Ibid. IV. B.

[22] Ibid. Glossary.

[23] ISO (International Organization for Standardization). Cleanrooms and associated controlled environments. Part 2: Specifications for testing and monitoring continued compliance with ISO 14644-1. International standard ISO 14644-2:2000(en). ISO, Geneva, Switzerland 2000.

[24] ISO (International Organization for Standardization). Cleanrooms and associated controlled environments. Part 3: Test methods. International standard ISO 14644-3:2005(en). ISO, Geneva, Switzerland 2005.

[25] European Commission. Enterprise and Industry Directorate. Manufacture of Sterile Medicinal Products. In: EudraLex. The Rules Governing Medicinal Products in the European Union. Volume 4. EU Guidelines to Good Manufacturing Practice. Medicinal Products for Human and Veterinary Use. European Commission, Brussels, Belgium 2008. Annex 1. 6.

[26] Ibid. 5.

[27] Ibid. 7.

[28] U.S. Department of Health and Human Services. Food and Drug Administration. Center for Drug Evaluation and Research (CDER). Center for Biologics Evaluation and Research (CBER). Office of Regulatory Affairs (ORA). Sterile drug products produced by aseptic processing – Current Good Manufacturing Practice. Guidance for Industry. FDA, Rockville, MD, USA 2004. IV. D. 2.

[29] European Commission. Enterprise and Industry Directorate. Manufacture of Sterile Medicinal Products. In: EudraLex. The Rules Governing Medicinal Products in the European Union. Volume 4. EU Guidelines to Good Manufacturing Practice. Medicinal Products for Human and Veterinary Use. European Commission, Brussels, Belgium 2008. Annex 1. 14.

[30] WHO (World Health Organisation). Good manufacturing practices for sterile pharmaceutical products. In: WHO Expert Committee on Specifications for Pharmaceutical Preparations. Forty-fifth report (WHO Technical Report Series, No. 961). WHO, Geneva, World Health Organization 2011. 4.7.5.

[31] ISO (International Organization for Standardization). Cleanrooms and associated controlled environments. Part 2: Specifications for testing and monitoring continued compliance with ISO 14644-1. International standard ISO 14644-2:2000(en). ISO, Geneva, Switzerland 2000.

[32] PDA (Parenteral Drug Association). Fundamentals of an environmental monitoring program. Technical Report No. 13. Revised. PDA, Bethesda, MD, USA 2014.

[33] U.S. Department of Health and Human Services. Food and Drug Administration. Center for Drug Evaluation and Research (CDER). Center for Biologics Evaluation and Research (CBER). Office of

Regulatory Affairs (ORA). Sterile drug products produced by aseptic processing – Current Good Manufacturing Practice. Guidance for Industry. FDA, Rockville, MD, USA 2004. IV. C.
[34] Ibid. Glossary.
[35] Ibid. X. B.
[36] Ibid. Glossary.
[37] WHO (World Health Organisation). Good manufacturing practices for sterile pharmaceutical products. In: WHO Expert Committee on Specifications for Pharmaceutical Preparations. Forty-fifth report (WHO Technical Report Series, No. 961). Geneva, World Health Organization 2011. 4.9.
[38] European Commission. Enterprise and Industry Directorate. Manufacture of Sterile Medicinal Products. In: EudraLex. The Rules Governing Medicinal Products in the European Union. Volume 4. EU Guidelines to Good Manufacturing Practice. Medicinal Products for Human and Veterinary Use. European Commission, Brussels, Belgium 2008. Annex 1. 19.
[39] U.S. Department of Health and Human Services. Food and Drug Administration. Center for Drug Evaluation and Research (CDER). Center for Biologics Evaluation and Research (CBER). Office of Regulatory Affairs (ORA). Sterile drug products produced by aseptic processing – Current Good Manufacturing Practice. Guidance for Industry. FDA, Rockville, MD, USA 2004. IV.
[40] European Commission. Enterprise and Industry Directorate. Manufacture of Sterile Medicinal Products. In: EudraLex. The Rules Governing Medicinal Products in the European Union. Volume 4. EU Guidelines to Good Manufacturing Practice. Medicinal Products for Human and Veterinary Use. European Commission, Brussels, Belgium 2008. Annex 1. 43

Chapter 9: Utilities

CHAPTER 9

Utilities

Abstract: Utilities are the blood who keeps alive and functional a pharmaceutical plant. Utility systems are very diverse and range from electricity to compressed air but they share the common fact of possessing points of use. They can be divided into "industrial" utilities which may interact with equipment but not with products and "pharmaceutical" utilities that may interrelate with both. These latter are critical and as such they have to be qualified and closely monitored. This is the only way for ensuring that they do not affect negatively the quality of the products. Utilities are normally tailor-made for each plant and as such a good study of their design is essential. Two utilities are particularly relevant: HVAC and water for pharmaceutical use. The HVAC system, in combination with the internal architecture, provides the controlled setting for the development of the pharmaceutical operations. Any failure puts at risk the production environment. The water for pharmaceutical use is a utility which provides water for cleaning but also water for compounding. This latter function turns water into a very particular starting material. It is obtained *in situ* and differently from other starting materials it is often used before formal sampling, testing and liberation by QC. This explains why it is one of the points of highest level of risk in a pharmaceutical plant. This chapter analyzes all these aspects and provides keys to the most effective approaches for protecting the quality of products.

Keywords: AHU, biofilm, compressed air, dehumidifier, dew point, distiller, dust exhaust, EDI, HVAC, lighting, nitrogen, passivation, pipework, P&IDs, point of use, RO, steam, storage, water for pharmaceutical use, welding.

INTRODUCTION TO THE PHARMACEUTICAL UTILITIES

Utilities are energies or fluids which are necessary for the functioning of equipment (*e.g.* electricity, gas, steam, compressed air, *etc.*) or for the appropriate development of the operations (*e.g.* lighting, HVAC, dust exhaust, *etc.*). By the collective name of utility systems (or simply, utilities) we design a rather quite heterogeneous group of systems that support production either directly or indirectly. Any factory can have several utilities and as such pharmaceutical plants too. However, from the GMP point of view only "pharmaceutical" or "critical" utilities count. That is, only utilities which may have an influence on the quality of the pharmaceutical products are required to meet predetermined specifications.

Physical contact with the product is usually considered the key factor in determining the criticality of a utility. Thus, for example, compressed air is critical when used to push stoppers into a filling machine (because it might

Jordi Botet

contaminate the stoppers, which in turn, might contaminate the products), but it is not critical when used just to activate a valve. In the first case compressed air is required to have pharmaceutical quality, whereas in the second its quality doesn't matter and appropriate pressure is its only requisite.

In a pharmaceutical plant, any utility susceptible of being critical must be considered as such. A quality risk assessment may help to determine it (Table **1**).

Table 1. Simplified example of quality risk assessment of utilities.

Topic	***E.g.* electricity**	***E.g.* compressed air**	
		pharmaceutical	**industrial**
Is it likely any contact between utility and product?	N. a.	Yes	No
Can this utility affect the quality of the product?	No	Yes (contamination)	No
Does a utility failure affect the manufacturing process?	Yes (equipment stop)	Yes (equipment stop)	
Key preventive measures	Install a generator. Qualify equipment to show that stop and restart do not affect the product	Qualify compressed air. Install a supplementary air-compressor. Qualify equipment to show that stop and restart do not affect the product	

A critical operation is *an operation in the manufacturing process that may cause variation in the quality of the pharmaceutical product* [1].

Thus the following utilities are normally considered "critical":

- Electrical supply (it is a particular case, but it should be ensured that critical equipment do not stop because an interruption on mains electricity supply);
- HVAC;
- Dust collection;
- Pharmaceutical water;
- Pharmaceutical steam;
- Pharmaceutical compressed air;

- Medicinal gases;
- Light (it should be considered critical because inadequate lighting can lead to inappropriate work).

Characteristics of the Utilities

In a utility system up to three parts or subsystems can be distinguished (Fig. **1**):

- Generation: The fluid/energy is produced in the same pharmaceutical unit (*e.g.* steam generation from mains water) or in a specific production factory (*e.g.* pressurized nitrogen in cylinders).
- Storage: When this is possible the fluid/energy is stored to be used when necessary.
- Distribution: The fluid/energy is supplied at the points of use. Utilities that can be stored have a closed network or loop, with return to storage, whereas those which cannot be stored have a unidirectional pipe or network which finishes at the use points. The existence of a distribution network is the most visible characteristic of a utility [2].

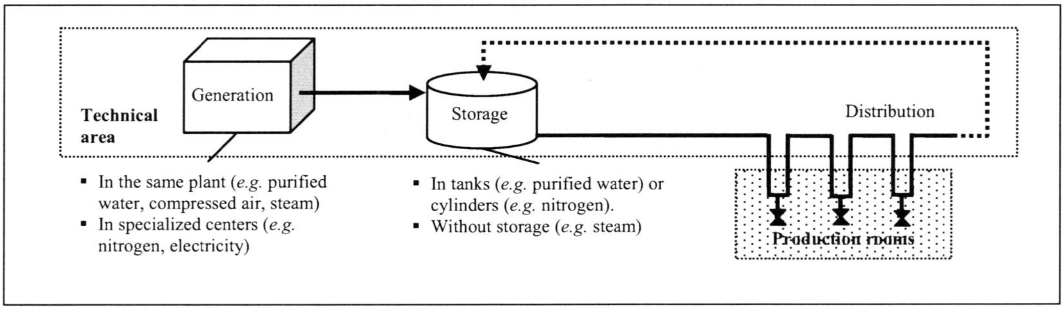

Fig. (1). Parts that compose a utility system.

In order to avoid recesses, the only elements of the system that are located inside the production zones are normally the use points, whereas the other elements are placed in technical zones. Pipework should be designed and sited to avoid the creation of recesses which are difficult to clean.

Any wet surface is prone to be colonized by microorganisms (unless protected by the addition of biocides) [3]. Colonies that adhere to a surface are known as "biofilm" (*i.e.* biological film). Some utility systems offer good possibilities for the development of biofilms which can contaminate the products and provoke the appearance of corrosion spots in metallic pipes. Several factors acting together allow the development of biofilm:

- Contamination of water by bacteria. This is a probable event because certain species such as *Pseudomonas* are ubiquitous and need very few nutrients in the water to survive;

- Passive dispersion of bacteria within the pipework due to the water flow;

- Active displacement of bacteria due to the existence of flagellated species;

- Secretion of extracellular polymers that allow sticking to the substrate and provide protection against biocides;

- Hides acting as "bridge heads" for the colonization of the pipes of a network (*i.e.* rough surface, small pits, death legs, cracks, non flash gaskets, *etc.*).

Pipework may be contaminated by bacteria which stick to surfaces protected from the water current, initially by electrostatic forces and, afterwards, by secretion of extracellular polymeric substances.

Cells start multiplying within a gelatinous matrix of polysaccharide. This is specifically the "biofilm" that protects their bacteria and captures others by electrostatic attraction or because they "fall" into it. A species like *Pseudomonas aeruginosa* may colonize a network in seconds and a mature biofilm can exist in a few hours. Bacteria can adhere to very different materials (steel, polymeric) even if they have been polished. The nutritional needs of bacteria are so restricted that any type of water can sustain a biofilm.

A mature biofilm is almost a "living tissue":

- Fixed bacteria – in comparison with free forms – are remarkably adapted (for instance, their wall has a different protein composition);

- Different species may coexist in the same biofilm and one can use the metabolism subproducts of the other. Besides the different enzymes produced can increase their metabolic capacity;

- The surface of the biofilm is occupied by aerobic bacteria, whereas anaerobic bacteria can develop in depth;
- The polysaccharide matrix contributes to seizing nutrients existing in water;
- Bacteria of a biofilm, due to the polysaccharides, have an increased resistance to sanitizing agents, in comparison with free forms.

As pipework is prone to contamination by bacteria when appropriate conditions exist, design and construction of pharmaceutical utility systems are extremely important. Although biofilms are mainly a problem in water piping, it should not be forgotten that water stagnation points in any pipe can be accessed by bacteria and become a contamination focus. This may happen, for instance, in utilities such as steam or compressed air, when there is water condensation in the lower parts of the system.

Pipework obviously is made to measure and this implies cutting and welding different parts with the corresponding risk of cracks, small pits, oxidation, *etc.* and this favors nesting of microorganisms and development of biofilms. This is why, as far as possible, pipework is built with prefabricated parts ("T", "L", *etc.*) or elements (valves, heat exchangers, pumps, gauges, *etc.*). This contributes in limiting the amount of welding performed *in situ*.

Dimensions of parts (pipes, ducts, valves, *etc.*) may be given in metric (DN) or Anglo-Saxon (NPS) units (Table **2**).

Table 2. Approximate equivalences between DN "Nominal Diameter" and NPS "Nominal Pipe Size".

ND (mm)	6	8	10	15	20	25	32	40	50	65	80	100	150	200
NPS (inch)	1/8	1/4	3/8	½	3/4	1	1 ¼	1 ½	2	2 ½	3	4	6	8

Utility systems, as they have been built, are represented in a P&ID ("Piping and Instrumentation Diagram") identifying any element with a reference or code. P&IDs show not only the items (instruments, pieces of equipment, valves, filters, pipes, *etc.*), but also their interrelations and the flow directions.

The elements which compose a utility system have to be identified with a tag containing the above mentioned reference or code. Fixed pipework should be labeled to indicate the contents and, where applicable, the direction of flow. Besides, points of use are recognized with the name of the utility and dangerous gases and liquids should be provided with non-interchangeable connections or adaptors for impeding mix-ups [4].

Pipework Building

Pharmaceutical utilities are built with materials adequate for product contact. The material of choice for the construction of pipework is 316L stainless steel. Polymeric materials are sometimes an alternative (need of water without metal, cost reduction, *etc.*). In any case, it is evident that the construction material influences the final characteristics of the pipework. The sulphur content in stainless steel has a marked influence on welding. Little differences in sulphur, as low as 0.001%, may produce different welding profiles, because the distribution of temperature depends on the content of sulphur ("Maragoni effect").

Additives modify the properties of polymeric materials, but they can be a source of contamination for the products in contact with the pipework too.

In comparison to stainless steel, polymeric materials have, generally speaking, the following advantages: low price, easy manipulation, and remarkable chemical resistance, but also the disadvantage of low heat dissipation and of not standing sterilization by heat. Vinyl polychloride (PVC), polypropylene (PP) and polyvinylidene fluoride (PVDF) are among the most frequently used polymeric materials.

Pipework should have a constant and regular gauge, inner pipe surfaces should be smooth (have an appropriate finish) and be free of irregularities (joints, cracks, pores, *etc.*), known colloquially as "bug traps", where products may accumulate and biofilms develop. A good surface is obtained by using materials of quality (because of their composition and finish) and by following the appropriate building procedures (Fig. **2**).

The requirement for material quality is usually fulfilled by getting certificates from suppliers concerning both materials and procedures (it must be remembered that smooth surfaces, free of irregularities, are not only obtained by using appropriate materials, but also as a result of their handling and, very particularly, of their welding). Parts should be protected during their transportation and storage before the construction of pipework. Welding quality is compromised by dirt and rust. Cutting can damage the pipe, especially if the construction material is stainless steel. It can create oxidation spots as a result of excess heating. An orbital cutting machine, with a sharp cutting edge, should be used [5].

Welding

Pipes after being cut at definite lengths are connected to the different elements and parts to build a network. This can be done in a permanent way by welding or by temporary sanitary connection.

(a) Stainless Steel

Nowadays the standard for building pharmaceutical permanent pipeworks of stainless steel is "tungsten inert gas (TIG) orbital welding". Its advantages derive from its characteristics:

- "Autogenous", that is, both parts are bonded by fusion, without adding external materials;
- It is made at controlled temperature with a non-consumable tungsten electrode;
- It is realized at controlled speed thanks to an automatic orbital welding system;
- It is performed within inert environment, usually argon. The welding head entirely encompasses the parts to be welded that are surrounded by argon. Should the stainless steel not be protected from oxygen (inside and outside of the pipe the content in oxygen should be under 500 ppm) during welding, chromium and carbon would be oxidized and give chromium carbide ("coking"), and this means reduced corrosion resistance.

Pipes to be welded should belong to the same manufacturing batch in order to ensure that they have exactly the same sulphur content. This allows for the production of smooth, regular and not oxidized (no visible coking) welds.

(b) Polymeric Materials

High frequency welding is considered for polymeric materials the equivalent of TIG orbital welding, because it is also autogenous (welding is achieved by thermofusion) and yields high quality unions. Instead, the union of polymeric parts by means of an adhesive is unacceptable for pharmaceutical use because joints are neither smooth nor regular and possess cracks and pores.

Cleaning and Passivation

When the construction of a pipework has been completed, it has to be cleaned with water and detergent to eliminate the residues of the welding process and of fatty dirt [6].

Besides, welded stainless steel parts have lost their protective layer of chromium oxide. To reconstruct this protective layer, the system is washed with an oxidizing solution (for instance a solution of nitric or citric acid with organic chelating agents). Then the chromium surface is oxidized and a new layer of chromium oxide appears. The system is finally washed with demineralized or purified water, so as to eliminate any trace of acid.

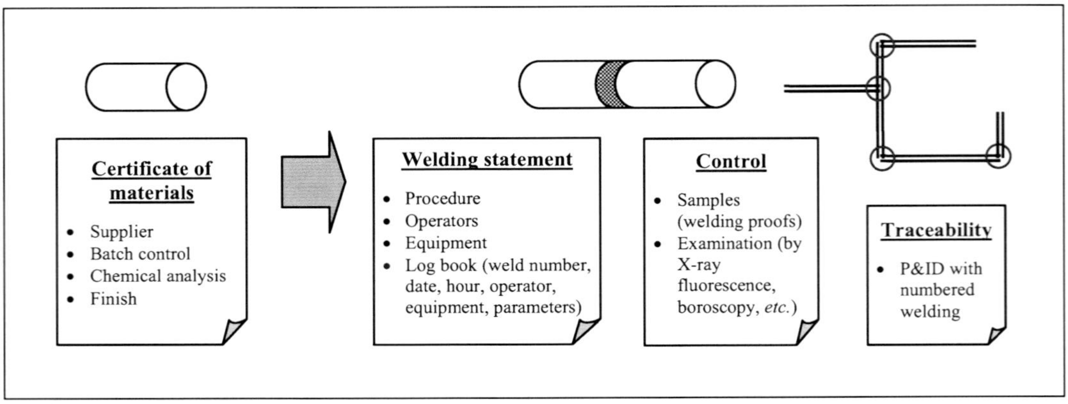

Fig. (2). Attestation of stainless steel pipework "quality" made by TIG orbital welding.

Pumps

Pumps are used to force liquids along pipework and to obtain the appropriate flow at the points of use. These pumps have to fulfill the same "hygienic" requirements as the other elements of the system in contact with the liquid:

- The construction material of the parts in contact with the liquid should satisfy the above-mentioned requirements. Usually they are made of stainless steel. Shaft seals must be of such a design as to isolate the liquid from the mechanical parts of the pump and avoid contamination;

- Material of parts contacting the liquids should have appropriate finish;

- A design ensuring absence of dead spaces and dead legs where liquid might stagnate (see chapter 10).

- In systems with several pumps operating alternately it is necessary to keep in mind that a stopped pump is a stagnation spot and this means risk of contamination.

Pumps used for liquids belong to two main types:

Centrifugal pumps, in which the movement of liquid is a consequence of the increase in energy produced by centrifugal force. They consist of an impeller, an intake at its centre and a casing surrounding the impeller. When the impeller rotates, the liquid is discharged by centrifugal force into the casing. The liquid leaves the impeller with higher velocity and pressure that it had when it entered. Centrifugal pumps are neither appropriate for viscous liquids nor for emulsions (risk of phase separation), but can be used for liquids with suspended solids.

Whereas, in positive-displacement pumps the liquid moves because of a change in volume. In this type of pumps, the displacement of a movable part within the body of the pump impels the liquid. The movement of the movable part may be rotational or alternative. Positive-displacement pumps can be used for viscous liquids and emulsions.

Filters

Filters are used to remove particles, both inert and viable, from liquids and gases Filters should neither shed fibers nor affect the product, either by removing ingredients from it ("extractables") or by releasing substances into it ("leachables"). Asbestos-containing filters, which had been used in the past, are not allowed anymore.

The integrity of the filter should be checked by an appropriate method such as bubble-point, diffusive-flow or pressure-hold test.

When a manufacturing process comprises filtration, the same filter should not be used for more than one working day unless such use has been validated.

Gas filters should be maintained dry, because condensates can cause blockage during use or allow for the growth of microorganisms. This problem can be prevented by using hydrophobic filters and by keeping them heated. Filters that serve as sterile boundaries (*e.g.* in a tank) or supply sterile gases should be integrity tested upon installation and periodically thereafter (*e.g.* end of use). Integrity tests are also recommended after activities that may damage the filter. Integrity test failures should be investigated, and filters should be replaced at appropriate, defined intervals [7].

Corrosion

Corrosion is an electrochemical process by which iron develops rust when air is damp [8]. See Tables **3** and **4**.

This may happen in a stainless steel pipework if the protective layer of chromium oxide is destroyed at a point as a result of defective welding or passivation, but also because of a biofilm ("biocorrosion").

Table 3. Iron corrosion.

The two components of the redox reaction of corrosion are the following:	• $O_2 + 2\,H_2O + 4\,e^- \leftrightarrow 4\,OH^-$ • $Fe \leftrightarrow Fe^{2+} + 2\,e^-$
1st. Iron is oxidized, initially to iron dihydroxide:	$2\,Fe + O_2 + 2\,H_2O \leftrightarrow 2\,Fe\,(OH)_2$
2nd. And, at once, to iron trihydroxide:	$2\,Fe\,(OH)_2 + \frac{1}{2}\,O_2 + H_2O \rightarrow 2\,Fe\,(OH)_3$

Iron trihydroxide, that has the typical color of rust, tends to come off and, consequently, new iron not yet oxidized is exposed. This is a non-limited process which can lead to the complete destruction of the element.

Table 4. Detection of iron oxidation with ferroxyl.

Existing oxidation can be exposed by means of the "ferroxyl" indicator, a solution of phenolphthalein and hexacyanoferrate (III) of potassium $K_3[Fe(CN)_6]$, capable of revealing tiny amounts of Fe^{2+}.	
Ion hexacyanoferrate (III) reacts with Fe^{2+} ions to produce a complex ion of an intense blue color ("Prussian blue"):	$Fe^{2+} + Fe(CN)_6^{3-} \rightarrow Fe(CN)_6^-$

Selection of Materials

Equipment should not present any hazard to the products. The parts of the production equipment that come into direct contact (production equipment) or indirect contact with the product (utility equipment of utility fluids coming into contact with products or production equipment) must not be reactive, additive or absorptive to such an extent that it will affect the quality of the product and thus present any hazard (Fig. **3**).

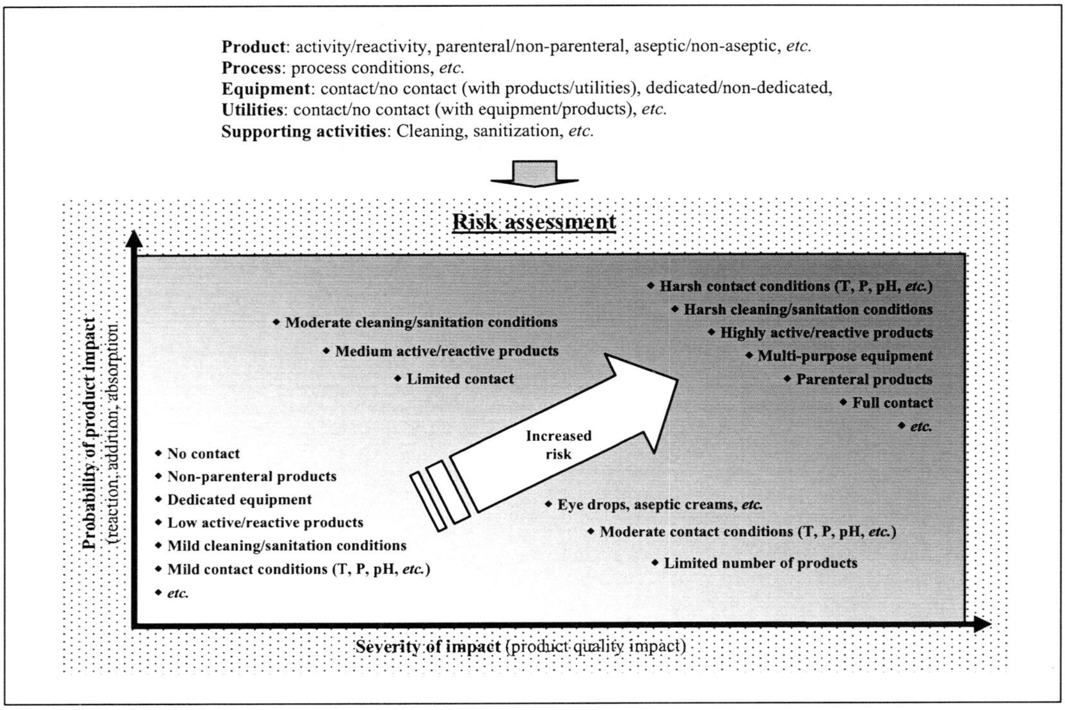

Fig. (3). Selection of materials for production and utility equipment.

ELECTRICAL SUPPLY

Electricity is an important utility, which cannot be treated like the other ones. Electrical supply should be appropriate in order not to affect negatively the quality of the products. Without it, a plant cannot work and GMP conditions disappear (environmental control, generation of adequate water, *etc.*). This is why, from a pharmaceutical point of view, it is necessary to show:

1st That back-up systems will ensure that the most critical equipment will not stop.

2nd That equipment will restart safely after a cut in electrical supply.

3rd That an alarm will inform operators of electrical failures (although a general failure is self-evident, a partial failure may affect just a part of the plant and stop a critical system).

4th That there will be procedures indicating what to do to protect the quality of products in case of electrical failure.

HVAC

HVAC is a commonly used acronym of "Heating, Ventilation, Air Conditioning". The HVAC system plays a very important role in a pharmaceutical plant because it controls the temperature (and sometimes the humidity too) of the air, supplies the rooms with fresh air, filters this air to eliminate suspended particles and defines room environments by creating pressure differentials [9].

The authentic heart of any HVAC system is the "air handling unit" (AHU) or units, because a complex system can possess more than one.

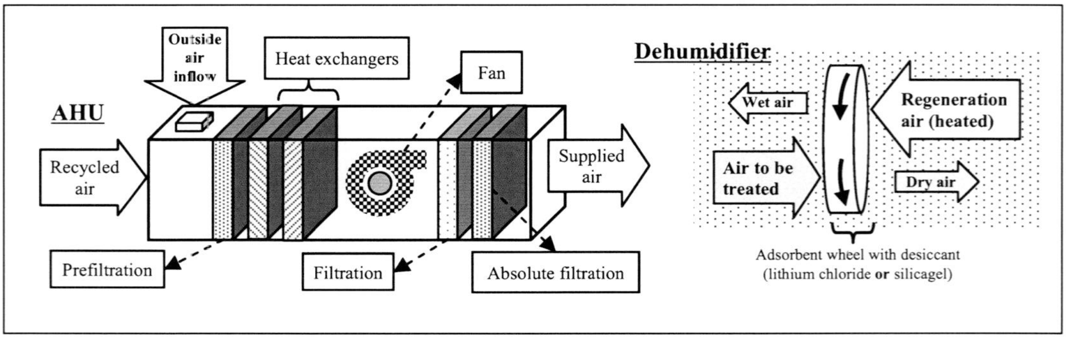

Fig. (4). Schematic representation of an AHU and a dehumidifier

An AHU can be composed of the following sections (Fig. **4**):

- Fan which impulses the air;
- Filters which retain solid matters suspended in the air. With the aim of increasing their efficiency filtration is double or triple (prefiltration, filtration and absolute filtration);
- Heat exchangers which warm or cool air (in most cases both types of exchangers are present to be able to regulate temperature during all the seasons of the year). Such an AHU can control air temperature but not humidity. This is only possible by adding a dehumidifier.

The AHU supplies air to the rooms through a net of tight ducts with smooth walls. Air is exhausted through another net of ducts and returns to the AHU to start again the cycle (in systems with air recycling) or is sent outside (in systems without recycling). To these basic parts it is possible to adjoin other elements like filtering units, additional fans or dehumidifiers (Fig. **4**).

Types of HVAC Systems

HVAC systems are designed and built on measure to handle particular conditions in each plant. However, they can be grouped in three principal types:

- Systems without recycling: In them there is a 100% renewal of air. Exhausted air from the rooms instead of returning to the AHU is sent outside by an additional fan. This approach has the advantage of excluding any risk of cross-contamination, but it entails throwing away air which has been conditioned. This energetic loss can be recovered by passing the air through a heat exchanger before being exhausted outside.
- Systems with recycling: In this case air exhausted from the rooms returns to the AHU to restart the cycle again. Anyway there is always some amount of air renewal because it is necessary to replace the inevitable loses and to ensure adequate ventilation.
- Systems with controlled humidity: In these systems humidity is maintained under a certain value because the AHU is complemented with a dehumidifier. Nowadays the most commonly used dehumidifiers are those working on the principle of the adsorbent wheel.

Air Filtration

Air is filtered in a three-staged process to eliminate suspended matters:

- Prefiltration through "gravimetric" filters which retain coarse particles and this way they protect the finer filters;
- Filtration through "opacimetric filters" of medium efficacy;
- Filtration through "Efficient Particulate Air Filters" (EPA) and "High Efficiency Particulate Air filters (HEPA)".

Efficacy (E) is the relation between amount of particles retained by the filter and amount of particles that reach it. Penetration (P) is the concentration of particles upstream divided by the concentration of particles downstream (Table **5**).

Table 5. Filter efficacy and penetration.

Efficacy (E) = 99.5%.	E = 1 – P	P = 1 – E	P% = 100 – E%
Penetration (P) = 100 – E%= 100 – 99.5 = 0.5%			

There are filters with even higher efficacy than HEPA which are known ULPA ("Ultra Low Penetration Air filters") used for very clean environments such as those required in the electronic industry [10].

Table 6. Classification of filters.

Class				Efficacy (%)			
Type	**Standard: EN 779**	**Standard: EN 1822**	**Standard: EUROVENT 4/4 e 4/5**	**Gravimetry** (Arrestance test) A_m (%)	**Opacimetry** (Atmospheric dust-spot efficiency test) E_m (%)	**DOP** (DOP Penetration test) % minimum: Global value	**DOP** (DOP Penetration test) % minimum: Local value (leak control)
Prefilters	**G-1**		EU-1	$A_m < 65$			
	G-2		EU-2	$65 \leq A_m < 80$			
	G-3		EU-3	$80 \leq A_m < 90$			
	G-4		EU-4	$90 \leq A_m$			
Filters	**F-5**		EU-5		$40 \leq E_m < 60$		
	F-6		EU-6		$60 \leq E_m < 80$		
	F-7		EU-7		$80 \leq E_m < 90$		
	F-8		EU-8		$90 \leq E_m < 95$		
	F-9		EU-9		$95 \leq E_m$		
EPA filters		**E10**	EU-10			85	
		E11	EU-11			95	
		E12	EU-12			99.5	
HEPA filters		**H13**	EU-13			99.95	99.75
		H14	EU-14			99.995	99.975

The classification of EPA, HEPA and ULPA filters (Table **6**) is based on the values for local particle collection efficacy and integral efficiency, which are assessed on the basis of the most penetrating particle size (MPPS) [11].

Qualification

See chapter 8.

DUST EXHAUST

When operations involve powdered substances it is necessary to take measures to avoid the liberation and dissemination of dust. HVAC systems are designed to control the liberation of particles during production, but not to cope with important quantities of dust. Then, it is necessary adding a forced exhaust at the point of liberation. This is obtained by installing a dust exhaust system. This system has to be adequately designed in order to absorb all dust, but also not to affect the pressure balances established by the HVAC system (Fig. 5).

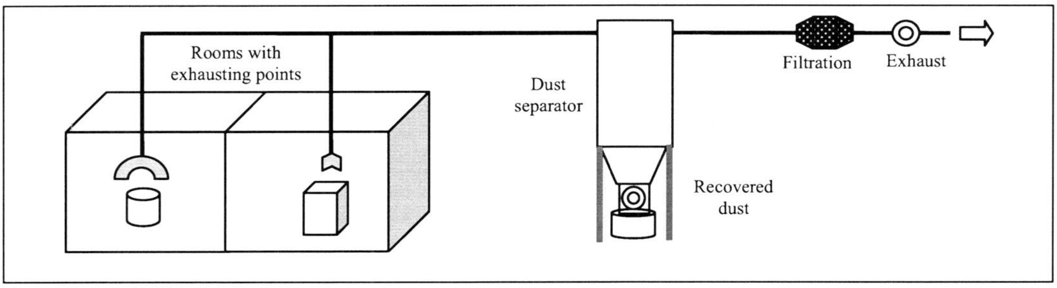

Fig. (5). Schematic representation of an exhausting system.

The qualification of this system is usually performed together with the clean rooms (see chapter 8).

a) Design qualification (DQ)

- Verify the compliance of the design with the requirements of the customer.
- Verify the compliance of the design with GMP/GEP.

b) Installation qualification (IQ)

- Collect and collate supplier documentation (operating instructions, maintenance requirements, P&ID drawings).
- Verify installed equipment (make, model) and its identification.
- Check installation of equipment, ducting and instrumentation to current engineering drawings and specifications.
- Check calibration of critical instruments (by collating calibration certificates). Usually there are no instruments requiring calibration, but calibration requirements should be seen in each case.
- Verify procedures (SOPs) connected to operation and maintenance.

- Verify operators' training.

c) Operational qualification (OQ)

- Verify the operation of equipment (according to operating instructions);
- Measure airflow rates.

d) Performance qualification (PQ)

- Verify that the connection of the system does not influence the environmental parameters of the clean rooms.
- Verify that when the system is disconnected there is no free flow of air between the rooms through ducting or between clean rooms and the outer environment.

WATER FOR PHARMACEUTICAL USE

In a pharmaceutical plant water can play different roles:

- Sanitary;
- Thermal fluid for heat exchangers (water has a high specific heat);
- Washing;
- Starting material.

Thus, quality requirements for water depend on its use the plant [12] (Table **7**).

Table 7. Summary of types of water in a laboratory and their utilization.

Type of water	Characteristics	Utilization
Obtained from the nature (river, well, *etc.*)	Non potable or doubtfully potable	• Sanitary (no risk of consumption) • In heat exchangers (no risk of contact with products)
Potable (mains) or obtained from the nature and treated to meet requirements	Potable	• Sanitary (risk of consumption) • Initial washing of equipment/containers for non parenteral pharmaceuticals

Type of water		Characteristics	Utilization
Water for pharmaceutical use	Purified (PW)	See below	• Production of non parenteral pharmaceuticals • Final washing of equipment/containers for non parenteral pharmaceuticals • Initial washing of equipment/containers for parenteral pharmaceuticals
	For injection (WFI)	See below	• Production of parenteral pharmaceuticals • Final washing of equipment/containers for parenteral pharmaceuticals.

Pharmacopeias define the characteristics of the different types of water for pharmaceutical use (Table **8**).

Table 8. Simplified summary of characteristics of potable water, PW and WFI.

Parameter	Potable water	Purified water (PW)	Water for injection (WFI)
Preparation	From natural water by adequate treatment.	From potable water by an adequate treatment.	From purified or potable water by distillation [Europe/WHO]. USP accepts also water prepared by reverse osmosis*.
Total aerobic microorganisms	<10 ufc/ml at 37°C/24 h <100 ufc/ml at 22°C/72h	≤100 ufc/ml at 30-35°C	≤10 ufc/100 ml at 30-35°C
Conductivity	N. a.	≤4.3 μS/cm (at 20°C) ≤1.1 μS/cm (at 20°C) [USP]**	≤1.1 μS/cm (at 20°C)
TOC (Total Organic Carbon)	N. a.	≤0.5 mg/l (ppm)	≤0.5 mg/l (ppm)
Bacterial endotoxins	N. a.	< 0.25 Units (only if water is used to prepare dialysis solutions)	< 0.25 Units
* WFI obtained by reverse osmosis outside of the USA is considered Highly Purified Water/HPW **Three stage determination: The first one requires ≤1.3 μS/cm (at 25°C), equivalent to ≤1.1 μS/cm (at 20°C)			

Water Systems

A pharmaceutical plant needs great amounts of water, in general, and of water for pharmaceutical use (purified or for injection) in particular. This is why waters for pharmaceutical use are normally prepared *in situ*.

The systems of water for pharmaceutical use are composed of different parts and in fact they can be named "generation, storage and distribution systems" referring to these parts (Fig. **6**).

Water for pharmaceutical use has to be obtained from potable water. Conventionally, it is often distinguished between pretreatment and treatment, the former preparing a water of an adequate purity for an efficient use of the latter. This distinction is, however, purely conventional. Sometimes it is also spoken of a polishing, when it is applied a final technology which eliminates the rests of impurity subsisting after treatment [13].

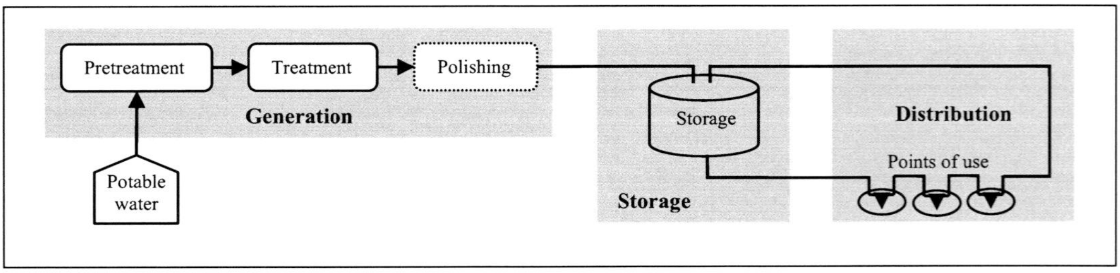

Fig. (6). Schematic representation of a system of water for pharmaceutical use.

Pretreatments

The most commonly used pretreatments are the following:

FILTRATION: The particles suspended in the water are retained by a porous material. Usually water entering the system is initially filtrated in a sand bed with the aim of retaining particles bigger than 10 μm. Filtering beds are simple and efficient, but have the disadvantage of a high risk of biofilm. They are protected by periodic countercurrent washing and disinfection. A particular case of filtering bed is constituted by activated coal, which thanks to its huge porosity retains chlorine and organic molecules that provide color and flavor to water.

CHEMICAL REDUCTION WITH METABISULFITE: This is an alternative to coal bed for the elimination of chlorine, which is transformed into chloride ion by the addition of sodium metabisulfite.

ION EXCHANGE: Ions contained in the water are exchanged by ions of the same electric charge which are linked to a resin. There are cationic resins which hold positive ions and anionic resins which have negative ions. Resins are presented in cartridges which can be easily substituted for regeneration. Ionic exchange resins are normally used to "soften" or "demineralize" water.

Water "softening" implies treatment with cationic resin to exchange cations responsible for hardness (calcium and magnesium) with sodium ions of the resin.

This resin can be regenerated with a solution of NaCl (brine).

Water "demineralization" requires two ionic exchange reactions (Table **9**). Water to be treated passes through a cationic resin, where cations (calcium, magnesium, sodium, *etc.*) are exchanged by the hydrogen ions of the resin. This cationic resin is regenerated with a solution of an acid. Afterwards, water flows through an anionic resin, where anions (chloride, sulphate, carbonate, bicarbonate, silicate, nitrate, *etc.*) are permuted by hydroxyl ions of the resin. The anionic resin is regenerated by a solution of sodium hydroxide.

As many resins are damaged by chlorine, water has to be previously treated with active coal or metabisulfite. Unprotected water and resin stagnation supposes risk of biofilm development.

Table 9. Ionic exchange reactions.

Cationic resin	Exchange reaction	$Ca^{2+} + 2\,NaR \rightarrow CaR + 2\,Na^{+}$ and $Mg^{2+} + 2\,NaR \rightarrow RMg + 2\,Na^{+}$	Water softening
	Regeneration (with NaCl)	$CaR + 2\,Na^{+} \rightarrow Ca^{+2} + 2\,NaR$ and $MgR + 2\,Na^{+} \rightarrow Mg^{2+} + 2\,NaR$	
	Exchange reaction	$NaCl + HR \rightarrow HCl + NaR$	Water demineralization
	Regeneration (with HCl)	$NaR + HCl \rightarrow NaCl + HR$	
Anionic resin	Exchange reaction	$HCl + ROH \rightarrow H_20 + RCl$	
	Regeneration (with NaOH)	$NaOH + RCl \rightarrow NaCl + ROH$	

DEGASIFICATION: Ion carbonate can be eliminated by acidification (pH $\approx$ 5), because it is transformed into CO_2 and liberated to the environment. The anion of the acid that has been added (*e.g.* sulphuric) is eliminated by reverse osmosis.

Treatments

Neither the group of treatments is well defined, but the following can be mentioned.

REVERSE OSMOSIS (RO): Water is purified by passage through semipermeable membranes against concentration gradient by application of pressure. Efficacy of RO is directly linked to the membrane characteristics (composition and disposition) and to the substances solved in the water. RO equipment consists of a series of pipes containing the membrane cartridges which are connected to a pressure pump in order to impulse the water through the membranes. Water has to be pretreated in order to eliminate suspended solids, hardness and oxidizers (mainly chlorine). Maintenance of RO equipment is relatively simple. There is limited need of reactives and can be automated (on-line conductivity measure allows detecting failures). Semipermeable membranes should be periodically sanitized.

ELECTRODIALYSIS (ED): In this process water is demineralized by migration of ions through membranes by action of an electrical field. Cations are attracted by the anode and anions by the cathode. Then selective membranes placed between the electrodes purify the water.

In order to impede depositions on the membranes the electrical field is alternatively inverted. Then this technology is known as **electrodialysis reversal (EDR)**. The inversion of electrical field makes unnecessary the use of chemicals to eliminate sedimentations on membranes, and this is clearly an advantage over RO. However, membranes should be periodically sanitized.

ELECTRODEIONIZATION (EDI): This technology also known as **continuous electrodeionization (CEDI)** combines ionic exchange and electrodialysis. Within EDI cells ions are captured by resins, but as water molecules are hydrolyzed (broken into hydrogen and hydroxyl ions) by action of the electric current, the ions which are obtained regenerate continually the resins. Ions are finally extracted through the membranes by the electric field. Thus, reactives for the regeneration of membranes are not necessary. EDI cells can have different configurations. Frequently EDI is used in combination with RO. EDI/RO produce high quality water and do not require many chemical reactives.

DISTILLATION: Distillation differs from other methods of water purification: water is separated from the impurities instead of the opposite. During distillation water changes of phases, passing from liquid to steam and again from steam to liquid. Impurities as they have a higher boiling point than that of water (100ºC) remain in the boiler, whereas water and some impurities with a boiling point equal or lower than that of water are turned into steam. When steam condenses water is only accompanied by some of those substances which boil at a lower temperature. Distillation is in fact the purification technology with the largest purification capacity, because it can effectively eliminate most of inorganic solids, all organic substances with higher boiling point than water, microorganisms and pyrogens. However, gases and organic substances of lower boiling point are not eliminated by distillation and have to be eliminated from water before or after distillation by means of other technologies. Distillation requires much energy, but it is the only procedure for obtaining water for injection which is accepted by the WHO and in Europe. In this type of water the contents of endotoxins is a critical factor. In order to impede that steam drag small water vesicles with endotoxins stills are provided with demisters, which only allow passage of steam. A well designed still should reduce the endotoxin contents of water at least in three logarithmic units. In pharmaceutical plants three types of stills are used. Two of them (multi-effect and steam compression stills) can be used both for obtaining water for injection and as source of steam.

- **Single-effect distillers**: Used for small amounts of water for injection. Steam generated in a boiler is condensed by passage through a heat exchanger (condenser). Basic elements in a still are the boiler, a demister for reducing pyrogens, a condenser and a water-level controller.

- **Multi-effect distillers**: They are used for great amounts. Steam produced in a chamber is used to heat up the water of the following chamber and thus obtaining more steam. Only the first chamber needs to be heated from outside, because the following ones are heated by the steam of the preceding chamber. Finally steam in the last chamber is condensed to yield water for injection. This chamber grading allows for an increased thermal efficiency.

- **Steam compression distillers**: Obtained steam is compressed to get a higher temperature and thus it can be used for the production of steam in a continuous cycle. These stills are used for very high amounts, because possess a higher thermal yield.

Storage and Distribution

High quality water is very "fragile" and has to be protected from contamination, but without addition of any product (*e.g.* chlorine) [14]. Four types of strategy are used:

1st Hot storage and distribution: Water is maintained at 80°C in the entire subsystem. This provides optimal security against contamination, but there is an important risk of scalding for operators.

2nd Hot storage and distribution at room temperature: Water is maintained at 80°C in the storage tank and is cooled for the points of use. This provides good security against contamination and protects operators, but heating and cooling requires significant amounts of energy.

(I) Generation subsystem	(II) Storage and distribution subsystem
1st Chlorination reservoir. 2nd Primary filtration (60 µm). 3rd Ionic exchange. 4th Degasification. 5th pH adjustment by addition of NaOH. 6th Double filtration (3 µm and 1 µm). 7th UV for microorganism control. 8th Soft water reservoir. 9th Two stage reverse osmosis.	1st PW reservoir. 2nd Impulsion group with two pumps. 3rd Heat exchanger. 4th UV for microorganism control. 5th Distribution loop to points of use.

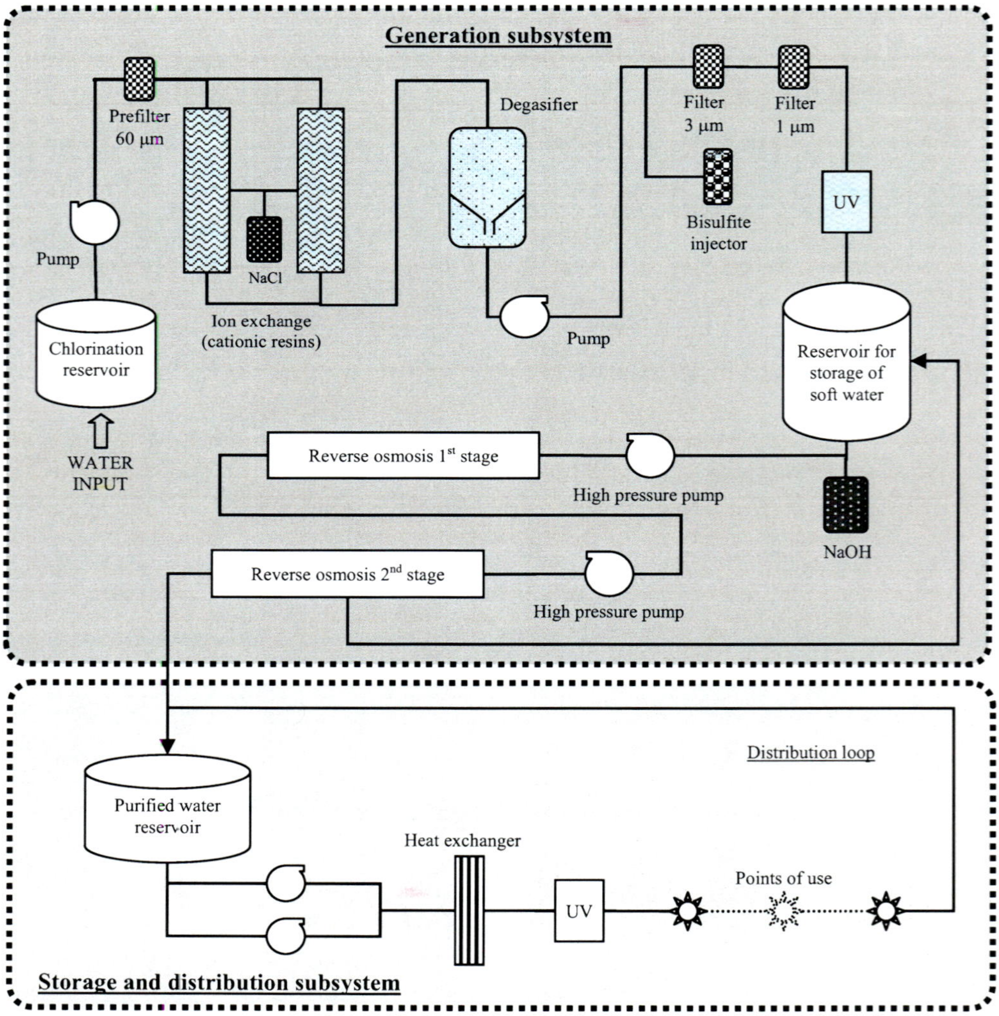

Fig. (7). Schematic diagram of a purified water system.

3rd Storage and distribution at room temperature: Water is at high risk of contamination and it has to be protected either with UV (ultra violet) or ozone. Temperature is monitored to impede excessive water warm up (< 25ºC).

4th Cold storage and distribution: Water is kept at a low temperature (around +10ºC) which does not favor microbiological growth.

Example of a Purified Water (PW) System

Fig. 7 shows the elements which compose the two subsystems.

Qualification

Waters for pharmaceutical use systems are qualified following a similar pattern of tests than those utilized for other systems, but with an important difference: sampling and analysis is much more extensive and requires establishing a detailed schedule [15, 16]. See Table **10**.

Table 10. Example of qualification of a system of water for pharmaceutical use: Schedule.

Element	Duration	Actions	Sampling/ Monitoring	Can water be used for production?
DQ	Indefinite	- Study of project documentation.	No.	No (no generation of water yet).
IQ	Indefinite	- Verification of installation of system as regards to the project documentation. - Preparation of procedures (SOPs).	No.	No (no generation of water yet).
OQ	2 weeks	- Verification of system operation (as described in the project). - Application of SOPs. - Intensive monitoring. - Verification of the quality of water. (a) Operation in "normal" conditions. (b) Operation in "stress" conditions.	Yes: **Phase 1.** (intensive)	No (water is obtained, but its quality is not established yet).
PQ	2 weeks	- Revision of SOPs. - Intensive monitoring. - Verification of the quality of water.	Yes: **Phase 2.** (intensive)	Yes (provided there were not detected anomalies).
	1 year	- Approval and implementation of SOPs. - Routine monitoring. - Verification of the quality of water. - Verification that the system performs adequately notwithstanding seasonal potable water variations.	Yes: **Phase 3.** (normal)	Yes (provided there were not detected anomalies).

Note: The previous example of purified water system is used for qualification too.

(A) Testing

IQ Tests

(1) Verification of the supplier documentation

(2) Installation revision regarding supplier P&IDs.

(3) Component identification and verification of their characteristics.

(4) Verification of dead legs.

(5) Verification of piping slopes.

(6) Verification of the calibration of critical instrumentation.

(7) Verification of welding.

(8) Verification of water-tightness (hydrostatic test).

(9) Verification of passivation and cleaning.

OQ Tests

(1) Verification of SOPs.

(2) Verification of start, stop and functionalities of equipment.

(3) Sanitization

(4) Electricity failure

(5) Water failure

(6) Pump failure

(7) Alarms and failure messages

(8) Simulation of a period of inactivity

(9) Simulation of maximal consumption

(10) Operation with low level of water

(11) Verification of operational parameters

(12) Analytical verification of water quality

The minimal duration of OQ is two weeks. The installation is carefully monitored verifying that critical parameters are within acceptance ranges, while water is sampled in order to verify analytically that PW meets specifications (**Phase 1**).

Qualification tests correspond to two situations. Functional tests in "normal" conditions are performed initially, followed afterwards by functional tests in "stress" conditions. The aim of the former is verifying that the system is able to produce quality PW, whereas the aim of the latter is verifying that worst case conditions do not affect this quality.

PQ Tests

(1) Verification of functional parameters

(2) Verification of specifications of water quality

(3) Revision and approval of system SOPs

Besides defining the system procedures (SOPs), the remaining sampling phases (**Phase 2** and **Phase 3**) are implemented. Water can already be used for production. The aim of PQ is verifying the appropriate operation and monitoring of the system under routine conditions, and demonstrating that the system is able to supply water for pharmaceutical use meeting requirements in spite of the seasonal variations of potable water input.

(B) Monitoring program (Fig. **8**)

Definition of the parameters to be monitored to ensure that the system is under control:

- Water level in the chlorination tank.

- Water flow.

- Differential pressure in the 60 μm filter.

- Hardness at the outlet of ionic exchange.
- Differential pressures in the 3 μm and 1 μm filters.
- Redox value after addition of sodium metabisulfite.
- Water level in the soft water tank.
- Water temperature prior to the 1st reverse osmosis stage.
- Water pressure prior to the 1st reverse osmosis stage.
- Water temperature prior to the 2nd reverse osmosis stage.
- Water pressure prior to the 2nd reverse osmosis stage.
- pH prior to the 2nd reverse osmosis stage.
- Conductivity at the 2nd reverse osmosis stage outlet.
- Water level in the PW tank.
- Water pressure at the loop pumping group outlet.
- Water pressure at the loop return (prior to the storage tank).
- Water flow at the loop return (prior to the storage tank).
- Water temperature at the loop return (prior to the storage tank).

(C) Sampling and analysis program (Fig. **8**)

Sampling points:

- PW generation subsystem,
  (1) Mains water inlet: PA-01
  (2) Chlorination tank outlet: PA-02
  (3) Ion exchange outlet: PA-03

(4) Degasification outlet: PA-04

(5) Sodium metabisulfite injector outlet: PA-05

(6) UV lamp outlet: PA-06

(7) 1st stage of reverse osmosis outlet: PA-07

(8) 2nd stage of reverse osmosis outlet: PA-08

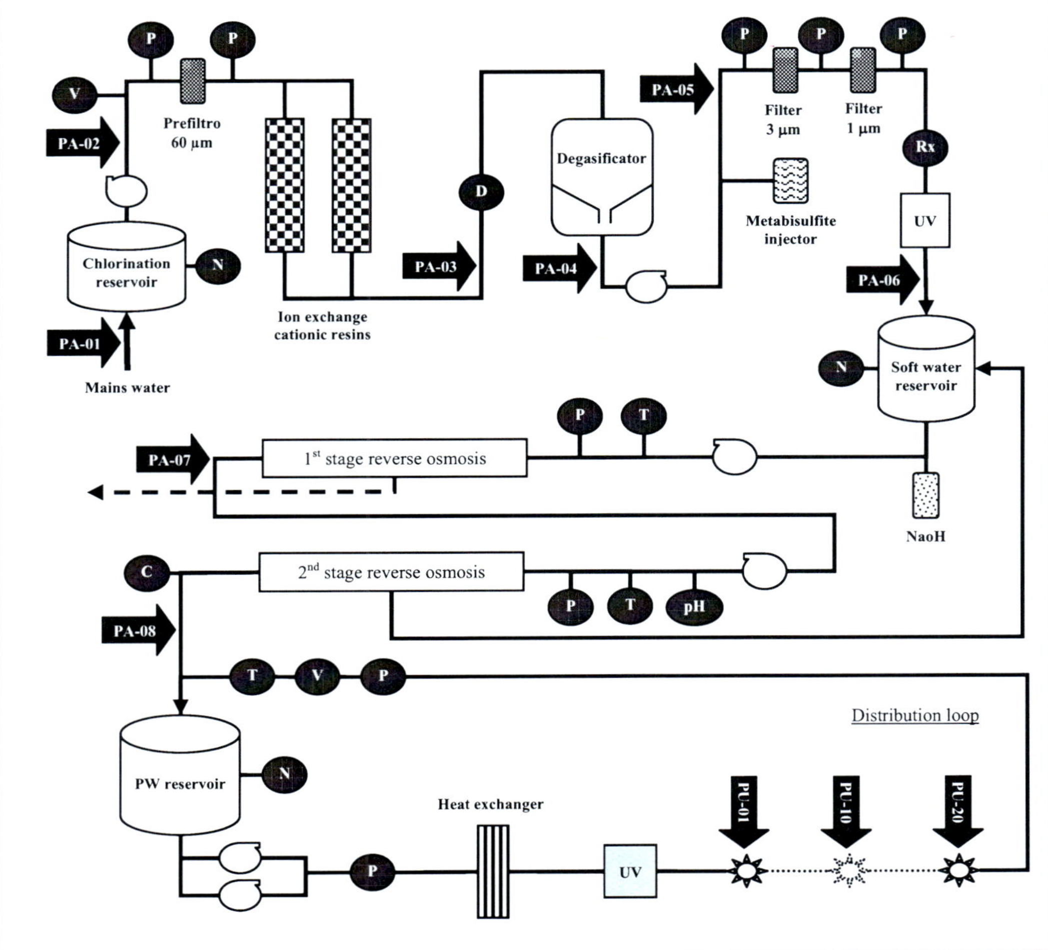

<u>Monitoring instrumentation:</u> **C**: conductivity; **D**: hardness; N: water level in reservoir; **P**: pressure; **pH**: pH; **Rx**: redox potential; **T**: temperature; **V**: flow.

Fig. (8). Monitoring and sampling points.

- PW storage and distribution subsystem,

All points of use (*e.g.* PU-01 through PU-20).

Sampling and analytical schedule:

Phase 1: Intensive sampling/monitoring of all the points, everyday during at least two weeks (Table **11**).

Table 11. Phase 1. Example of sampling/analytical program.

Sampling point		Weekday						
		Monday	Tuesday	Wednesday	Thursday	Friday	Saturday	Sunday
#1	Mains water inlet (PA-01)	P-C/M	P-C/M	P-C/M	P-C/M	P-C/M	P-C/M	P-C/M
#2	Chlorination tank outlet (PA-02)	P-C/M	P-C/M	P-C/M	P-C/M	P-C/M	P-C/M	P-C/M
#3	Ion exchange outlet (PA-03)	P-C/M	P-C/M	P-C/M	P-C/M	P-C/M	P-C/M	P-C/M
#4	Degasification outlet (PA-04)	P-C/M	P-C/M	P-C/M	P-C/M	P-C/M	P-C/M	P-C/M
#5	Sodium metabisulfite outlet (PA-05)	P-C/M	P-C/M	P-C/M	P-C/M	P-C/M	P-C/M	P-C/M
#6	UV lamp outlet (PA-06)	P-C/M	P-C/M	P-C/M	P-C/M	P-C/M	P-C/M	P-C/M
#7	1st stage of RO outlet (PA-07)	P-C/M	P-C/M	P-C/M	P-C/M	P-C/M	P-C/M	P-C/M
#8	2nd stage of RO outlet (PA-08)	P-C/M	P-C/M	P-C/M	P-C/M	P-C/M	P-C/M	P-C/M
#9	Point of use P-01	P-C/M	P-C/M	P-C/M	P-C/M	P-C/M	P-C/M	P-C/M
#10	Point of use P-02	P-C/M	P-C/M	P-C/M	P-C/M	P-C/M	P-C/M	P-C/M
#11	Point of use P-03	P-C/M	P-C/M	P-C/M	P-C/M	P-C/M	P-C/M	P-C/M
---	---	P-C/M	P-C/M	P-C/M	P-C/M	P-C/M	P-C/M	P-C/M
Full analysis: P-C: physico-chemical analysis + M: Microbiological analysis								

Phase 2: During the 2 weeks of this phase it is followed the same intensive sampling and monitoring program of phase 1 and SOPs are applied and, if necessary, improved.

Phase 3: This phase consists in a sampling plan scattered along one year. Samples are taken following a simplified program (in comparison to the one followed during the previous two phases). The objective is designing a sampling chronogram capable of evaluating the quality of the water generated by the system. This chronogram (with minor modifications) will be used later on for routine monitoring (Table **12**).

Table 12. Phase 3. Example of sampling/analytical program.

Sampling point		Weekday				
		Monday	**Tuesday**	**Wednesday**	**Thursday**	**Friday**
#1	Mains water inlet (PA-01)	P-C/M		P-C/M		P-C/M
#2	Chlorination tank outlet (PA-02)		P-C		M	
#3	Ion exchange outlet (PA-03)	M		P-C		
#4	Sodium metabisulfite injector outlet (PA-05)		M		P-C	
#5	UV lamp outlet (PA-06)			M		P-C
#6	1st stage of reverse osmosis outlet (PA-07)	M		P-C		
#7	2nd stage of reverse osmosis outlet (PA-08)		M		P-C	
#8	Point of use P-01			M		P-C
#9	Point of use P-02	M		P-C		
#10	Point of use P-03		M		P-C	
---	---	---	---	---	---	---

STEAM

Steam or vapor, water in gas state, is a very popular utility in the pharmaceutical industry, because it conveys energy in a dependable and efficient manner and transfers rapidly its energy when condensing.

Two kinds of steam can exist in a pharmaceutical plant:

- Non pharmaceutical steam, produced in boilers, is used when there is no contact with the products (mainly in heat exchangers). Water is mixed with additives to protect boilers and piping from corrosion and impede precipitations. This steam is also known as "industrial steam" or "service steam".

- Pharmaceutical steam is obtained in steam generators or as a subproduct of a multieffect still and is used when there is contact with products (real or potential). In this case it is not possible to add substances to the water and consequently, it is necessary to use water having already been submitted to purification treatments. Pharmaceutical steam is also known as "pure steam" (PS) or "clean steam" (CS). This kind of steam is used:

- In steam sterilizers (autoclaves);
- In SIP (sterilization in place) systems;
- For sterilization of pipe-works (mainly of water, but also of other fluids).
- As humidifier in HVAC systems.

Characteristics of Steam

High evaporation enthalpy: Saturated steam at atmospheric pressure has high vaporization enthalpy or latent heat of change of state (2,257 kJ/kg). See Fig. (**9**).

Purity: It refers to the presence of other substances different from water. Thus, for instance, if the water used for the generation of steam contains volatile substances (amines, hydrazines, *etc.*) or endotoxins, they could be carried away with steam.

Non condensable gas: If steam contains other gases (chiefly air) this can put at risk a sterilization process, because gas would not condensate and liberate a high quantity of heat while condensing. Besides, this gas may have isolation effect in certain points and impede contact between steam and product.

Saturation: Saturated steam shows a direct relation between pressure and temperature. Consequently, processes could be controlled simply by temperature measurement, because to each temperature corresponds a given pressure.

Quality: Defined as "% of saturation", it shows the quantity of steam (water gas) in relation to the total (water gas + water liquid). This is very important because only saturated steam (100% of saturation) has maximal latent heat. Water droplets possess isolating effect and make difficult adequate transfer of heat. The quality of a given steam can be determined by a calorimeter, because the temperature of saturated steam depends exclusively of its pressure. Besides, liquid water wets wrapping of products submitted to sterilization, with the consequent risk of losing its isolating properties.

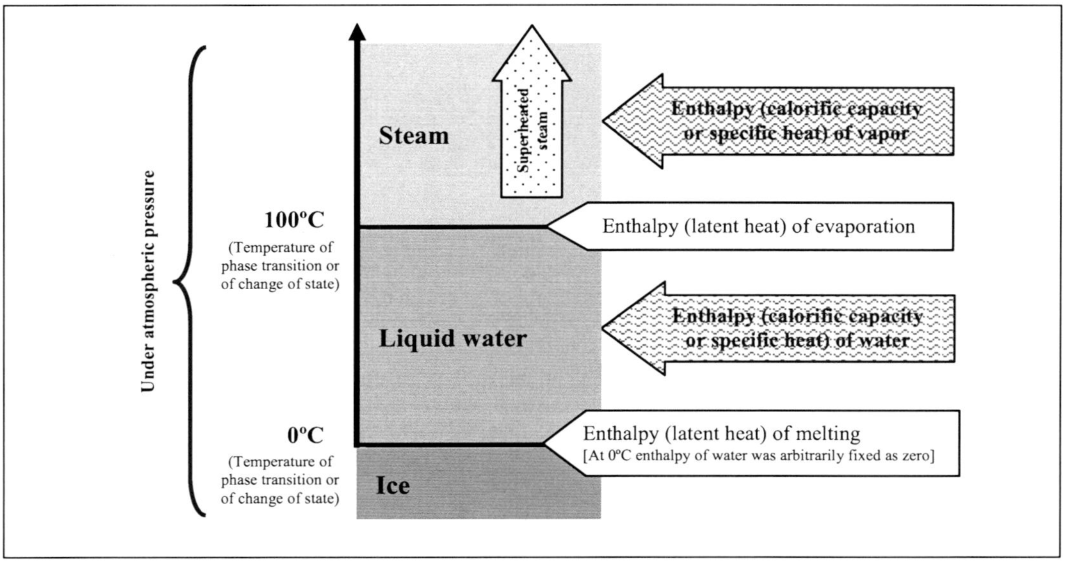

Fig. (9). States of water: Changes in energy.

Superheating: Steam can be "superheated", that is, it can acquire higher temperature than the one corresponding to its pressure. Steam temperature, for a given pressure, above its saturation temperature, expresses its level of superheating. With reference to saturated steam superheated steam shows important differences:

1st It has to cool until attaining its evaporation enthalpy. Consequently the amount of heat liberated by superheated steam is relatively small, at least in comparison with the evaporation enthalpy. If superheating is small, it is easily yielded before condensing, but if steam is strongly superheated the process is much slower.

2nd Superheated steam neither has uniform temperature, nor are directly related temperature, pressure and specific calorific capacity. This means that at a given pressure it is possible to find superheated steam at different temperatures.

Steam in Humid Sterilization

As it has been explained, the efficacy of superheated steam is lesser than that of saturated steam, because the liberated thermal energy by superheated steam (specific heat) is minor than that liberated by condensation (latent heat). Thus, sterilization requires saturated steam, of high quality, pure and free of non condensable gases (Fig. **10**).

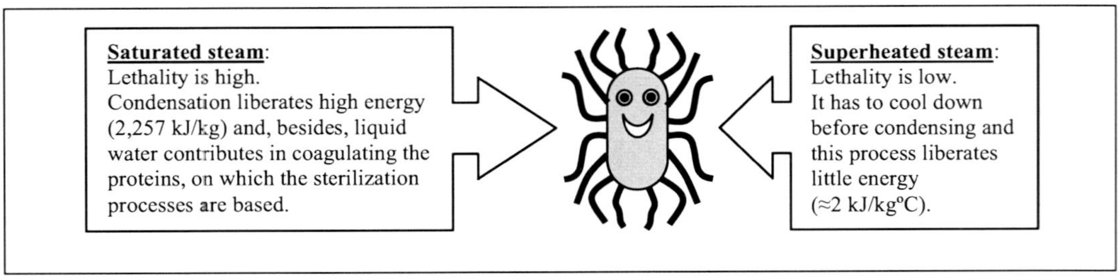

Fig. (10). Steam for sterilization.

Condensed steam used for sterilization should meet the specifications of WFI.

Steam Systems

They are relatively simple, because they are composed of a steam generator and pipework for the transportation towards the points of use. It is necessary, however, taking into account that as a consequence of the inevitable cooling there will be condensation and accumulation of liquid water in the colder points of the system. There, biofilms might appear and contaminate steam with endotoxins (the microorganisms themselves would die by steam action). Thus, it is necessary to design a system where condensates are drained. This can be done, on one hand, by adequate slope of piping (at least 1%) and, on the other, by condensate traps in the points of likely condensation [17].

Qualification

a) Design qualification (DQ)

- Verify the compliance of the design with the requirements of the customer.
- Verify the compliance of the design with GMP/GEP.

b) Installation qualification (IQ)

Collect and collate supplier documentation:

- ✓ operating instructions,
- ✓ maintenance requirements,
- ✓ P&ID engineering drawings,

- ✓ Calibration requirements (list of instruments, indicating those considered critical).

- Verify installed equipment (make, model) and its identification.
- Check installation of equipment, piping and instrumentation to current engineering drawings and specifications.
- Check calibration of critical instruments (by collating calibration certificates).
- Verify materials of construction (by collating supplier certificates).
- Verify welding, passivation and cleaning documentation (as appropriate).
- Verify the slope of piping.
- Verify SOP connected to operation and maintenance.
- Verify operators' training.

c) Operational qualification (OQ)

- Verify the connection and disconnection of equipment.
- Verify messages (failure and alarms).
- Verify analytical parameters of condensed steam according to a sampling schedule.
- Verify the quality of the steam.

d) Performance qualification (PQ)

- Verify operational parameters (temperature, pressure, *etc.*).
- Verify analytical parameters of condensed steam (during this step, the scheduled sampling program is less intensive, and prefigures the monitoring sampling used during the following routine operation of the system).

Absolute pressure measures are those that take "absolute vacuum" as a reference, whereas relative measures take into account atmospheric pressure.

Relative Pressure (Bar r) = Absolute Pressure (bar a) – Atmospheric Pressure

As atmospheric pressure varies in relation to height and meteorology, it is taken as a reference value of 1 atmosphere = 1.01325 bar (0 bar r = 1.01325 bar a).

COMPRESSED AIR

Air at a higher pressure than atmospheric is frequently used in pharmaceutical plants, where two kinds of it can exist:

Industrial or non pharmaceutical compressed air: This air should not come into contact with products (*e.g.* when it is used to operate pneumatic valves or pistons). It has no purity requirements and only the adequate pressure is needed.

Pure or pharmaceutical compressed air: This air can come into contact with products or with materials contacting products. Consequently, it has definite purity requirements [18].

Characteristics of Compressed Air

Humidity: Air always contains some amount of humidity. This content in water, known as absolute humidity, is expressed in g/m³ (grams per cubic meter of air). The maximum amount of humidity depends on temperature and pressure. Thus, the saturation point is reached when air contains the maximal possible quantity of water steam at the existing pressure and temperature. Cool air can contain less water steam than warm. This means that as the air temperature diminishes, the quantity of water it can contain diminishes too. A reduction in air temperature of 11ºC means a reduction of 50% in humidity content (Fig. **11**).

When air is cooled, relative humidity increases up to a certain temperature known as "dew point", when air reaches the saturation point. Increased cooling (below this point) will turn into condensation of exceeding air steam. Thus, dew point can be defined as the temperature (at a given pressure) at which water steam starts condensing. Consequently, the dew point of compressed air should be lower than minimal room temperature in order to impede condensation of water, since this water would accumulate in the lower parts of the system (*e.g.* points of use). This water is damaging because it causes erosion of piping, it can create corrosive solutions, it presents risk of microbial contamination and it may freeze and damage the system.

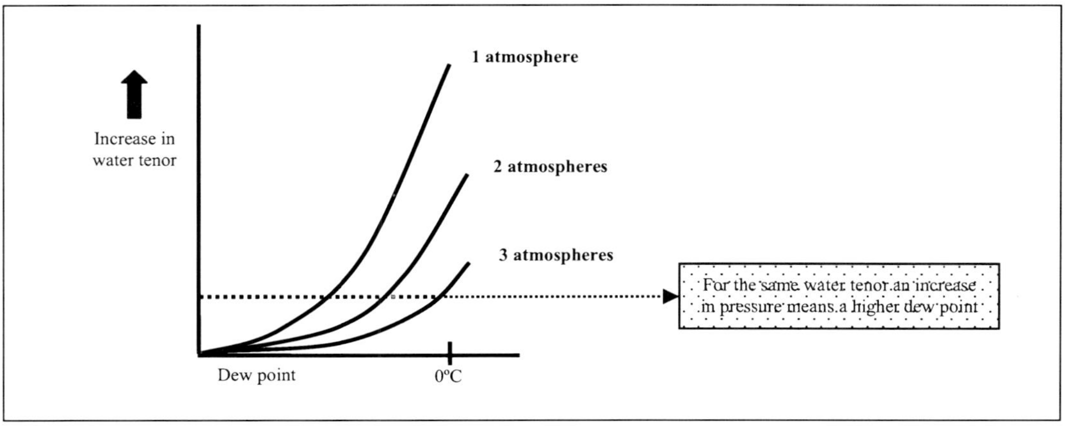

Fig. (11). Relation of dew point with pressure.

For the compressed air of a pharmaceutical production unit, it is usually enough to have a dew point of around -8°C. Other specialized applications of air may require a lower dew point.

Particle contents: Air exhausted by a compressor has always suspended particles, both endogenous (attrition, wear, oxidation) or exogenous (environmental dust). Generation of particles is highest when starting the compressor. Strokes which attain the distribution line cause liberation of particles too.

In the pharmaceutical industry the acceptable concentration of particles in compressed air follows the same criteria than the air of clean areas. This has the advantage of linking the purity requirements for compressed air to the cleanliness level of the area.

Oil content**:** In this case "oil" is meant as a mixture of hydrocarbons possessing 6 or more than 6 carbon atoms. If the compressor is lubricated air will probably always have some traces of lubrication oil. This is why, when compressed air may be considered critical it is required using dry (oil-free) compressors. However, even using this type of compressors, air can contain hydrocarbons coming from the environment and this is why air is normally filtered through high absorptive filters.

Compressed Air Systems

Compressed air is prepared by compression of environmental air by means of a compressor and is supplied to the points of use by a pipe network [19] (Fig. **12**).

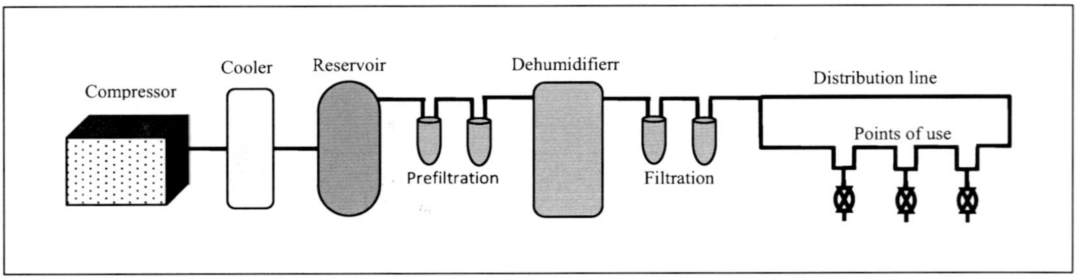

Fig. (12) Schematic representation of a compressed air system

Compressor: This is the basic element of the system. It compresses the atmospheric air to a given working pressure. Air captured by the compressor should be free of contamination (far from sources of contamination and filtered). It has already been mentioned that a lubricated compressor suffices largely for an industrial system, since filtration controls the build-up of emulsions of oil-water-solid matters in piping. However pharmaceutical air requires oil-free compressors.

Cooler: It diminishes the temperature of the air supplied by the compressor below its dew point. It is a heat exchanger (air/water) which eliminates as much as 75% of the air humidity and particles too. Water has to be drained to impede being dragged by the air draft.

Reservoir: It allows for the stabilization of the pressure in the system and also avoids the continual operation of the compressor.

Dehumidifier: It exists only in systems which require compressed air with a very low dew point. Dehumidifiers based on desiccation have divided solids (silicagel, activated alumina, zeolites) capable of adsorbing/absorbing water.

Filters: They allow for the elimination of solid matters generated as a consequence of the friction of the mechanic parts and of air against the system walls. Good quality equipment and building materials allow for the diminishing of the particle number, but elimination can only be guaranteed by the installation of batteries of filters with diminishing pore size. At the start of the line are installed coarse filters (1 to 5 µm), whereas those situated near the points of use are much finer. For aseptic applications they should be of 0.1 or 0.2 µm. Any gas coming in direct contact with the product (*e.g.* those used in the filling or filtering process) has to be submitted to sterilizing filtration. The integrity of the critical air filters should be verified after use.

Distribution line: It conveys compressed air to the points of use. Air does not affect materials, but the particles which are dragged can erode or corrode materials. This is why stainless steel is the recommended material, because it ensures good performances (durability, resistance, inertness, welding, *etc.*). The points of use are usually provided with regulators with manometer in order to better adjust supplied pressure. A loop with interconnections allows for a diminution in the loss of charge.

Demand: It is evident that a good knowledge of the compressed air needs is essential. In the simplest cases (few use points) this is not difficult, but when there are long distribution lines with many use points, this can be much more complicated. It is very practical to prepare a chart with needs and usage schedules. The approach should be similar to that used in defining water systems.

For existing systems, a measure of the air demand can be obtained by measuring use point airflow (installation of flowmeters). It is possible to get an indication on air demand by studying stop and functioning schedules of the compressor. It is very important taking into account that measures often do not supply a real estimate of demand because of:

- leaks (air leaking across cracks in the system can be significant);
- inadequate use of the system (*e.g.* use points adjusted to a pressure higher than necessary).

In older systems, installation of new compressors is a way to cope with increased demands for air, but sometimes a reconfiguration of the system proves to be a simpler and more efficient solution.

It is necessary to remember that an overdimensioned compressor is often inefficient and it is better to replace it with smaller compressors that can operate according to demand.

Qualification

a) <u>Design qualification</u> (DQ)

- Verify the compliance of the design with the requirements of the customer.
- Verify the compliance of the design with GMP/GEP.

b) Installation qualification (IQ)

- Collect and collate supplier documentation:
  - ✓ operating instructions,
  - ✓ maintenance requirements,
  - ✓ P&ID engineering drawings,
  - ✓ calibration requirements (list of instruments, indicating those considered critical).
- Verify installed equipment (make, model) and its identification.
- Check installation of equipment, piping and instrumentation to current engineering drawings and specifications.
- Check calibration of critical instruments (by collating calibration certificates).

c) Operational qualification (OQ)

- Verify the connection and disconnection of equipment.
- Verify messages (failure and alarms).
- Verify operational parameters at the use points (pressure, supply).
- Verify the air quality (particle content [20], moisture [21], hydrocarbons [22] and microbiology [23]).

NITROGEN (AND OTHER MEDICINAL GASES)

Usually these gases are not prepared in the pharmaceutical plants, but supplied in pressurized cylinders which are filled in special plants.

Gas systems are very simple, because they consist of distribution lines connected to the cylinders by means of a manometer and a regulator in order to control the supply pressure. According to the needs, systems can be more complex with several cylinders, filters, *etc.*

An alternative to nitrogen cylinders is the separation of nitrogen from the air by special equipment [24].

LIGHTING

From the pharmaceutical point of view light:

- should not affect products and, thus, it is necessary to use special lamps when manipulating photosensible products.
- should be sufficient to allow for the adequate development of operations.
- should be designed in order to allow for an agreeable work environment ("visual comfort").

Luminaries of the pharmaceutical areas should not be sources of contamination. They should be tight to impede dust collection and particle liberation. This is why they should preferably be installed to allow for maintenance from the technical zone above the false ceiling. When this is not possible luminaries are serviced from the same production areas, but in this case maintenance should be realized when there is no production and once works are finished it is necessary to perform the adequate cleaning or even disinfection.

Guidelines on security and hygiene provide orientation on the minimal illumination standards. In pharmaceutical units, however, specifications are usually higher. Thus, for example:

- Secondary rooms and passage areas (like corridors): 100 Lux;
- Rooms where plain activity is developed (*e.g.* changing rooms): 300-500 Lux;
- Rooms where complex operations are performed: 500-1,000 Lux.

For these required values of illumination, it is necessary to take into account that measurements for passage areas and rooms should be performed at ground level, whereas for working areas and rooms, by convention, it is considered that the working horizontal plane is placed at a height of 0.85 m from ground.

Minimum required values should exist at any point of the area or room at any moment. Consequently, it is necessary to increase the planned illumination value (that is, the initial average illumination), in order to ensure this minimum required value at each point and to cope with deterioration of light sources.

Working areas may be illuminated by means of localized illumination sources, completing general illumination. Some national regulations, for instance, establish that the relationship between localized and general illumination level or between the levels of two contiguous rooms should be between 1 and 5 (maximum). This means that, if the illumination of a working point is of 500 Lux, the average level of illumination must not be less than 100 Lux.

The capacity of illumination to render the true color aspect of objects, as defined by the color reproduction index (CRI or Ra), with a maximum value of 100, should be higher than 80 for works with high visual requirements.

See chapter 8 for qualification.

NOISE

Sound is an acoustic sensation produced by a rapid change in air pressure. This change is caused by the vibration of an object, which causes vibration of the air around it. Thus, a succession of pressure and depression areas, known as an acoustic wave, is created. When the sound wave reaches the ear, sound is perceived because the wave causes the tympanum to vibrate. See Table **13**.

Table 13. Parameters which characterize sound.

Frequency (f)	It is expressed in Hertz (Hz) and it is the number of vibrations per unit of time	**f = 1/T**
Period (T)	It is the duration of the vibration, expressed in seconds (s).	
Wave length	It is the distance travelled by a wave during a period	
Intensity	It is the acoustic pressure. The human ear can measure tiny pressure deviations, of around 0.00002 Pa (2 x 10^{-5} Pa), up to 20 Pa.	
Sound level" (L_p)	It describes in a practical way the intensity of sound. It is expressed in decibels (dB). **L_p = 20 x log (P** [air pressure in Pa]/**P_0** [reference pressure: 2.x 10^{-5} Pa])	

Disagreeable and uncomfortable sounds to the ear are known as "noise". It is necessary to point out that the impression of "sound strength" as perceived by the ear varies with the frequency. For frequencies between 1,000 and 6,000 Hz sounds seem to be much stronger, although acoustic pressure levels are the same.

Thus, a sound of 40 dB, with a frequency of 100 Hz is perceived as less powerful than a sound of 40 dB with a frequency of 1,000 Hz.

Table 14. Noise exposure limit values (Europe: Directive 2003/10/EC).

Value	$L_{Eq, 8h}$	P_{peak}
Exposure limit values	**87 dB(A)**	**200 Pa**
Upper exposure action values (the employer has to take provisions aimed at reducing exposure, signs have to be placed, workers have to wear hearing protectors and workers are granted health surveillance)	**85 dB(A)**	**200 Pa**
Lower exposure action values (workers have hearing protectors available and are informed and trained on risk protection)	**80 dB(A)**	**112 Pa**

Filters are used to take into account this peculiarity of the ear. They consider the sound levels according to the frequency. The most commonly used filter is the "A". Thus, it is possible to have sound levels, which are considered (from the physiological point of view) and expressed in dB (A).

The acoustic pressure level of a noise is proportional to its "sound strength", but also to its duration. Consequently, it is possible to distinguish between a "day limit exposition level" ($L_{Eq,\ 8\ hours}$) and an "acoustic pressure peak value" (P_{peak}) [25]. See Table **14**.

See chapter 8 for qualification.

CONCLUDING REMARKS

Utilities constitute a heterogeneous group of systems characterized for distributing a fluid or energy to points of use. They are necessary for the manufacturing operations and although often they do not participate, properly speaking, in the production processes they can affect seriously the quality of the products. When this is the case, they have to meet preestablished requirements of purity. These pharmaceutical utilities require watchful design, installation and qualification, because usually they participate, in a more or less important degree, in the processes without previous sampling and testing by QC control. This means that their quality has to be ensured by qualification and by careful routine monitoring to guarantee that they are kept "in state of qualification" and thus, they perform as purported.

CONFLICT OF INTEREST

The author confirms that this chapter contents have no conflict of interest.

ACKNOWLEDGEMENT

Declared None.

REFERENCES

[1] WHO (World Health Organization). WHO Good manufacturing practices for pharmaceutical products: main principles. In: WHO Expert Committee on Specifications for Pharmaceutical Preparations. Forty-eigth report (WHO Technical Report Series, No. 986). WHO, Geneva, Switzerland 2014: Annex 2

[2] PIC/S (Pharmaceutical Inspection Convention. Pharmaceutical Inspection Co-Operation Scheme). Inspection of utilities. Aide-memoire PI 009-3. PIC/S, Geneva, Switzerland 2007.

[3] Clontz L, Wagner C. (editors). Biofilm control in drug manufacturing. PDA, Bethesda, MD, USA 2012.

[4] ISPE (International Society of Pharmaceutical Engineering). Good Engineering Practice. ISPE Good Practice Guide, Tampa, Florida, USA 2008.

[5] PIC/S (Pharmaceutical Inspection Convention. Pharmaceutical Inspection Co-Operation Scheme). Aide-memoire. Inspection of utilities. PI 009-3. PIC/S, Geneva, Switzerland 2007.

[6] Tuthill A H. Fabrication and post-fabrication cleanup of stainless steels. Chemical Engineering, September 1986, 1-5.

[7] FDA (U. S. Food and Drug Administration). Guide to inspections of high purity water systems. FDA, Inspection Technical Guides, 7/93. FDA, Rockville, MD, USA 1993.

[8] Avery R E, Keith Raney R. Rouging in stainless steel equipment for hygienic services. EJPPS, 13 (1) 2008, 21-24.

[9] ISPE (International Society of Pharmaceutical Engineering). Heating, Ventilation, and Air Conditioning (HVAC). ISPE Good Practice Guide, Tampa, Florida, USA 2009.

[10] WHO (World Health Organization). WHO Guidelines on good manufacturing practices for heating, ventilation and air conditioning systems for non-sterile pharmaceutical dosage forms. In: WHO Expert Committee on Specifications for Pharmaceutical Preparations. Forty-fifth report (WHO Technical Report Series, No. 961). WHO, Geneva, Switzerland 2011: Annex 5.

[11] CEN (European Committee for Standardization). High efficiency air filters (EPA, HEPA and ULPA). Part 1: Classification, testing, marking. Standard EN 1822-1: 2009. CEN, Brussels, Belgium 2009.

[12] EMA (European Medicines Agency). Note for guidance on quality of water for pharmaceutical use. CPMP/QWP/158/01 Revision. EMEA/CVMP/115/01 Revision. EMA, Committee for Proprietary Medicinal Products (CPMP). Committee for Veterinary Medicinal Products (CVMP), London, UK 2002.

[13] ISPE (International Society of Pharmaceutical Engineering). Water and steam systems. ISPE Baseline Pharmaceutical Engineering Guides, 2nd edition, Tampa, Florida, USA 2011.

[14] FDA (U. S. Food and Drug Administration). Guide to inspections of high purity water systems. FDA, Inspection Technical Guides, 7/93. FDA, Rockville, MD, USA 1993.

[15] ANVISA (Agência Nacional de Vigilância Sanitária). Guia de qualidade para sistemas de purificação de água para uso farmacêutico. Brasília 2013.

[16] WHO (World Health Organization). WHO Good manufacturing practices. Water for pharmaceutical use. In: WHO Expert Committee on Specifications for Pharmaceutical Preparations. Forty-sixth report (WHO Technical Report Series, No. 970). WHO, Geneva, Switzerland 2012. Annex 2.

[17] ISPE (International Society of Pharmaceutical Engineering). Water and steam systems. ISPE Baseline Pharmaceutical Engineering Guides, 2nd edition, Tampa, Florida, USA 2011.

[18] ISO (International Organization for Standardization). Compressed air. Part 1: Contaminants and purity classes. International standard ISO 8573-1:2010(en). ISO, Geneva, Switzerland 2010.

[19] ISPE (International Society of Pharmaceutical Engineering). Commissioning and qualification. ISPE Baseline Pharmaceutical Engineering Guides, Tampa, Florida, USA 2001.

[20] ISO (International Organization for Standardization). Compressed air. Part 4: Test methods for solid particle content. International standard ISO 8573-4:2001(en). ISO, Geneva, Switzerland 2001.

[21] ISO (International Organization for Standardization). Compressed air. Part 3: Test methods for measurement of humidity. International standard ISO 8573-3:1999(en). ISO, Geneva, Switzerland 1999.

[22] ISO (International Organization for Standardization). Compressed air. Part 2: Test methods for oil aerosol content. International standard ISO 8573-2:2007(en). ISO, Geneva, Switzerland 2007.

[23] ISO (International Organization for Standardization). Compressed air. Part 7: Test method for viable microbiological contaminant content. International standard ISO 8573-7:2003(en). ISO, Geneva, Switzerland 2003.

[24] ISPE (International Society of Pharmaceutical Engineering). Process gases. ISPE Good Practice Guide, Tampa, Florida, USA 2011.

[25] The European Parliament and the Council of the European Union. Directive 2003/10/EC of 6 February 2003 on the minimum health and safety requirements regarding the exposure of workers to the risks arising from physical agents (noise). Official Journal of the European Union L 42/38 of 15.02.2003.

Chapter 10: Equipment

CHAPTER 10

Equipment

Abstract: Equipment plays an active role in a pharmaceutical unit by conveying, transforming and protecting from the environment materials and products. Pharmaceutical equipment should observe hygienic rules in its design, construction, installation, utilization and maintenance, as stated by GMP. As most equipment is controlled by computerized systems, it is necessary restricting access to them and ensuring that these can provide the same level of safety than operators (in fact higher). Equipment is as varied as existing operations and technical approaches for performing them, but it can be practically distributed into several groups. The first one is represented by weighing/measurement equipment. The second one is very large and comprises preparation equipment which is basically defined by the physical type of dosage form (liquid, semi-solid, solid). A third group would include secondary packaging equipment. Then a fourth group would be constituted by the booths, cabinets, benches and RABS, which provide limited protected operational environments. And finally we could still mention a fifth group collecting up other varied items of equipment. With the exception of disposable equipment, it is essential securing appropriate cleaning. Qualification, maintenance, calibration and, as required, requalification are essential activities for ensuring appropriate equipment performance.

Keywords: Access control, audit trail, BSC, cleaning, closed systems, computerized systems, materials of construction, dead leg, drainage, isolator, labeling, PLC, qualification, RABS, requalification, sanitary connection, sanitary design, SCADA, smooth surfaces, UDAF.

FUNCTION OF EQUIPMENT IN A PHARMACEUTICAL PLANT

Whereas internal architecture plays passive role providing overall protection and the physical frame for the processes, equipment actively transforms input materials (or products) into output materials (or products) or, simply transports them. Equipment is supported by the adequate utilities. Furthermore, equipment should also protect materials and products from contamination and minimize the risk of error and mix-up. These latter objectives are met by appropriate design, construction, and installation.

Additionally, there is also a specialized type of equipment known by the general name of "measuring instrumentation" which determines process parameters. These instruments can be either parts of manufacturing equipment or self-standing pieces of equipment. Thus, for instance, dosage machines or packaging lines are usually combined with weighing devices, whereas in weighing areas scales are basic items of equipment for weighing materials. It is important to emphasize that

Jordi Botet

pharmaceutical manufacturing control implies parameter monitoring and this usually requires measuring. This is why it can be said that product quality is impossible if there are no quality measures.

From the logistical point of view equipment can either be "dedicated" (used for a single product or for a specific group of products) or simply "multi-product" (used for different products, as necessary). In the first case, cross-contamination usually is not a major concern, but it should not be neglected, however, because degraded residues or bioburden from one batch might contaminate the following one. In the second case, cross-contamination is always lurking. Thus, ensuring proper cleaning is always a priority. In order to overcome this problem disposable equipment has been proposed, but for economical reasons, it still remains limited to particular cases [1].

GMP REQUIREMENTS FOR EQUIPMENT

Here are summarized the essential conditions for equipment as indicated in GMP:

(1) Design and construction: Equipment should be designed and built to be appropriate for its function and to minimize the risk of contamination and errors. It should be of adequate size and make easy the operations (production, cleaning and maintenance).

(2) Absence of dead spaces: Equipment should not have hollows where dust, dirt and materials can accumulate and promote microbial proliferation. These points, known as dead spaces, can be limited by good design and construction of equipment. The golden rule of sanitary design is avoiding them.

(3) Absence of threads, bolts or rivets: Grooves and flutes are in general dead spaces and, as such, should be eliminated from critical parts of equipment (that is, from surfaces contacting products).

Screwed pipe connections are not acceptable. If necessary, connections can be made in two ways (never threaded fittings!):

- Permanent connections: welding without additional material (autogenously) and in an inert atmosphere to avoid oxidation (TIG orbital welding). See chapter 9.

- Temporary connections: sanitary fittings (triclamp® system or equivalent).

(4) Adequate radius of internal corners: Angles and corners should have sufficient radius to ensure that materials will not accumulate there and that they will accessible for cleaning.

(5) Smooth surfaces: Critical parts of equipment should be free of both microscopic irregularities ("bug traps") and macroscopic ones.

(6) Full (100%) drainage: Equipment should be self-draining. It must be designed to avoid stagnation spots (Fig. **1**).

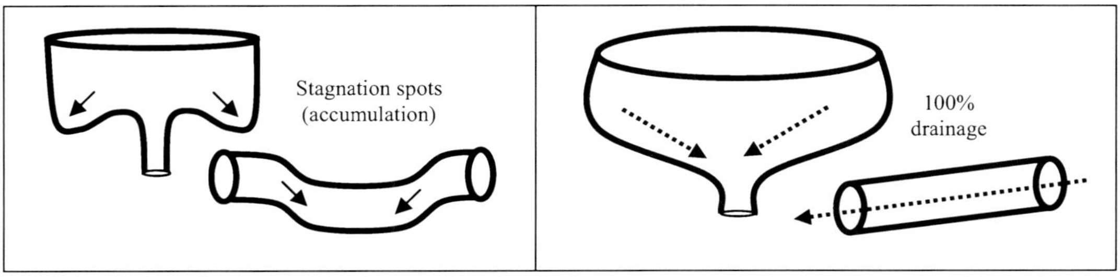

Fig. (1). Self draining equipment.

(7) Dead leg control: Dead spaces created by the blind branch of a pipe are known as "dead legs". In the main pipe liquids flow, but in a dead leg they stagnate. Thus, products can accumulate there and deteriorate, not to mention the possibility of biofilm growth. Materials within a dead leg escape from the action of cleaning or sanitizing agents. This is why equipment should be free of dead legs (Fig. **2**).

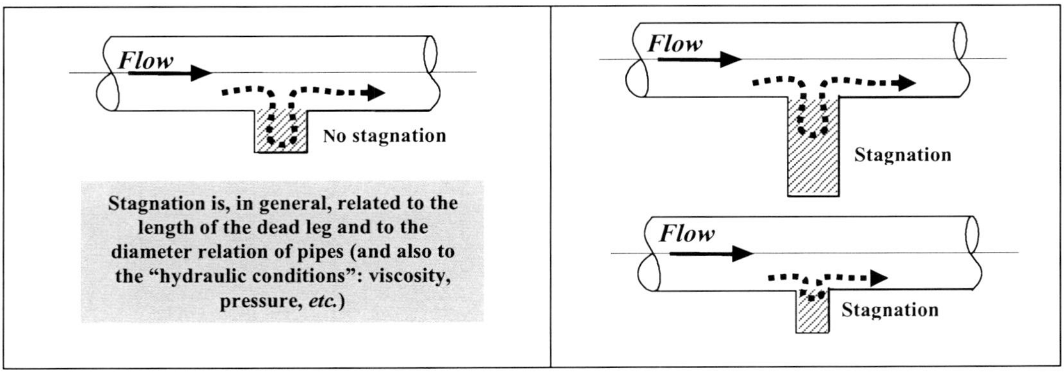

Fig. (2). Dead leg concept.

If any blind branch of a pipe was a dead leg, then, all instruments or valves should be considered as such. Traditionally, however, it is thought that what really matters is not the existence of a blind branch, but the stagnation produced in this piece of pipe.

Practical experience has led to the definition of several rules, basically empirical, for determining if a side unused pipe can be considered a dead leg (Fig. **3**).

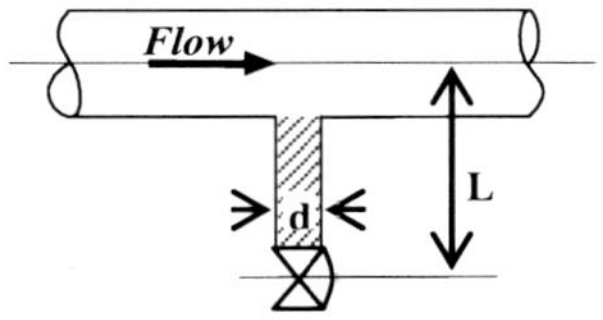	**6 d rule:** The distance (L) from the axis of the main pipe to the center of the valve must not be greater than 6 times the branch diameter [**L < 6 d**]. *It should be pointed out that this was developed for hot 75-80° circulating systems. With colder systems (65-75°C), any drops or unused portion of any length of piping has the potential for the formation of a biofilm and should be eliminated if possible or have special sanitizing procedures* [2].
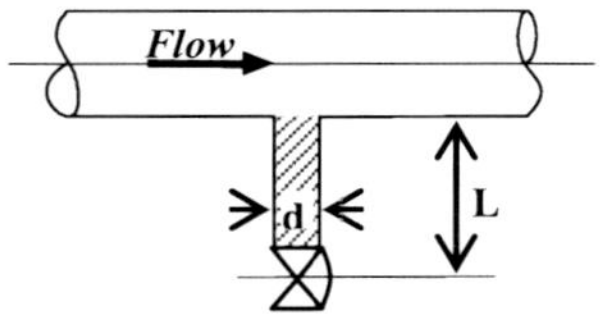	**1.5 d rule:** The distance (L) from the wall of the main pipe to the centre of the valve must not be bigger than 1.5 times the diameter of the branch (**L < 1.5 d**) [3].

Fig. (3). Dead leg: examples of measuring rules.

It is important to remember that dead legs are not exclusively the result of poor design and construction (Fig. **4**). They can also appear as a result of the connection of equipment to pipework. In fact, usually, dead legs do not appear in pieces of equipment designed by specialists but as a consequence of connecting the water hoses used for production (tank filling, *etc.*) or cleaning. Inadvertently, a hose may remain full of water or any other product, for several days.

Even if the above mentioned rules are taken into account in the design of a loop or network, dead legs might appear while connecting pieces of equipment. These stagnation spots may act as contamination sources both for the piece of equipment and for the whole loop or network (should the point of use valve be opened).	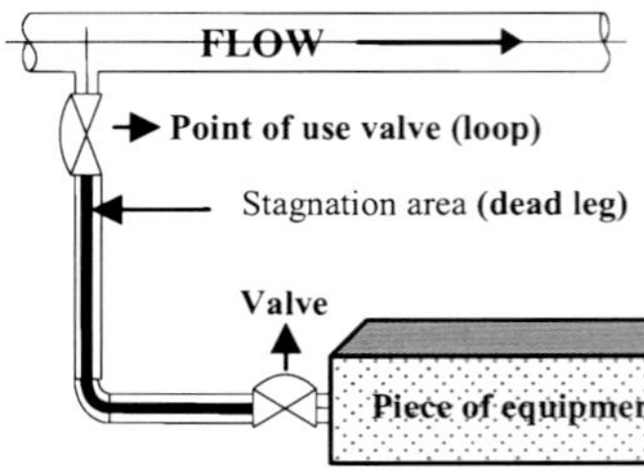

Fig. (4). Extended concept of dead leg.

Technical progress in design and construction of the pieces used for making piping and equipment has led to a large choice of self-draining parts, without significant dead legs (Fig. **5**).

(8) <u>Flush gaskets</u>: A non-flush gasket means a risk of dead space (Fig. **6**).

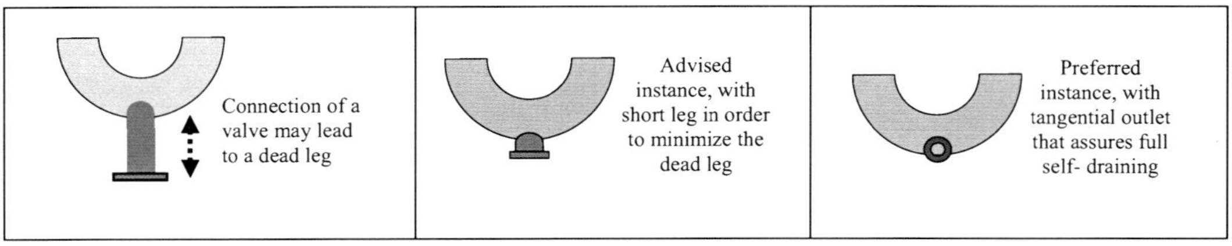

Fig. (5). Valve connections.

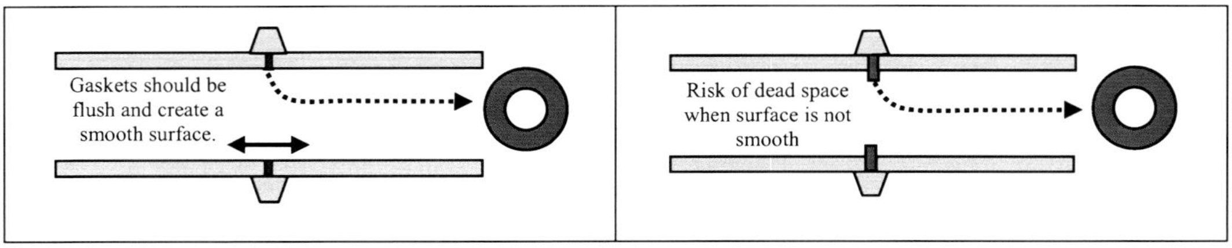

Fig. (6). Dead space.

(9) "Closed systems": The use of closed equipment ensures both the protection of the products from contamination and of the operators/environment from harmful products (provided there is no leakage). This is, however, only true as far as equipment remains closed. Their loading and unloading remains a critical operation and precautions should be taken to control contamination and this is why equipment can be complemented with closed transfer systems.

(10) Easy cleaning: The design and layout of equipment should impede build-up of dust and dirt and allow for effective cleaning. In fact cleaning, washing, and drying of equipment can be not only inefficient but turn into sources of contamination.

This is why there should exist detailed cleaning procedures, which should be validated (taking into account all the intervening items of equipment, the cleaning methods, the use of detergents or solvents and all the involved products) [4]. Nevertheless, manual cleaning is difficult to validate because of the intrinsic variability introduced by operators and thus, the use of "clean in place" (CIP) systems is highly advisable. These systems work on reproducible programs which are readily validated.

(11) Easy sanitization/sterilization: The design of equipment should allow for effective sterilization (including accessory fittings such as valves, pipes, filters, pumps, *etc.*). This is usually performed by steam and in some cases by hydrogen peroxide or dry heat. Equipment should allow for easy sanitization/sterilization. This is why "sterile in place" (SIP) systems are advisable.

(12) Conveyor belt: Conveyor belts should not pass through a partition separating clean rooms of grade A or B and clean rooms of lower air cleanliness (grade C or D), except if the belt itself is ceaselessly sterilized, such as in an sterilizing tunnel.

(13) Materials of construction: Materials used for product contact must follow the general rule of not affecting them and not being affected by them.

Production equipment should not present any hazard to the products. The parts of the production equipment that come into contact with the product must not be reactive, additive, or absorptive to an extent that would affect the quality of the product [5].

(14) Double-tube sheet heat exchangers: Heat exchangers used for product contact should have a double wall in order to exclude the possibility of product contamination in case of utility fluid leakage (usually it is non-pharmaceutical water or steam, as it is supposed they are not going to come into contact with the product). An alternative solution, but not advised because of control difficulties (unless there is an automatic monitoring system), may be the installation of a manometer. A utility fluid leakage would be detected through loss of pressure [6].

(15) Air vent filters: They should be hydrophobic and validated for their designed service life (to be replaced at defined intervals). They should be accessible for in-place periodical integrity testing and after end of use (or whenever there is any doubt about their integrity). A typical problem with vent filters is water condensation which can lead to filter blocking and biofilm growth. To keep vent filters dry they can be heated [7].

(16) Separation of substances required for operation: Any auxiliary substance required for equipment operation (*e.g.* lubricants, coolants, *etc.*) or process (*e.g.* cleaning, pest control products, *etc.*) should never come into contact with products or materials contacting products. Whenever feasible, these substances should minimize the risk of toxicity (*i.e.* they should be of food grade) [8].

(17) Equipment installation: Equipment should be appropriately located and installed to be adequate for the operations, and for cleaning and maintenance. It should minimize any risk of contamination and error.

(18) Equipment should be appropriately identified: Equipment and appropriate parts (piping, valves, instruments, filters, *etc.*) should be labeled with a tag marked with an identification code or number, which will be used in the documentation of batches in order to ensure traceability (Fig. **7**).

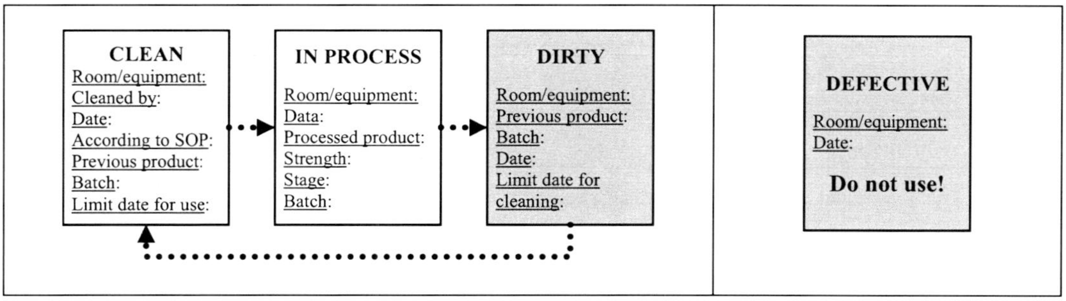

Fig. (7). Room and equipment labeling to show their situation.

Rooms and equipment (both production equipment and packaging lines) should be labeled during process in order to show their situation and, thus, to avoid cross-contamination: clean (ready to be used), batch in process, dirty (waiting to be cleaned) or defective [9]. Production and quality control areas should be free of faulty equipment. If it is impossible to withdraw them from these areas, they should be labeled as defective to avert use [10]. Usually labels use colors to indicate status (red: dirty/defective; green: ready for use; yellow or white: in process).

MAINTENANCE OF EQUIPMENT

Whenever possible, equipment should be installed so as to enable maintenance and repair from a technical zone. Equipment procedures (SOPs) should describe precautions to be taken to avoid product contamination when an intervention is unavoidable (change of format, adjustment, emergency stops, etc). Whenever an intervention may have contaminated equipment parts and this may suppose a hazard for products the successive use of equipment should be authorized by a supervisor after the appropriate cleaning/disinfection. See Fig. (**8**).

Manufacturing equipment and their related utilities should be maintained to suit its intended purpose.

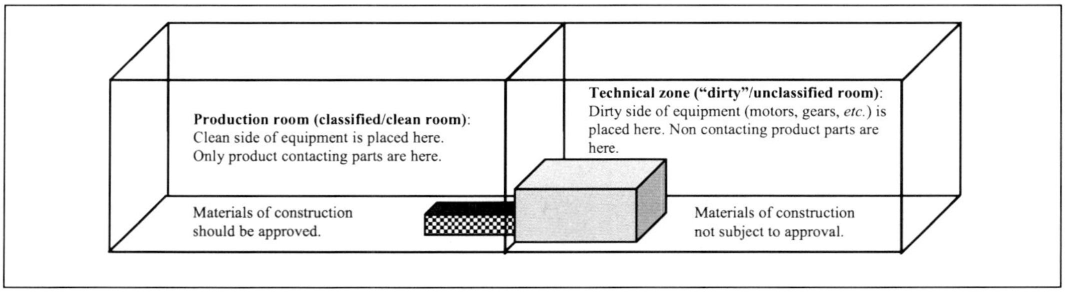

Fig. (8). Equipment reparation and maintenance from outside the production zone.

Weighing and measuring instruments of the production and quality control areas should be of the adequate measuring range and precision, they should be periodically maintained and calibrated and they should be verified daily or before any use [11].

COMPUTERISED CONTROL SYSTEMS

A process is controlled by means of its variables. Automated process control is obtained by using control devices, which read inputs (variable values), compare these values with established set points and generate outputs (actions to match the input values to the set point values).

PLCs (programmable logic controllers) and SCADA systems are commonly used to control processes. Personal computers combined with remote hardware can be used too.

Programmable Logic Controllers (PLCs) are microprocessors used for the automatic control of processes.

Inputs/outputs can be digital or analogue. Digital or discrete signals act like a switch (I/O), while analogue signals have a full value range. In both cases signals are sent by using voltage or current, but whereas digital signals identify specific ranges as "on" or "1" and "off" or "0", analogue signals read a magnitude that is proportional to the process signal.

PLCs can be modular (having a limited number of connections built in for inputs and outputs) or rack-style (having processor modules with separate I/O modules, which may occupy many racks, having a great number of discrete and analogue inputs and outputs). There are more inputs than outputs (usually three times more) for the sake of better control.

PLC programs are stored in the PLC either in battery-backed-up RAM or in some other non-volatile flash memory.

A **SCADA** (Supervisory Control and Data Acquisition) system is a software package used for monitoring and controlling. The SCADA system gathers information and controls field equipment with Remote Terminal Units (RTUs) or with PLCs and formats information to enable an operator to supervise and change set points. Field information is conveyed to the master station by a communication infrastructure.

The master station of a small SCADA system is made up of a single PC, whereas a larger system may be composed of several servers.

The information provided by the SCADA system is shown to the personnel in the form of graphical diagrams. Thus, operators are presented with schematic representations of the system being controlled.

A "computerized system" is *a system including the input of data, electronic processing and the output of information to be used either for reporting or automatic control* [12].

From the GMP point of view the rule of thumb is that computerized systems should provide the same security level than manual operations. It is not necessary adding that in practice well designed and validated systems provide higher reliability [13, 14].

As it is well known, computerized systems are composed of hardware and software. Hardware should be sited in adequate conditions in order to protect it from external interferences. *A written detailed description of the system should be produced (including diagrams as appropriate) and kept up to date. It should describe the principles, objectives, security measures and scope of the system and the main features of the way in which the computer is used and how it interacts with other systems and procedures* [15].

Software determines how hardware will act and thus it is highly critical.

"Electronic record" *means any combination of text, graphics, data, audio, pictorial, or other information representation in digital form that is created, modified, maintained, archived, retrieved, or distributed by a computer system* [16].

"Electronic signature" *means a computer data compilation of any symbol or series of symbols executed, adopted, or authorized by an individual to be the legally binding equivalent of the individual's handwritten signature* [17].

Electronic records and signatures should provide the same reliability than their traditional counterparts on paper and thus, both can be used in production [18].

The main requirements for automated process control systems in order to ensure reliability can be summarized as follows:

(A) **Validation**: The system has to be validated to verify that it operates as specified and changes should be made in a controlled manner and validated [19].

Validation should be considered as a part of the complete life cycle of a computerized system. This cycle includes the stages of planning, specification, programming, testing, commissioning, documentation, operation and monitoring (including modification control) [20].

When a manual system is replaced by a computerized system both systems should be run in parallel during a certain time, in order to validate performance [21].

(B) **Accessibility and safety of recorded data**: The system has to be able to provide recorded process data in a humanly understandable form. Recorded data should be safely archived (*i.e.* with a back-up system) and retrieved during its retention period.

There should be validated procedures describing how to proceed if the system fails or breaks down. In case of failure the corrective actions should be recorded. There should be a procedure for recording and analyzing errors and applying corrective actions.

(C) **Access control and identification of operators**: Only authorized people can access the system and operators are identified by their electronic signatures (which provide the same identification security as a handwritten signature). Signed electronic records should contain information associated with the signature regarding the following data:

(1) The name of the signer;

(2) The date and time of the signature; and

(3) The significance of the signature (*e.g.* review, approval, responsibility, authorship, *etc.*).

Signatures should be linked to their respective electronic records to make certain that they cannot be cut away, copied, or transferred.

Each electronic signature shall be unique to one individual, with well verified identity. It should not be reused by anyone else or reassigned to another person. The entry of critical data by an authorized person requires verification by a second person equally authorized.

Electronic signatures can be based on biometric identifications or not. "Biometrics" *means a method of verifying an individual's identity based on measurement of the individual's physical feature(s) or repeatable action(s) where those features and/or actions are both unique to that individual and measurable* [22].

Electronic signatures that are not based upon biometrics shall:

(1) Employ at least two distinct identification components such as an identification code and password.

(i) When an individual executes a series of signings during a single, continuous period of controlled system access, the first signing shall be executed using all electronic signature components; subsequent signings shall be executed using at least one electronic signature component that is only executable by, and designed to be used only by, the individual.

(ii) When an individual executes one or more signings not performed during a single, continuous period of controlled system access, each signing shall be executed using all of the electronic signature components.

(2) Be used only by their genuine owners; and

(3) Be administered and executed to ensure that attempted use of an individual's electronic signature by anyone other than its genuine owner requires collaboration of two or more individuals.

(b) Electronic signatures based upon biometrics shall be designed to ensure that they cannot be used by anyone other than their genuine owners [23].

Personnel using electronic signatures composed of identification codes combined with passwords should make use of controls for ensuring integrity and security. These controls should comprise:

(a) Maintaining the uniqueness of each combined identification code and password, such that no two individuals have the same combination of identification code and password.

(b) Ensuring that identification code and password issuances are periodically checked, recalled, or revised (e.g., to cover such events as password aging).

(c) *Following loss management procedures to electronically deauthorize lost, stolen, missing, or otherwise potentially compromised tokens, cards, and other devices that bear or generate identification code or password information, and to issue temporary or permanent replacements using suitable, rigorous controls.*

(d) *Use of transaction safeguards to prevent unauthorized use of passwords and/or identification codes, and to detect and report in an immediate and urgent manner any attempts at their unauthorized use to the system security unit, and, as appropriate, to organizational management.*

(e) *Initial and periodic testing of devices, such as tokens or cards, that bear or generate identification code or password information to ensure that they function properly and have not been altered in an unauthorized manner* [24].

(D) **Audit trail**: The date and time of the entries of data and of the actions should be recorded. Record changes must not conceal previously recorded data. They should provide data audit trails with information on the date and time of the entries of data by the operators and on the creation, modification and deleting of records. New records should not delete old ones. This information should be kept at least during the specified retention time.

The system should record the identity of operators entering or confirming critical data. Authority to amend entered data should be restricted to nominated persons. Any alteration to an entry of critical data should be authorized and recorded with the reason for the change. Consideration should be given to building into the system the creation of a complete record of all entries and amendments (an "audit trail") [25].

(E) **Personnel training**: Computerized systems should be managed and used by personnel possessing adequate education, training and experience.

MANUFACTURING EQUIPMENT

Pharmaceutical manufacturing equipment is as varied as the dosage forms that are produced and packaged [26, 27]. Therefore, classifying satisfactorily equipment is as difficult as classifying dosage forms (see chapter 1). Here, thus, manufacturing equipment is described in a very general form taking into account the operations which are performed for obtaining the three groups of dosage forms that exist if they are simply considered from the physical point of view. Specialized dosage forms might require special equipment, which is not considered here. See Fig. (**9**).

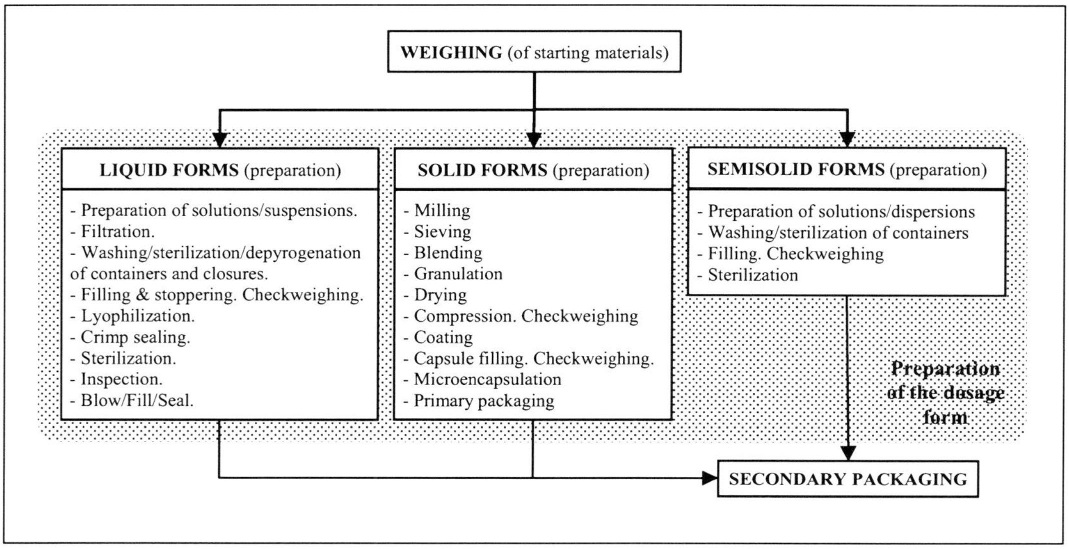

Fig. (9). Manufacturing operations.

Weighing

Any production process starts with the weighing of the starting materials which requires a weighing area. Here equipment is constituted by weighing instrumentation (besides weighing booths).

Liquid Forms

The preparation of these forms is usually relatively simple (Table **1**). However, the manufacture of parenteral forms is more complex because of the need of sterilization/depyrogenation and aseptic handling (Table **2**).

Table 1. Production of liquid non sterile forms.

Operation	Equipment
Preparation of solutions/dispersions	Tanks (with temperature control and stirring)
Filtering	Filters (with pumps, pressure gauges and integrity tester)
Cleaning of containers and stoppers	Container washing machine. Stopper washing machine.

Table 1: contd...

Dosing into containers and stoppering	Container filling, check weighing and stoppering machine
Fixing of labels on the containers	Labeling machine

Solutions/suspensions are prepared in tanks with stirring, temperature control, *etc.*

Then they are usually filtered either for clarification or sterilization and this requires besides filters pumps and other tanks.

Non sterile liquids are usually filled in containers and closures which come already clean from validated vendors (although it is not very practical they are sometimes washed in the plant), but sterile parenteral forms require special containers (vials, ampoules, syringes, cartridges) which are either received ready for use or are washed/sterilized/depyrogenated in the plant and this requires special equipment. Ophthalmic sterile non-parenteral forms are usually filled in plastic containers which are either received ready for use or prepared in place with BFS equipment (blow/fill/seal) [28, 29].

Table 2. Production of liquid sterile forms.

Operation	Equipment
Preparation of solutions/dispersions	Tanks (with temperature control and stirring)
Filtering	Filters (with pumps, pressure gauges and integrity tester)
Cleaning of containers and stoppers	Washing, (siliconization), sterilization and depyrogenation machines
Dosing into containers and stoppering	Filling, check weighing and stoppering machines
Lyophilization	Lyophilizers
Crimp sealing	Crimp sealing machines
Particle inspection	Particle inspection machines
Fixing labels on the containers	Labeling machine
Container forming and filling	Blow/fill/seal machines

Filling equipment varies according to the technology used for dosage and the number of filling heads.

Filled containers are stoppered and also can be checkweighed in line [30]. Stoppered parenteral containers are usually crimp sealed either then or after lyophilization (in case of lyophilized products). Crimp sealing generates particles and this is why this operation has to be completely separated from filling.

Sterilization of sterile products (parenteral or not) is performed either by sterilizing filtration and then aseptic processing or by terminal sterilization which requires steam sterilizators (in case of parenterals) or radiation sterilizators (in most cases of ophthalmics). Other sterilization methods are less frequent.

Parenterals have to be inspected for particulates and this can be performed manually by trained personnel or by automatic equipment.

Solid Forms

Conversely, the production of solid forms is usually rather complex [31]. The first steps are normally milling, sieving and blending. The order of these steps depends on the characteristics of the starting materials. Often they can be performed more than once (*i.e.* sieving of the starting material and after granulation, blending of a part of the starting materials and then addition of the other). See Table **3**.

There are very different types of milling, sieving and blending equipment. The mix of powders (or granules) can be used for filling capsules but if it is necessary producing pills normally this requires the preparation of granulates which are then compressed. These tablets can be coated too. Sometimes capsules are filled with granulates instead of mixtures of powder (or granules). All these operations are performed with specialized equipment. In particular, granulates can be prepared in very complex equipment (fluid beds, specialized granulators, *etc.*).

Table 3. Production of solid forms.

Operation	Equipment
Milling	Grinders/Milling machines
Sieving	Sieving machines
Blending	Blenders (mixers)
Granulation	Dry granulators
	Humid mixing, granulating and drying machines
	Fluid bed granulators
Desiccation	Drying chambers
Capsule filling	Capsule filling machines
Compression (tableting)	Compressing machines
Coating	Coating pans

Table 3: contd...

Primary packaging	Blistering, stripping machines
	Container filling machines
	Sachet filling machines

Microcapsules are obtained in liquid media and this requires tanks, pumps, *etc.*

The primary packaging of solid forms is variable too (tubes, sachets, pill-boxes, *etc.*) but blister packaging is very popular and predominates.

Semi-Solid Forms

These forms are rather complex to obtain too. The different phases (W and O) are prepared in separated reactors and then mixed to obtain the emulsions. The most common forms, like ointments and creams, are filled in tubes or similar containers; whether other specialized forms like the aerosols require specialized containers. Filling machines are much specialized, in particular those required for preparing spray containers. Some semi-solid forms are required to be sterile. For practical reasons the product is prepared to ensure a low bioburden and then the finished tubes are sterilized by radiation. See Table **4**.

Table 4. Production of semi-solid forms.

Operation	Equipment
Preparation of solutions/dispersions	Tanks (with T control and stirring)
Filtering	Filters (with pumps, pressure gauges and integrity tester)
Cleaning of containers and stoppers	Washing machines
Dosing into containers and stoppering/closing	Container filling, checkweighing and stoppering/closing machines

Secondary Packaging

Once the different dosage forms are safely packaged into their primary packaging container (*e.g.* blister, vial, tube, *etc.*) they can be put into the secondary packaging (box, directions for use, *etc.*) to obtain the finished product. In this last manufacturing step the product is isolated within its primary packaging. Consequently secondary packaging rooms do not require any particulate environmental control, just (and very important) temperature monitoring and measures against cross-contamination, understood in this case as product mix-up.

ENVIRONMENTAL PROTECTIVE EQUIPMENT

Manufacturing is performed with equipment installed in environmentally controlled rooms (particles, temperature, humidity, pressure, *etc.*). Sometimes, however, it is necessary to perform certain operations in a secluded special type of controlled environment.

This can be obtained inside specialized booths or cabinets or by means of RABS.

UDAF Booths/Cabinets

When it is necessary to protect materials or products from contamination, operations can be realized under UDAF (unidirectional air-flow). Often a part of a clean room has an integrated UDAF, where are performed the most critical operations. A first example of this are clean rooms classified grade B, but with a part of them separated by plastic strips which is classified grade A. A second example may be provided by weighing rooms which are usually classified grade D, but which include a UDAF classified grade C, where weighing is performed. In these cases parts provided with UDAF can be built into the room with HEPA filters installed on the ceiling and separated by plastic curtains from the rest of the room. When there is no need of extended UDAF areas it is possible to install there a piece of equipment providing this type of environment: a UDAF booth or cabinet. This equipment can be movable or be fixed in place.

UDAF booths/cabinets, which traditionally had been known as "laminar flow" booths/cabinets, thanks to their type of air-flow provide a high-quality environment and, thus, manipulated products are protected from contamination, but the operator is not protected, because the air-flow after colliding with the product might be deflected towards the operator. This situation is inacceptable in case of hazardous products and then a biological safety cabinet should be used.

Restricted Access Barrier System (RABS)

The acronym RABS is used for designing an ensemble of devices conceived for separating aseptic processes from operators. Previously we have already seen how personnel, regarding contamination, are the enemy number one of pharmaceutical quality. RABS constitute, then, another approach for overcoming this problem.

Although the principles for developing RABS are the same used for designing class III BSCs (isolators), it should be born in mind that RABS possess doors and the principle of separation is less strict. They are in fact small clean rooms where equipment is placed, but personnel are excluded. In isolators the process of internal sanitization has to be validated, whereas in RABS the internal environment is validated like that of a clean room.

Initially RABS were simply thought as parts of a clean room where aseptic filling was performed and which were separated from the operator by a glass or plastic panel. Operators could manipulate the process through openings provided with gloves and sleeves (gauntlets). However, RABS gained progressively sophistication to come close to isolators.

Although RABS have doors, in principle, they should only be opened for preliminary adjusting of equipment.

During the aseptic process they should remain closed, thus turning a RABS into practically an isolator.

Therefore, a RABS might be characterized as follows:

- Rigid separation wall;
- UDAF providing a class ISO 5/grade A environment in the critical area;
- Sterilization in place (SIP) or sterilization in an autoclave and aseptic transfer and assembling *in situ*;
- Aseptic ingress of items which are necessary for working;
- Use of gloves + sleeves or half-suits;
- Sanitization of all the surfaces without direct contact with the product;
- Clean room environment of class ISO 7/grade C at least. As an additional measure of protection (especially when doors should be opened) both clean room and critical area might possess the same level of classification (ISO 5/grade A).

From the aforementioned considerations it is evident that RABS are effective whenever their doors remain closed during the process. This is why there should be a procedure describing the actions to be taken if doors are to be open (*i.e.* some containers tumbled over and a piece of equipment got stuck or needs adjustment). The following points should be considered:

- Controlled opening of the door;
- Recording of the door opening (reason, time which remained opened, responsible which authorized it, *etc.*);
- While the door remains open there should be an outbound steady flow of air, to impede entrance of contamination;
- Sanitization of surfaces which are not in contact with the product;
- After the intervention work will be resumed only when the critical area will reach again environmental class ISO 5/grade A.

Biological Safety Cabinets (BSC)

BSC are a particular kind of booths designed primarily to protect operators (and environment) from hazardous microorganisms and materials. According to their characteristics they belong to three classes which offer different performances (Fig. **10**). Closed cabinets of class III are more commonly known as isolators and have a very wide use ranging from sterility testing or aseptic production to the manipulation of hazardous substances or microorganisms.

Class/ Subclass		Characteristics	Operator protection	Product protection	Used with	Schematic representation
I		Open front booth. Exhaust air is HEPA filtered and sent into the room or outside.	Yes. Front flow > 0.7 – 1.0 m/s.	No.	Biologic agents (groups 1, 2 and 3).	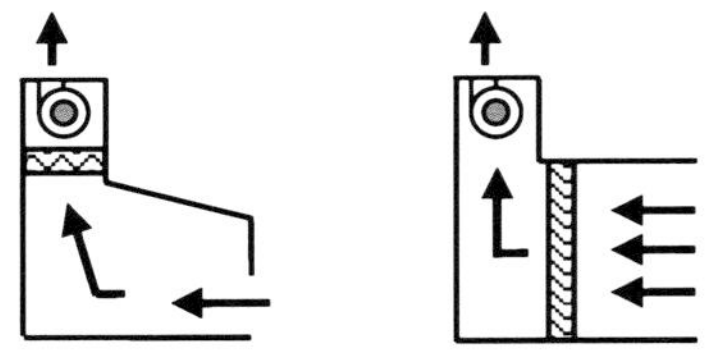
II	A1	70% of air is recycled. 30% of air is exhausted outside after HEPA filtering.	Yes. Front flow ≥ 0.4 m/s.	Yes. UDF: 0.25 – 0.60 m/s.	Biologic agents (groups 1, 2 and 3). Subclass B2 is also suited for hazardous and radioactive substances.	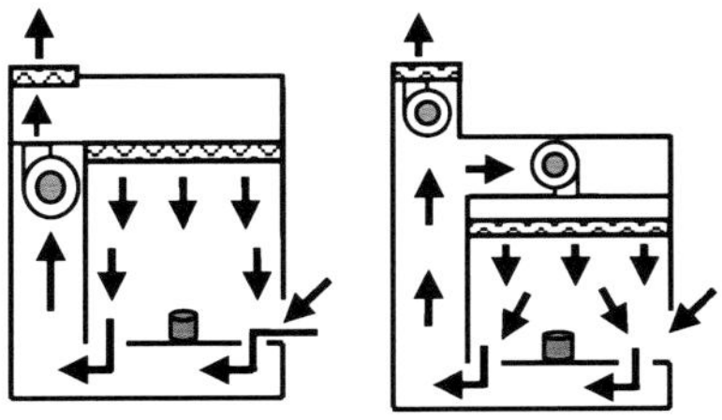 Model with one fan; Model with two fans
	A2	Like A1 but higher frontal airflow speed.				
	B1	30% of air is recycled. 70% of air is exhausted outside after HEPA filtering.				
	B2	No air recycling. Air is exhausted outside after HEPA filtering.				

Contd Fig. (10)

III	Closed enclosure (total contention). Air is supplied and exhausted through HEPA filters. They are known as isolators	Yes. Front flow ≥ 0.7 m/s (with a glove removed).	Yes. With or without UDF.	Biologic agents from groups 1, 2, 3 and 4. Suited for hazardous and radioactive substances.	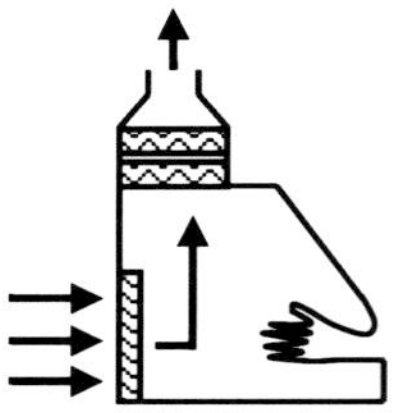

Fig. (10). Classes of BSC.

HAZARD ANALYSIS OF EQUIPMENT

Quality risk analysis is an essential tool to understand how a piece of equipment operates, which are its weak points, which is the better approach for writing the related procedures, how operators should be trained, how to develop qualification, *etc.*

This can be practically done by a baseline hazard analysis using "primary hazard analysis" (PHA). Afterwards, when more knowledge has been gathered, it is possible to use other more complex tools and estimate risk. See chapter 3 for more details.

This analysis (Table **5**) has to be specifically done for each type of equipment, but as this is not possible here, below is given a general draft to be simply taken as a rough model.

Table 5. Simplified model of PHA for a piece of equipment: identification of quality hazards.

Hazard	#	Cause	Preventive measures
Contamination (external)	1	Open equipment	Use of closed equipment/Segregate equipment within a booth or RABS
	2	Dirty environment	Equipment sited in a clean room
	3	Dirty operators	Use adequate clothing/Train operators
	4	Decomposition of materials of construction of tools/equipment	Use only approved materials of construction.
	5	Microbial contamination	Qualify sanitization procedure.
	---	---	---
Cross-contamination	1	Airborne dust	Provide dust exhaust/Provide adequate separation between products (different rooms, pressure cascades, airlocks, *etc.*).

Table 5: contd...

	2	Presence of dead spaces/legs	Use only equipment designed, built and installed according to GMP.
	3	Incomplete drainage	
	4	Inadequate cleaning	Validate cleaning procedures.
	---	---	---
Environmental contamination	1	Open equipment	Do not use open equipment for hazardous products or place it within an isolator.
	2	Contaminated exhausting air	Provide sure exhaust (*e.g.* HEPA filtration, incineration).
	---	---	---
Error/mix-up/substitution	1	Inadequate use of equipment by operator	Train operators/Supervise critical operations/Prepare clear SOPs/Monitor process/Restrict access to equipment.
	2	Equipment failure	Qualify equipment/Provide maintenance and calibration/Periodical requalification of equipment (as necessary)/Monitor process.
	---	---	---
Material/ Product alteration	1	Reactivity of materials of construction	Use only approved materials of construction.
	2	Inadequate process temperature	Determine and monitor adequate temperature range.
	---	---	---

MAINTENANCE AND CALIBRATION

See chapter 2 for detailed information on these topics.

QUALIFICATION

The organization of the qualification master plan (QMP) and its related testing (DQ, IQ, OQ and PQ) were described in chapter 2. Here are just given some complementary hints [32]. For practical reasons equipment can fall in four groups (Fig. **11**):

1st - Weighing equipment: Weighing is a very important operation in pharmaceutical manufacturing (*e.g.* weighing is required for ascertaining the quantities that are sampled, for measuring the quantities of starting materials, for controlling production operations, for estimation of yields, for checking dosage, for scrutinizing boxes of finished product.).

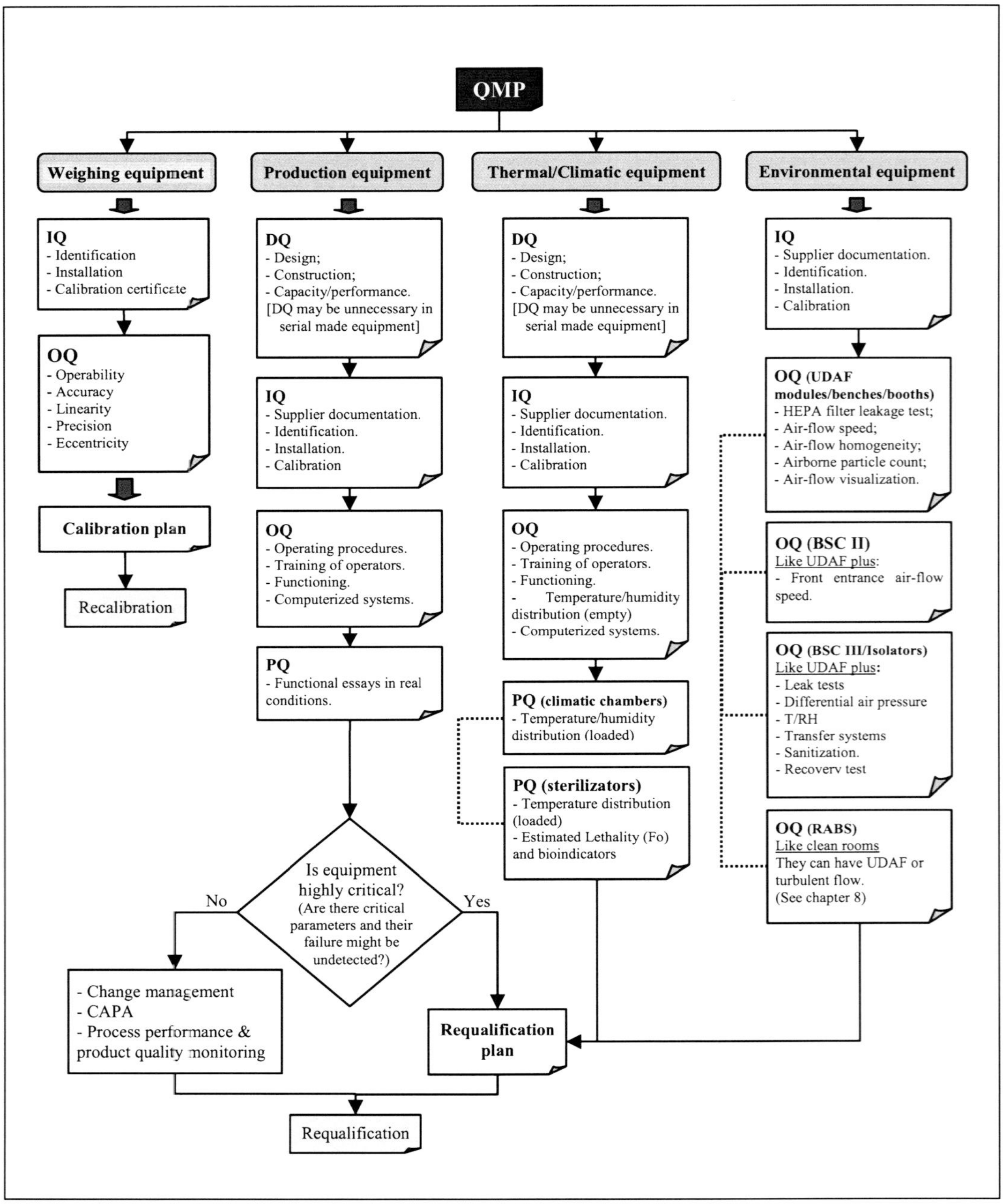

Fig. (11). Schematic representation of the organization of the qualification.

2nd – <u>Production equipment</u>: It is so varied that it is only possible to provide general orientation.

3rd – Thermal/climatic equipment: This group can be subdivided into two kinds. On the one hand devices which use high temperature, either for heating (stoves) or for sterilizing (autoclaves, ovens and SIP systems).

On the other devices which use low temperature (climatic chambers, freezers, refrigerators, and cold chambers). Although this equipment might be also considered "production equipment", it is so particular, that it is better to treat it separately.

4th - Environmental equipment: This group is composed by pieces of equipment that are installed within clean rooms in order to provide a separated environment in terms of particle contamination for the production operations.

The objective of UDAF modules/benches/booths is providing a localized class ISO 5/grade A environment.

Biological safety cabinets are used basically to protect operators from the materials which are manipulated (class I) and also to keep these materials uncontaminated (class II). Isolators (class III) provide a completely separated environment (aseptic or not). RABS, as it was previously discussed, can vary in design, but in principle they should be treated as small clean rooms, installed within a big clean room, and which keep operations separated from the operators.

Weighing Equipment

Scales are submitted to initial qualification (IQ and OQ), to permanent verification and to periodical recalibration [33].

Installation Qualification (IQ)

- Confirmation of make and model and identification (fixed tag with its code).
- Verification that the supplier provided operation and maintenance instructions.
- Verification that standard weights are available.
- Verification of appropriate location, leveling and connection.
- Verification of the certificate of calibration and that a label has been stuck.

Operational Qualification (OQ)

- Verification of the assembly, checking, utilization, cleaning, and calibration procedure.
- Verification that operators are adequately trained.
- Verification of equipment functioning (switch on/off, messages, alarms, realization of foreseen functions, working parameters, printing reports, *etc.*).
- Verification of accuracy, linearity, precision, eccentricity.

Permanent Verification

- Check of leveling (every day before starting weighing).
- Automatic internal calibration (every day before starting weighing).
- Verification with standard weights (every day for highly critical balances; once/twice a week for less critical balances).

Periodical Recalibration

It is often realized once a year (or twice for very critical balances). See chapter 2.

Production Equipment

Pieces of equipment used in the manufacture of pharmaceutical products are submitted to IQ and OQ.

DQ is mainly realized for tailor-made equipment.

PQ is performed when it is necessary testing the equipment with (real or placebo) materials or products. Often OQ and PQ are realized together [34, 35].

Design Qualification (DQ)

- Verification that the design (material/product flows, protection from contamination, cleanability, separation from service parts and fluids, lack of dead spaces/legs, *etc.*) corresponds to GMP/GEP.
- Verification that parts in contact with products are adequate (materials of construction, finishes, sanitary connections, *etc.*).

- Confirmation that capacity and performances correspond to the user requirements specification (URS).

Installation Qualification (IQ)

- Gather and evaluate the supplier documentation.
- Confirm make and model and identification (fixed tag with its code).
- Verify the appropriate putting in place.
- Check the calibration certificates.
- Check the certificates of the materials of construction.

Operational Qualification (OQ)

- Verify the procedure/s (assembling, checking, utilization, cleaning, maintenance and calibration).
- Verify that operators are adequately trained.
- Verify equipment while functioning (start/stop, alert messages, alarms, working parameters, realization of foreseen functions, protection mechanisms, *etc.*).
- Verify computerized systems (access control, traceability, filing and retrieving of data, report printing, *etc.*).

Performance Qualification (PQ)

- Verify equipment functioning with authentic or mock materials/products and in true processing conditions (*e.g.* connected to other items of equipment, real production speed, *etc.*).

Thermal/Climatic Equipment

DQ is usually realized for tailor-made pieces of equipment. IQ, OQ and PQ are performed for all items. OQ and PQ are normally performed together. For these items it is essential to proof that within the chamber there are no significant differences in temperature both when empty and loaded. OQ and PQ require specialized equipment provided with wire probes. These probes are placed in points of the chamber homogeneously distributed, including worst case points (*i.e.*

for the OQ the coldest or warmest points; for the PQ the points of the load where penetration of heat is more difficult, like big containers with liquid or big parcels).

Design Qualification (DQ)

- Verify that the design (material/product flows, protection from contamination, cleanability, *etc.*) corresponds to GMP/GEP.

- Confirm that capacity and performances correspond to the user requirements specification (URS).

Installation Qualification (IQ)

- Gather and evaluate the supplier documentation.

- Confirm make and model and identification (fixed tag with its code).

- Verify the appropriate putting in place.

- Check the calibration certificates.

Operational Qualification (OQ)

- Verify the SOPs referring to the operation of equipment (assembling, checking, utilization, cleaning, maintenance, calibration).

- Verify that operators are adequately trained.

- Verify equipment functioning (start, stop, alert messages, alarms, realization of functions, parameters, protection mechanisms, *etc.*).

- Verify the homogeneity of distribution of temperature (sterilizators, ovens and systems for sterilization in place) and of temperature and humidity (RH) in the chamber.

- Verify computerized systems (access control, traceability, filing and retrieving of data, report printing, *etc.*).

Performance Qualification (PQ)

- Verify the homogeneity of distribution of temperature or of temperature and RH with loaded chamber.

- For sterilizators it is verified that the programmed lethality (F_0) is obtained and that bioindicators when are incubated show no growth.
- For steam sterilization of tissues the Bowie and Dick test.

Environmental Equipment

In most cases neither DQ nor PQ are necessary.

Installation Qualification (IQ)

- Gather and evaluate the supplier documentation.
- Confirm make, model and identification (fixed tag with its code).
- Verify the appropriate putting in place.
- Check the calibration certificates.
- Check ergonomy (for isolators).

Operational Qualification (OQ)

UDAF Modules/Benches/Booths

- Count airborne particles.
- Verify the integrity and tightness of HEPA filter/s (filter leakage test).
- Measure airflow (airflow velocity and homogeneity).
- Visualize airflow (airflow pattern).
- Measure lighting and noise.

BSC Class II

Besides the above mentioned tests:

- Measure the airflow speed at the front entrance.

BSC Class III (Isolators)

Besides the tests which are performed for UDAF modules/benches/booths:

- Test leaking of the isolator chamber and of the gloves, sleeves, half-suits.
- Measure the air ΔP between isolator chamber and clean room.
- Check the transfer systems (clean room–isolator chamber–clean room).
- Verify the sanitization of the isolator chamber.
- Realize recovery test.
- Measure temperature.
- Measure relative humidity (as appropriate).
- Measure lighting and noise.

RABS

See chapter 8 for information on clean room tests.

MONITORING OF PRODUCTION EQUIPMENT

The system of "Process performance & product quality monitoring" is mainly thought for the verification of the quality of the products, but it allows also for the detection of changes in the performance of equipment (*i.e.* capability, yield, deviations, *etc.*).

REQUALIFICATION

Generally speaking it can be said that periodical requalification is only necessary for very critical equipment (*e.g.* thermal/climatic and environmental equipment). Other equipment is requalified either because required by the change monitoring system or because process monitoring detects that it might be going out of control.

CLEANING VALIDATION

What it is and why it is imperative?

Defective cleaning of equipment is the hallmark of contamination. Materials and products processed in "dirty" equipment can be contaminated by three types of items which should be considered separately because they have different origins:

- Active substances: Cross-contamination derived from the presence of residues of previously prepared products. Contamination can be produced by the product itself or by their products of degradation (important point: are there products of degradation?). It has to be pointed out that the hazard is normally caused by the active substances of the products (APIs) because excipients are in principle inactive. If residues of these active substances are transferred to another product they might provide it with undesired pharmacological properties.

- Microorganisms: Products and equipment surfaces contain microorganisms which can contaminate the next products (important points: is bioburden an important concern for the product? does the composition of the product favor the growth of microbes?)

- Chemicals: If cleaning/sanitizing agents are used in the cleaning process and they are not eliminated during the final rinsing they will contaminate the next products.

Therefore, it is indispensable proving that any remainder of previous products on the surfaces of equipment will be so insignificant that they will not affect the properties of the following products [36].

Cleaning validation is documented evidence that an approved cleaning procedure will remove all traces of the previous product used in the equipment [37].

Validation takes for granted that residues of product which remain on the surfaces of equipment and tools are incorporated in a homogeneous manner in the following batch of product which is prepared in this equipment. Thus, the contamination of a product will be the sum of all the partial contaminations produced in each item of equipment or tool used in the manufacturing process. In the validation of cleaning procedures should only be considered the detergents/sanitizers which are not volatile, because those which evaporate quickly (*e.g*. ethanol) do not leave residues.

Approach

First of all it is necessary to point out that validation concerns a specific cleaning procedure for an item or model of equipment (Fig. **12**).

Use of Equipment

In dedicated equipment cleaning validation consists basically in determining if after cleaning remain on the equipment significant amounts of residues of the product itself or of its products of degradation and also evaluating if there is significant microbiological contamination.

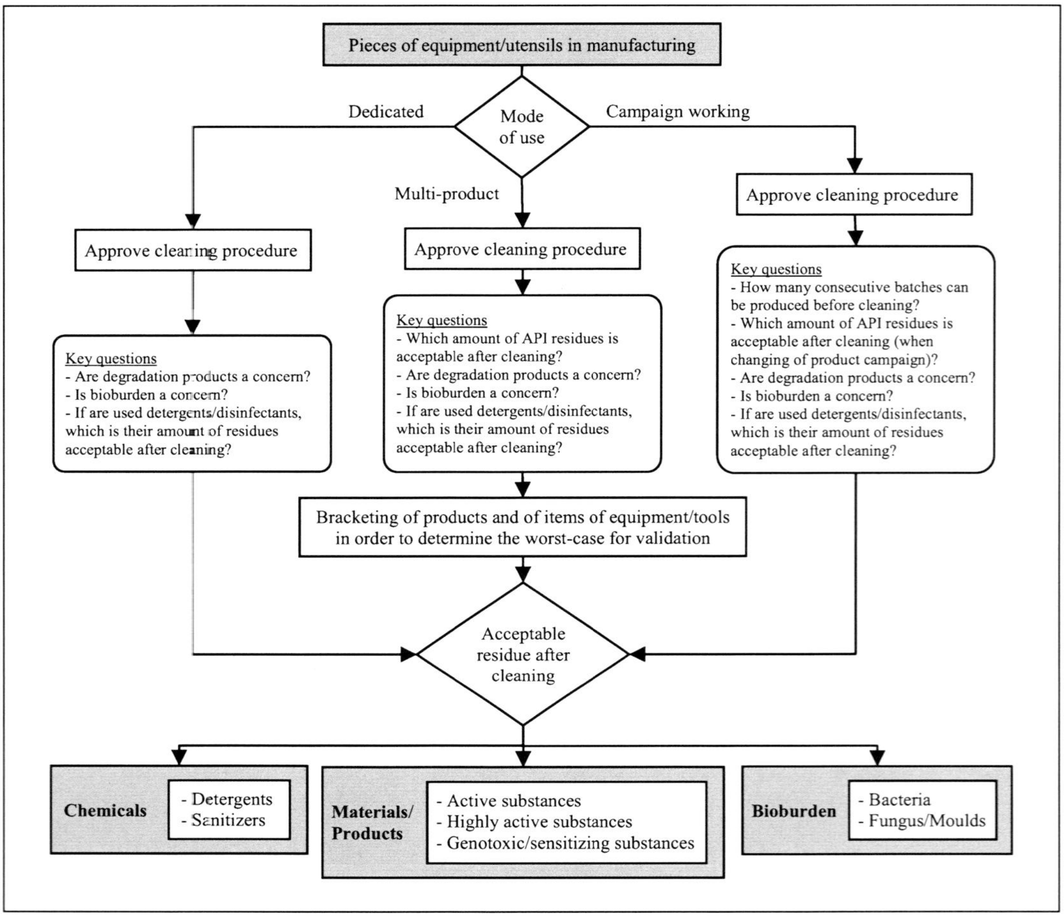

Fig. (12). Cleaning validation rationale.

In <u>multiproduct equipment</u> it should be validated that the approved cleaning procedure is effective in cleaning all the products which are manufactured with this equipment. As this is normally not workable, a risk study of the intervening products and items of equipment will allow for choosing a worst case. It is accepted that only the worst case will be validated, on the assumption that if the cleaning procedure is appropriate for the most difficult product to clean, then it will also work for the other easier products.

In case of <u>campaign working</u> the aim of cleaning validation is showing that a determinate number of batches of the same product can be produced with the same equipment, one after the other and not doing intermediate cleaning, without affecting the quality of the product. Attention to the change of product campaign!

Cleaning Intervals

When validating the cleaning procedures it is necessary to consider three types of time intervals. In the validation of a cleaning procedure should be considered all of them (Fig. **13**).

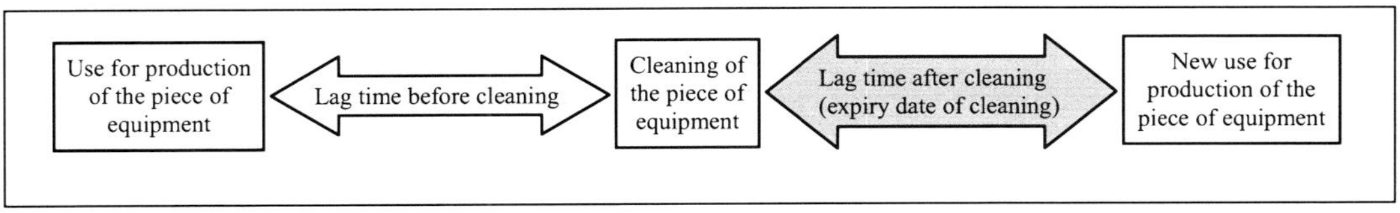

Fig. (13). Cleaning validation approach I (lag times).

(1) From completing the production process to starting the cleaning of equipment: Cleaning validation should ensure that the cleaning procedure is correct within a maximal interval of time established between use of equipment and cleaning. This interval should be based on logistic considerations and risk analysis, and validated.

(2) Expiry date of cleaning: The intent is establishing how long clean equipment can lay fallow (but kept in adequate conditions described in written) and maintain its adequate proprieties for considering it clean and adequate for starting production. This interval should be based on logistic considerations and risk analysis, and validated. Once a piece of equipment surpasses the period which was shown adequate after validation it should be cleaned anew.

(3) Maximal working interval: In campaign working with the same product often it is not necessary cleaning equipment after each batch. Thus, the pieces of equipment will keep producing for a determinate number of batches without cleaning. This interval will be established according to the results obtained in the cleaning validation and will be established in order to impede the generation of degradation products and microbiological contaminations. The priority of performing campaign validation will be decided for each piece of equipment according to the manufacturing requirements. In each case it will be determined the worst case corresponding to the campaign equipment. See Fig. (**14**).

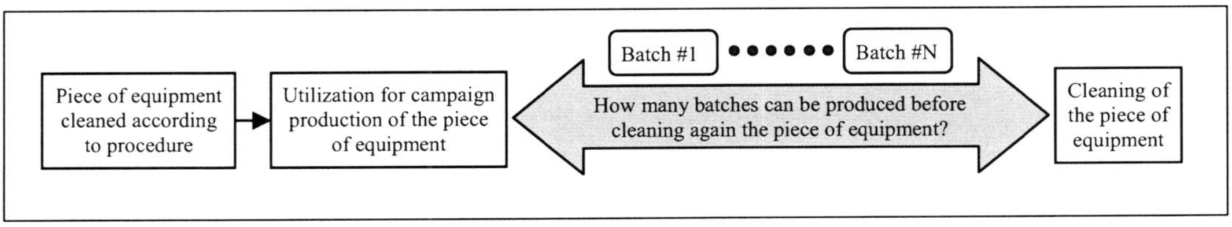

Fig. (14). Cleaning validation approach II (batch series in campaign production).

Bracketing

Cleaning procedures for products and processes which are very similar do not need to be individually validated. A validation study of the "worst case" may be considered acceptable. There should be a justified validation program for this approach referred to as "bracketing", addressing critical issues relating to the selected product, equipment or process [38].

The worst case is usually constituted by the product containing the API less soluble which is produced in the piece/s of equipment to be validated. Other topics which should be taken into account are the adherence of the API to the surfaces of equipment, its potency or toxicity, *etc.* After determining the worst case for each item of equipment, new products will be analyzed to see if they suppose a new worst case and it is necessary modifying the validation.

In order to determine the worst case a risk analysis tool, Risk ranking and filtering (RRF), which was described in chapter 3, is very useful because it allows for identifying and integrating all the factors (Table **6**) contributing to the global risk:

- Which product is processed before cleaning (solubility, therapeutic dose, adsorption to surfaces, degradation, batch size, *etc.*);
- Which product is processed after cleaning (therapeutic dose, batch size, *etc.*);
- Characteristics of the production process (humidity, powder, concentration at a point, *etc.*);
- Characteristics of the equipment (contact surface, qualities of its surface, dedication or not, *etc.*);
- Characteristics of the cleaning process (automatic, manual, time between utilization and cleaning, *etc.*);
- Cleaning/sanitizing intervals;
- Use of chemicals (toxicity, concentration, *etc.*).

It is evident that different equipment requires separated validation, but when validating a process where slightly different equipment is involved it is necessary to take into account the pieces of equipment with the most differentiated design.

In case of introducing new equipment a revision of the risk assessment is required. This would allow evaluating its impact on the validation plan and, if necessary, to modify it.

The cleaning procedure is validated after production of worst case products. If there are products possessing a particular method of cleaning, they should be validated separately.

Table 6. Simplified example of evaluation of factors which contribute in building the global risk.

HAZARD	RISK	
	Components	**Factors**
API contamination	PRODUCT BEFORE CLEANING (P1)	Solubility
		Toxicity/Activity (Therapeutic single dose)
		Quantity. Batch size
		Physical characteristics: Adsorption to surfaces, humidity, granulometry
		Existence of products of degradation
	EQUIPMENT/TOOLS	Dedicated/multi-product
		Size (surface coming into contact with the product)
		Characteristics of surface: polished, soft, irregular
		Materials of construction: Stainless steel, silicone, natural products (latex, cotton, *etc.*).
		Design: Accessibility, pipes, gaskets, *etc.*
		Product dispersion: Regular/irregular (concentration in certain points).
	FABRICATION PROCESS	Presence of humidity, degree of dispersion of the product, duration of the process.
		Time of equipment use between two cleaning runs (dedicated equipment/campaign working).
	CLEANING PROCESS	Mode of cleaning: Manual, semi-automatic, automatic (CIP).
		Lag time between cleaning and use.
		Temperature.
		Lag time between utilization for production and cleaning (how long it remains dirty).
	PRODUCT AFTER CLEANING (P2)	Quantity: Batch size.
		Maximum daily dose.

Table 6: contd…

Residues of chemicals	PRODUCT USED	Toxicity: DL_{50}.
		Quantity: Concentration.
	EQUIPMENT	Surface extension.
		Surface characteristics.
		Materials of construction: Stainless steel, silicone, natural products (latex, cotton, *etc.*).
		Design: Accessibility, pipes, gaskets, valves, *etc.*
	CLEANING PROCESS	Mode of cleaning: Manual, semi-automatic, automatic (CIP).
		Temperature.
Microbiological contamination	PRODUCT BEFORE CLEANING (P1)	Physical characteristics: Adsorption to the surfaces, humidity, granulometry.
		Origin: Natural, synthetic.
		Antimicrobial activity: Yes/no.
	FABRICATION PROCESS	Room temperature/high temperature.
		Humidity: Dry or wet process.
		Closed system/Open system with manual intervention.
	EQUIPMENT/TOOLS	Surface extension.
		Surface characteristics.
		Building materials: Stainless steel, silicone, natural products (latex, cotton, *etc.*).
		Design: Accessibility, pipes, gaskets, valves, *etc.*
	CLEANING PROCESS	Mode of cleaning: Manual, semi-automatic, automatic (CIP).
		Temperature: at room temperature, warm, steam.
		Time of equipment use between two cleaning runs (dedicated equipment/campaign working).
		Lag time between cleaning and use.
		Expiry date of cleaning.
		Lag time between utilization for production and cleaning (how long it remains dirty).
		Drying time.
	CHEMICALS	Detergent/disinfectant.
		Concentration.

Acceptance Criteria for Residues After Cleaning

In case of not detecting residues or detecting them but not being able to quantify them, for the calculation it will be used the detection limit as residue (Fig. **15**).

Visual Revision

The first criterion to be met is that visual inspection does not detect remains on the surfaces of equipment. Visual sensitivity is very high (4-20 $\mu g/cm^2$).

Active Substances

This is a debatable point in cleaning validation. Admitting that, even if it is so small that it cannot be quantified, there will always be some remains of the product before cleaning (P1) in the product after cleaning (P2) the key question is: which amount of these remains may be considered acceptable? The logical approach is considering a critical parameter of P1 and quantifying its presence in P2. This presence should be low enough for not having any relevant effect.

Even accepting that boundaries between them are not always well-defined, in a practical way it is possible to consider three different situations:

a) In multi-product facilities residues containing active substances of P1 can be transferred to P2. As the products, generally speaking, do not possess high activity, it is possible to consider a global maximal amount of P1 in P2 or, in a more technical way, a maximal amount of the minimal therapeutic dose of P1 in P2. Not more than 0.1% of the minimal therapeutic dose of the previous product should appear in the following product.

b) In highly active substances it has been proposed to use the "Permitted (or Acceptable) Daily Exposure" (**PDE/ADE**), which is the dose that is unlikely to cause an adverse effect if an individual is exposed at or below this dose every day for a lifetime.

   This PDE is determined for every substance by means of the existing data from clinical or toxicological studies performed in order to obtain a "no-observed-effect-level" (**NOEL**), which is the highest tested dose at which no critical effect is observed. In this context, critical means that there has not been observed any negative impact on health (in a toxicological study) or therapeutic effect (in a clinical study). Once NOEL has been determined, its lowest value is used to calculate the PDE, which is obtained dividing the NOEL by security factors [39].

c) It is necessary to exclude from this approach the substances which posses a genotoxic or sensibilizing potential and, thus, require a particularized approach. For genotoxic substances it is possible to apply the "Threshold of Toxicological Concern" (TTC). For APIs it has been established a TTC of 0.15 µg/person/day.

When threshold values are not supported by scientific data (*e.g.* allergenic potential from highly sensitizing materials) or when risk cannot be adequately controlled by operational and/or technical measures, it is necessary to use dedicated equipment in the manufacture of these high risk medicinal products.

Chemicals

It is indispensable to establish maximal limits of residues of detergents/sanitizers on the equipment after cleaning. In case of introducing a new chemical it will be necessary to perform risk analysis to determine its impact on the validation plan.

Bioburden

Maximal acceptable limits of microbiological contamination after cleaning should also be established. In order to avoid contamination, when validating a cleaning procedure it is necessary taking microbiological samples before those used for chemical studies and choose different places for sampling.

MC (ppm) = F x (TSD/MDD)

MC (Maximum Carryover): Maximal quantity of contaminant (API) per weight unit in the following batch (in ppm)
TSD (Therapeutic Single Dose): Minimal therapeutic dose of the previous product (in µg)
MDD (Maximum Daily Dose): Maximal daily dose of the following product (in g)
F (fraction of the TSD) = 0,001

MACO (µg) = MC (ppm) x MBS (Kg) x 1000

MACO (Maximum allowable carryover): Maximal quantity of contaminant (API) allowed in the entire following batch.
MBS (Minimum Batch Size): Smallest size of batch (in Kg)

Qs (µg/cm^2) = MACO (µg)/S (cm^2)

Qs: Maximal quantity of contaminant (API) which is allowed per surface unit (µg/cm^2)
S: Total surface (in cm^2) of the common items of equipment which intervene in the manufacturing process of the product which creates the contamination (previous product) and of the product which is contaminated (following product). It refers to the surface which is in direct contact with the product.

Fig. (15). Calculation of the maximal acceptable residue of contaminant.

Revalidation

A revalidation of the cleaning process is indicated when modifying the cleaning procedures, or after 5 years from the validation, or in case of cleaning problems.

Practical development of the validation of cleaning procedures

Is it Necessary to Validate?

The necessity of validation of a cleaning procedure should be evaluated in whichever of the following cases (Table **7**):

- Introduction of a new process;
- Modification of an existing process;
- Introduction of a new product;
- Introduction of a new item of equipment or tool;
- Change in cleaning intervals.

Table 7. Is it necessary to validate?

Reason for validation	Description	Is there a worst case?	Is validation required?
(1) New process □		□ Yes/□ No	□ Yes/□ No
(2) Modification of a process □		□ Yes/□ No	□ Yes/□ No
(3) New product □		□ Yes/□ No	□ Yes/□ No
(4) New item of equipment/tool □		□ Yes/□ No	□ Yes/□ No
(5) Change in cleaning intervals □		□ Yes/□ No	□ Yes/□ No

Bracketing to Establish the Worst Case

It is basic to gather information on the products, their activity and the size of their batches (Table **8**).

Table 8. List of products which are fabricated in the plant.

Product	Dosage form	Active principle	TSD (Therapeutic Single Dose)	MDD (Maximum Daily Dose)	BS (Batch size/s)
Product #1	df	aaaa	nn	dd	ss
Product #2	df	aaaa	nn	dd	ss
...	...	...	...	...	...

And evidently, it is necessary to see which equipment is used for each product (Table **9**).

Table 9. Table relating products with equipment.

Product	Pieces of equipment/tools being used in the fabrication of the product							
	A	B	C	D	E	F	G	H
Product #1	✓			✓	✓	✓		✓
Product #2	✓		✓	✓				✓
Product #3		✓	✓	✓				✓
Product #4	✓			✓	✓			✓
Product #5	✓		✓		✓	✓	✓	✓

Then, the worst case product is determined by risk analysis (RRF) taking into account the characteristics of each one of the products which are involved, as it has been previously described.

The cleaning validation of the product (P1) which has been chosen as worst case (because of its characteristics) has to be combined with the worst case of cleaning. This latter is represented by the biggest batch size of P1followed after cleaning by the fabrication of the smallest size of a product (P2) with a high daily dose.

Organization of the Validation

The elements which are to be taken into account are the following:

(a) The product fabricated before cleaning (P1). See Table **10**:

Table 10. Characterization of the product to be cleaned (P1).

Name of the product	API	Dosage form	Batch size (BS)	Therapeutic single dose (TSD)
P1	nnn	ddd	xx **kg**	yy **µg**

(b) The new product fabricated after cleaning (P2). See Table **11**:

Table 11. Characterization of the product to be prepared after cleaning (P2).

Name of the product	API	Dosage form	Minimal batch size (MBS)	Maximal daily dose (MDD)
P2	mmm	ddd	xx **kg**	yy **g**

(c) The pieces of equipment involved in the fabrication of both products (P1/P2). See Table **12**:

Table 12. Surface of equipment to be considered in the validation.

Pieces of equipment/tools used for P1	Pieces of equipment/tools used for P2	Surface (cm^2)	S = Total surface of equipment intervening in the fabrication of P1 and P2 (cm^2)

(d) The cleaning process: Is it manual or automatic? Does it use chemicals? *Etc.*

Establishment of Validation Criteria

There should be pre-established criteria for the following topics: analytical methods, sampling (points/methods), cleaning intervals, acceptation limits (visual revision, microbiological contamination and residues of API/detergent).

Analytical Methods

Sampling procedures (do they ensure appropriate recovery of residues?) and analytical methods (are they specific and sensitive? is their limit of detection/quantification adequate?) should be validated.

Sampling Points

They should be chosen to meet two kinds of requirements. Firstly, it is necessary to obtain representative samples of the surfaces of equipment which come into contact with the products. Secondly, the worst case parts of the equipment should be included in the sampling plan (*i.e.* parts where products are likely to accumulate, parts difficult to clean because of the structure of equipment, *etc.*).

The inclusion of pictures of the pieces of equipment showing the exact localization of the sampling points is very useful.

Cleaning Intervals

Risk analysis is useful in evaluating the likely influence of the products and equipment on these intervals (*i.e.* expected growth of microorganisms, degradation of the rests of product, conditions of storage of equipment, efficiency of the cleaning procedure in eliminating the product, *etc.*). Once this has been taken into account it is usually the logistics of production which dictate the validation needs regarding intervals. Thus, if it is evident that equipment will never remain inactive more than two-three days, why validating a lag period of more than one week? Then, in the case exceptional of exceeding the validated period the equipment should be cleaned anew.

Acceptation Limits

(a) Visual revision: The first criterion to be met is visual inspection. There should not be detected product remains on the surfaces of equipment. In case of detecting dirty surfaces, the piece of equipment should be considered not compliant and inquiries should be made for determining the causes of the failure (incorrect application of the cleaning procedure, incomplete disassembling of the parts to be cleaned, *etc.*) and apply the appropriate corrective/preventive measures.

(b) Microbiological contamination: Alert and action limits are established for the counting of bacteria and moulds on the surfaces of equipment, obtained by two different sampling methods (Rodac plates and rinsing).

(c) Residues of chemicals: For detergents and sanitizers the maximal amount which is accepted to remain in the equipment and be transferred to the following product is 10 ppm of each one, considering the worst case. This latter appears when the product prepared after cleaning has the smallest batch size (in kg) of those produced in the pieces of equipment which are validated, because in this situation the concentration of contaminant (detergent/disinfectant) is maximal.

(d) Residues of API: There should be applied the most stringent of the following two criteria:

- Not more than 0.1% of the minimal therapeutic dose of the previous product should appear in the following product.

- Not more than 10 ppm of previous product can contaminate the following one.

The maximal residue of contaminant (API) should be calculated considering as worst case that the product manufactured after cleaning in the piece of equipment which is validated corresponds to the smallest batch size prepared and possesses the maximal daily dose. In this situation the concentration of contaminant will be maximal.

Sampling Methods

After performing the visual revision are taken samples according to the established plan (regarding quantity, procedure, points, *etc.*).

As a rule of thumb validation will be performed by analyzing the results of several runs, usually three, in which will be studied the critical parameters corresponding to the worst case chosen. However, according to experience and to risk analysis it is possible to reduce the number of cleanings to be realized (except in the initial validation) and realize the validation by means of a matricidal approach where can intervene several worst case products and/or different models of equipment. Also as a result of risk analysis it may be considered necessary validating the surroundings of the pieces of equipment (floor and walls) regarding microbiology. As a general rule, surfaces considered non critical (floors, walls, tables, computers, *etc.*) do not require cleaning validation, but are included in the environmental monitoring plans.

Results

(1) Regarding residues of API (Table **13**)

Table 13. Determination of the maximal quantity of API of P1 per surface unit of equipment (Qs).

Product to be cleaned (P1)		**Next product (P2)**		**Equipment**
Batch size **(BS)**	Therapeutic single dose **(TSD)**	Minimum batch size **(MBS)**	Maximum daily dose (**MDD**)	Total surface of equipment common to P1 and P2 (**S**)
--- kg	--- µg	--- kg	--- g	--- cm^2

<table>
<tr><td rowspan="2">MC: Maximum carryover (ppm) of P1 into P2.</td><td>• 1st criterion: <0,1% TSD in MDD
[F= Acceptable fraction of TSD = 0,001]</td><td>MC = F x TSD/MDD</td><td rowspan="2">The more restrictive is chosen as MC</td></tr>
<tr><td colspan="2">• 2nd criterion: ≤ 10 ppm of P1 into P2</td></tr>
<tr><td>MACO: Maximum allowable carryover (µg) of P1 into P2</td><td colspan="3">MACO = MC x MBS x 1000</td></tr>
<tr><td>Qs: Maximal quantity of P1 API per surface unit (µg/cm²)</td><td colspan="3">Qs = MACO/S</td></tr>
</table>

Verification of the results obtained in the validation (Table **14**):

Table 14. Verification of the results of sampling for cleaning validation (API remains).

Sampling				Result	Visually clean?	Qs	Correct?
#	Description	µg	surface (cm^2)	µg/cm^2		µg/cm^2	

(2) Regarding residues of chemicals (Table **15**)

Table 15. Determination of the maximal quantity of detergent/sanitizer per surface unit of equipment (Qs).

Surface of equipment cleaned (S)	Chemicals used	Product to be fabricated after cleaning (P2)	
		Denomination	Minimum batch size (**MBS**)
--- cm^2	---	---	--- cm^2
MC: Maximum carryover of chemicals into P2.	• Criterion ≤ 10 ppm	**MC = 10**	
MACO: Maximum allowable carryover (µg) of P1 into P2	**MACO = MC** x **MBS** x **1000**		
Qs: Maximal quantity of API of P1 accepted per surface unit (µg/cm^2)	**Qs = MACO/S**		

Verification of the results obtained in the validation (Table **16**):

Table 16. Verification of the results of sampling for cleaning validation (chemicals remains).

Sampling				Result	Qs	Correct?
#	Equipment	µg	surface (cm^2)	µg/cm^2	µg/cm^2	

(3) Regarding bioburden (Table **17**)

Table 17. Example of acceptance limits for bioburden.

Type of criterion	Sampling	Surface in contact with product?	Bacteria		Fungus and moulds	
			Alert limit	Action limit	Alert limit	Action limit
General criterion after cleaning	Rodac plates/25 cm^2	Yes	n. a	20 cfu	n. a	4 cfu
		No (floor)	n. a	40 cfu	n. a	8 cfu
	Rinsing 1 m^2	Yes	n. a	8000 cfu	n. a	1600 cfu
Criterion for campaign production	Rodac plates/25 cm^2	Yes	50 cfu	100 cfu	10 cfu	20 cfu
		No (floor)	100 cfu	200 cfu	20 cfu	40 cfu

Verification of the results obtained in the validation (Table **18**):

Table 18. Verification of the results of sampling for cleaning validation (bioburden).

Equipment:							
Sampling by Rodac plates				Sampling by rinsing			
Sample No.	Localization	Result (cfu)	Correct?	Sample No.	Localization	Result (cfu)	Correct?

Approval and Acceptance of Risk

Completed the validation, direct or indirect (when exists equivalence with a case already validated), of the cleaning procedure it should be verified that the final risk level is acceptable. If this is not the case the procedure should be modified and the validation repeated.

Revalidation of the Cleaning Procedures

Based on risk analysis regarding modifications:

- In the cleaning process (procedure, detergents, sanitizers, concentrations).
- In the structure of equipment and tools.
- In the automatic cleaning systems (CIP).

- In the products which are manufactured in the equipment, in their batch volumes or in the duration of the campaign.

Every now and then (*e.g.* every year/every two years, depending on the criticality level) the cleaning procedures should be verified in order to proof that they are still acceptable and the corresponding procedure and report will be written.

CONCLUDING REMARKS

Equipment plays a key role in production, but at the same time it can affect negatively materials and products by passively allowing their contamination or by actively contributing to their contamination. Initial qualification and, when necessary, requalification allows for ensuring that equipment is safe for the products. However, equipment can be a source of cross-contamination if it is not adequately cleaned. Single-use equipment would solve this problem, but this is not a realistic solution in most cases. Dedicated equipment could solve this problem, but with two limitations. On one hand this is often a too expensive solution and on the other, dedicated equipment does not exclude problems derived from contamination by degradation products or by microbial growth in case of inappropriate cleaning. Thus, in most cases technicians have to cope with multi-use equipment and provide an adequate validation of the cleaning procedures.

CONFLICT OF INTEREST

The author confirms that this chapter contents have no conflict of interest.

ACKNOWLEDGEMENT

Declared None.

REFERENCES

[1] PDA (Parenteral Drug Association). Application of single-use systems in pharmaceutical manufacturing. Technical Report No. 66. PDA, Bethesda, MD, USA, 2014.

[2] FDA (U. S. Food and Drug Administration). Guide to inspections of high purity water systems. FDA, Inspection Technical Guides, 7/93. FDA, Rockville, MD, USA, 1993. IX.

[3] WHO (World Health Organization). WHO Good manufacturing practices. Water for pharmaceutical use. In: WHO Expert Committee on Specifications for Pharmaceutical Preparations. Thirty-ninth report (WHO Technical Report Series, No. 929). WHO, Geneva, Switzerland, 2005. Annex 3. 6.5.3.

[4] WHO (World Health Organization). WHO Good manufacturing practices for pharmaceutical products: main principles. In: WHO Expert Committee on Specifications for Pharmaceutical Preparations. Forty-eighth report (WHO Technical Report Series, No. 986). WHO, Geneva, Switzerland, 2014. Annex 2. 13.12.

[5] Id. 13.9.

[6] FDA (U. S. Food and Drug Administration). Guide to inspections of high purity water systems. FDA, Inspection Technical Guides, 7/93. FDA, Rockville, MD, USA, 1993. VI.

[7] WHO (World Health Organization). WHO Good manufacturing practices. Water for pharmaceutical use. In: WHO Expert Committee on Specifications for Pharmaceutical Preparations. Forty-sixth report (WHO Technical Report Series, No. 970). Geneva, World Health Organization, 2012. Annex 2. 6.4.3.

[8] WHO (World Health Organization). WHO Good manufacturing practices for pharmaceutical products: main principles. In: WHO Expert Committee on Specifications for Pharmaceutical Preparations. Forty-eighth report (WHO Technical Report Series, No. 986). WHO, Geneva, Switzerland, 2014. Annex 2. 14.3.

[9] Ibid. 16.6.

[10] Ibid. 13.10.

[11] Ibid. 13.5.

[12] European Commission. Good manufacturing practices. Medicinal products for human and veterinary use. The rules governing medicinal products in the European Union. Volume 4. Brussels. Glossary.

[13] U.S. Department of Health and Human Services. Food and Drug Administration. Center for Drug Evaluation and Research (CDER). Center for Biologics Evaluation and Research (CBER). Center for Devices and Radiological Health (CDRH). Center for Food Safety and Applied Nutrition (CFSAN). Center for Veterinary Medicine (CVM). Office of Regulatory Affairs (ORA). Part 11, Electronic Records; Electronic Signatures — Scope and Application. Guidance for Industry. Pharmaceutical CGMPs. FDA, Rockville, MD, USA, 2003.

[14] PIC/S (Pharmaceutical Inspection Convention. Pharmaceutical Inspection Co-Operation Scheme). Good Practices for Computerised systems in regulated "GXP" environments. Guidance PI 011-3. PIC/S, Geneva, Switzerland, 2007.

[15] European Commission. Health and Consumers Directorate General. Computerised Systems. In: EudraLex. The Rules Governing Medicinal Products in the European Union. Volume 4. Good Manufacturing Practice. Medicinal Products for Human and Veterinary Use. European Commission. Brussels, Belgium, 2010. Annex 11. 4.

[16] US National Archives & Records Administration. Federal Register. Code of Federal Regulations (CFR). Title 21 (Food & drugs). Part 11. Section 11.3.b.6.

[17] Id. 11.3.b.7.

[18] ISPE (International Society of Pharmaceutical Engineering). GAMP: A risk-based approach to compliant electronic records and signatures. ISPE, Tampa, Florida, USA, 2005.

[19] Gough J, Nettleton D. Risk-based software validation. PDA Bethesda, MD, USA 2006.

[20] WHO (World Health Organisation). Supplementary guidelines on good manufacturing practices: validation. In: WHO Expert Committee on Specifications for Pharmaceutical Preparations. Fortieth report (WHO Technical Report Series, No. 937). WHO, Geneva, Switzerland, 2006. Annex 4 (Appendix 5: Validation of computerized systems).

[21] ISPE (International Society of Pharmaceutical Engineering). GAMP: A risk-based approach to GXP process control systems. Second edition. ISPE, Tampa, Florida, USA 2011.

[22] US National Archives & Records Administration. Federal Register. Code of Federal Regulations (CFR). Title 21 (Food & drugs). Part 11. Section 11.3.b.3.

[23] Ibid. Section 11.200.

[24] Ibid. Section 11.300.

[25] European Commission. Health and Consumers Directorate General. Computerised Systems. In: EudraLex. The Rules Governing Medicinal Products in the European Union. Volume 4. Good Manufacturing Practice. Medicinal Products for Human and Veterinary Use. European Commission. Brussels, Belgium, 2010. Annex 11. 10.

[26] Rosetto Y (editor). φ41. Pharmacotechnie industrielle. I.M.T. Editions, Tours, France, 1998.

[27] Le Hir A, Chaumeil JC, Brossard D. Pharmacie galénique. Bonnes pratiques de fabrication des médicaments. 9th Edition. Elsevier Masson, Issy-les-Moulineaux, France, 2009.

[28] ISPE (International Society of Pharmaceutical Engineering). Sterile manufacturing facilities. Baseline pharmaceutical engineering guides. Second edition. ISPE, Tampa, Florida, USA, 2011.

[29] Lysfjord J. Practical aseptic processing: Fill and finish. Volume I and II. PDA Bethesda, MD, USA 2009

[30] PDA (Parenteral Drug Association). Recommended practices for manual aseptic processes. Technical Report No. 62. PDA, Bethesda, MD, USA, 2013

[31] ISPE (International Society of Pharmaceutical Engineering). Oral solid dosage forms. Baseline pharmaceutical engineering guides Tampa, Florida, USA, 2009.

[32] WHO (World Health Organisation). Supplementary guidelines on good manufacturing practices: validation. In: WHO Expert Committee on Specifications for Pharmaceutical Preparations. Fortieth report (WHO Technical Report Series, No. 937). WHO, Geneva, Switzerland, 2006. Annex 4 (Appendix 1: Validation of heating, ventilation and air-conditioning systems. Appendix 6: Qualification of systems and equipment).

[33] Council of Europe. European Directorate for the Quality of Medecines & Healthcare. OMCL Network of the Council of Europe. Qualification of Equipment. Annex 8: Qualification of balances. Quality management document. PA/PH/OMCL (12) 77 7R. 2013.

[34] ISPE (International Society of Pharmaceutical Engineering). Commissioning and qualification. ISPE Baseline Pharmaceutical Engineering Guides. ISPE, Tampa, Florida, USA, 2001.

[35] PIC/S (Pharmaceutical Inspection Convention/Pharmaceutical Inspection Co-Operation Scheme). Validation Master Plan, Installation and Operational Qualification, Non-sterile Process Validation, Cleaning Validation. Recommendations PI 006-3. PIC/S, Geneva, Switzerland, 2007.

[36] WHO (World Health Organisation). Supplementary guidelines on good manufacturing practices: validation. In: WHO Expert Committee on Specifications for Pharmaceutical Preparations. Fortieth report (WHO Technical Report Series, No. 937). WHO, Geneva, Switzerland, 2006. Annex 4 (Appendix 3: Cleaning validation).

[37] European Commission. Directorate General for Health and Food Safety. Qualification and Validation. In: EudraLex. The Rules Governing Medicinal Products in the European Union. Volume 4. EU Guidelines to Good Manufacturing Practice for Medicinal Products for Human and Veterinary Use. European Commission, Brussels, Belgium, 2015. Annex 15: Glossary.

[38] WHO (World Health Organisation). Supplementary guidelines on good manufacturing practices: validation. In: WHO Expert Committee on Specifications for Pharmaceutical Preparations. Fortieth report (WHO Technical Report Series, No. 937). WHO, Geneva, Switzerland, 2006. Annex 4 (Appendix 4: Analytical method validation). 4.1.4.

[39] European Medicines Agency (EMA). Committee for Medicinal Products for Human Use (CHMP), Committee for Medicinal Products for Veterinary Use (CVMP). Guideline on setting health based exposure limits for use in risk identification in the manufacture of different medicinal products in shared facilities. EMA/CHMP/CVMP/SWP/169430/2012. EMA, London, 2014.

CHAPTER 11

Products

Abstract: The application of the lifecycle model to the pharmaceutical products has modified existing approaches to quality assurance. The quality of a product is not simply the outcome of a GMP-compliant manufacturing, but the result of a GMP-compliant lifecycle. Product development means devising a formula and a manufacturing process, but most importantly, understanding thoroughly the product. This, known as quality by design, goes from defining its quality target profile to identifying the quality attributes of the starting materials and the quality parameters of the manufacturing process. Critical variables are the hallmark of a product during its lifecycle. They are identified and studied during the development stage and knowledge on them is increased during the product's lifetime. Technological transfer means confirming that what worked in the development center will also work in the manufacturing plant, but also increasing and improving knowledge on the critical variables under industrial-scale conditions. Validation means verifying that the production process can be successfully controlled by means of the critical variables and that if these remain within proven acceptable ranges the process can be deemed under control and consequently yielding quality products. Thus, by monitoring critical variables each batch can be considered concurrently validated. The application of the above described approaches will enhance the level of quality insurance of the new products, but what happens with legacy ones? The model can be usefully applied to these latter too by using the same principles but proceeding step by step in a reverse approach, from knowledge to development instead of development to knowledge.

Keywords: Analytical validation, commercial manufacturing, computerized systems validation, CPP, CQA, critical variable, DAME, design space, development, discontinuation, DoE, evaluation, monitoring, PAT, process validation, proven acceptable range, QbD, QTPP, RTRT, technological transfer.

PRODUCT LIFECYCLE

Following the lifecycle model described in chapter 2, Fig. (**1**) shows the four lifecycle stages of a pharmaceutical product (*i.e.* development, technological transfer, manufacturing and discontinuation).

Although the phases of a product life-cycle have always been recognized, only recently they have acquired their fully developed outline. Besides, nowadays these stages are purely seen as different faces of the same reality and, consequently, it is acknowledged that they have to be considered in a global way because together they build quality.

Jordi Botet

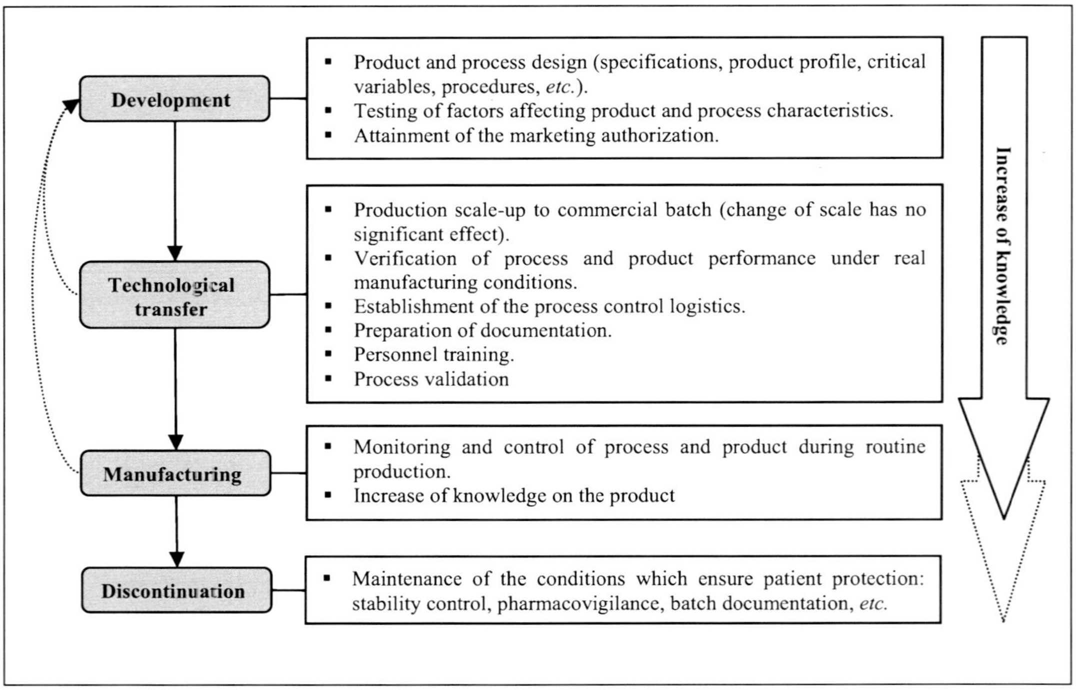

Fig. (1). Product life-cycle.

New approaches came as a consequence of understanding that in practice there are not and may not exist two separated parts in the life of a product and of its manufacturing process (the first one devoted to obtaining knowledge and the second one of simple exploitation of this knowledge), because the process of increasing of knowledge is a never ending one and this includes manufacturing too.

Development

The aim of pharmaceutical development is to design a quality product and its manufacturing process to consistently deliver the intended performance of the product...

It should describe the knowledge that establishes that the type of dosage form selected and the formulation proposed are suitable for the intended use [1].

Periods

Fig. (**2**) shows the periods of development and the standards which are applied (GLP and GCP). Postapproval studies (standard: GCP) and control (standard:

GVP) are also included to get a better understanding of the matter. For comparative purposes manufacturing (standard: GMP) is also incorporated.

Development is composed of three periods, which can be partially superposed. The total duration of this first stage of a product life-cycle is very variable but it is generally considered that usually averages ten years.

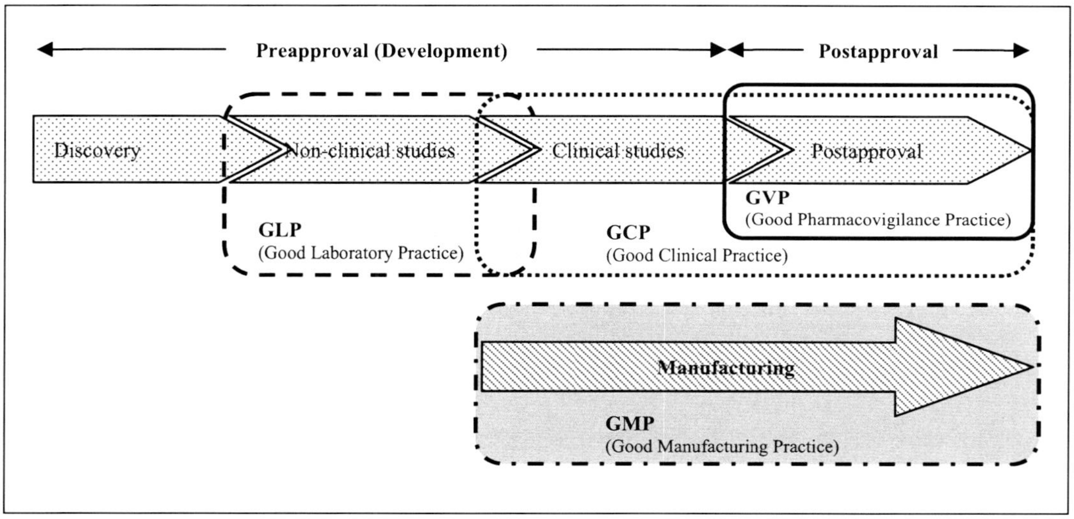

Fig. (2). Pharmaceutical development periods.

The period of discovery of an active molecule is very variable. In large research centers it is the result of the examination of huge quantities of candidates. It is well known that only a few of the molecules which are analyzed show interesting pharmacological effects. And from these latter it is necessary to eliminate those which show toxic side-effects. Only these rare molecules which are thus selected can pass to the second period of development. Another approach is starting with natural products of well-known effects in order to isolate the active principle and use it or a derivative with improved properties.

The non-clinical period is composed of toxicological and pharmacological studies developed in animals or in-vitro. Pharmakinetic and biodisponibility tests can also start. The former study the behavior of the molecule in the organism (*i.e.* its distribution, transformation, effect and elimination), whereas the latter determine how quickly and at what concentration the active principle is available to the organism, verifying, for instance, the evolution of its concentration in blood along the way (Fig. **3**).

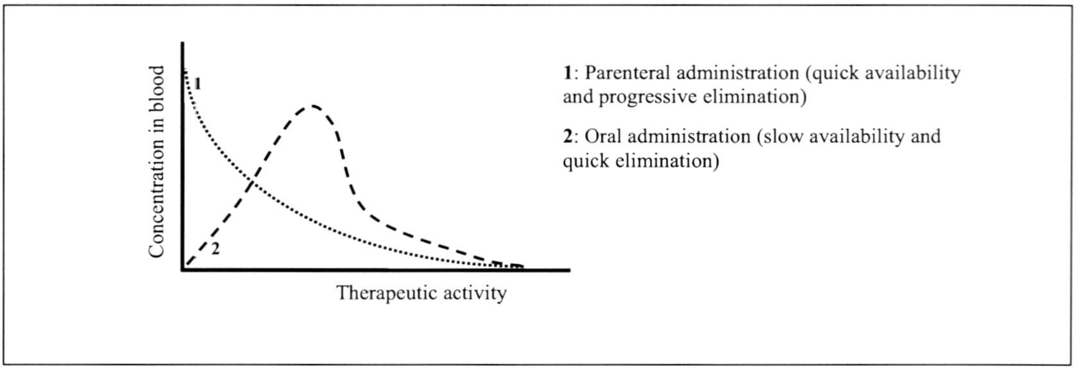

Fig. (3). Biodisponibility profile.

The period of clinical studies involve assays in human beings. It is divided into four phases (in fact phase IV is outside from development because it starts after approval and is realized during the period of commercial manufacturing of the product, but for practical purposes it is better consider it here):

- **Phase I**: It demonstrates tolerance and pharmacokinetics.
- **Phase II**: It confirms the relation dose-effect.
- **Phase III**: Large scale studies are realized, frequently in diverse centers for verifying the efficacy of the new product on hundreds of patients.
- **Phase IV**: The medical product has already been authorized and commercialized. Now the studies are of pharmacovigilance (when a product is authorized it has been studied on a limited number of patients, whereas after being commercialized, the number of patients is very high, consequently, it is necessary to go on monitoring its behavior). Additional clinical studies may appear necessary.

It has to be kept in mind that clinical studies require a quality pharmaceutical product. This is why GMP is applied to the preparation of pharmaceuticals under development already from period 3 onward.

GMP applies to all manufacturing of bulk and finished product [2, 3].

To ensure the quality of the non-clinical studies realized in the laboratory they are realized under GLP (Good Laboratory Practice) regulations. See chapter 12.

Finally, clinical studies need to be realized within a quality frame and this is why a GCP (Good Clinical Practice) has been developed [4-6]. Most of these studies are performed during the period of clinical studies to release a new product, but they can be also carried after registration to obtain complementary data or to test new applications.

After registration of a product it is necessary to keep on identifying, quantifying, evaluating and preventing risks associated to its use and this is covered by Good Pharmacovigilance practices (GVP). See chapter 12.

Quality Design

The development of a drug product means not only determining a dosage form, a formula, a preparation procedure and specifications, but also creating a quality product (Fig. **4**). This is expressed as "quality by design" (QbD) [7] which can be defined as *a systematic approach to development that begins with predefined objectives and emphasizes product and process understanding and process control, based on sound science and quality risk management* [8].

The dosage forms of new products are developed by research, but also thanks to previous knowledge and manufacturing experience. The starting point of a development process is defining the "Quality Target Product Profile" (QTPP) which can be defined as *a prospective summary of the quality characteristics of a drug product that ideally will be achieved to ensure the desired quality, taking into account safety and efficacy of the drug product* [9].

In practice this means establishing:

- Dosage form;
- Active principle and dose;
- Specifications that make sure and effective the drug product;
- Aspect and properties;
- Characteristics.

The result of development is establishing a manufacturing procedure and defining the specifications of the starting and packaging materials, of the intermediate products (if they exist) and of the finished product. A quality design means that it is possible to correlate the characteristics of the finished product with the properties which are specified for the starting materials and with the set of parameters of the manufacturing process. This connection between manufacturing process and finished product properties (*i.e.* between inputs, process and outputs) should exist both regarding starting materials (*e.g.* temperature and stirring ↔ crystal size) and the medicinal product itself (*e.g.* humidity ↔ tablet hardness).

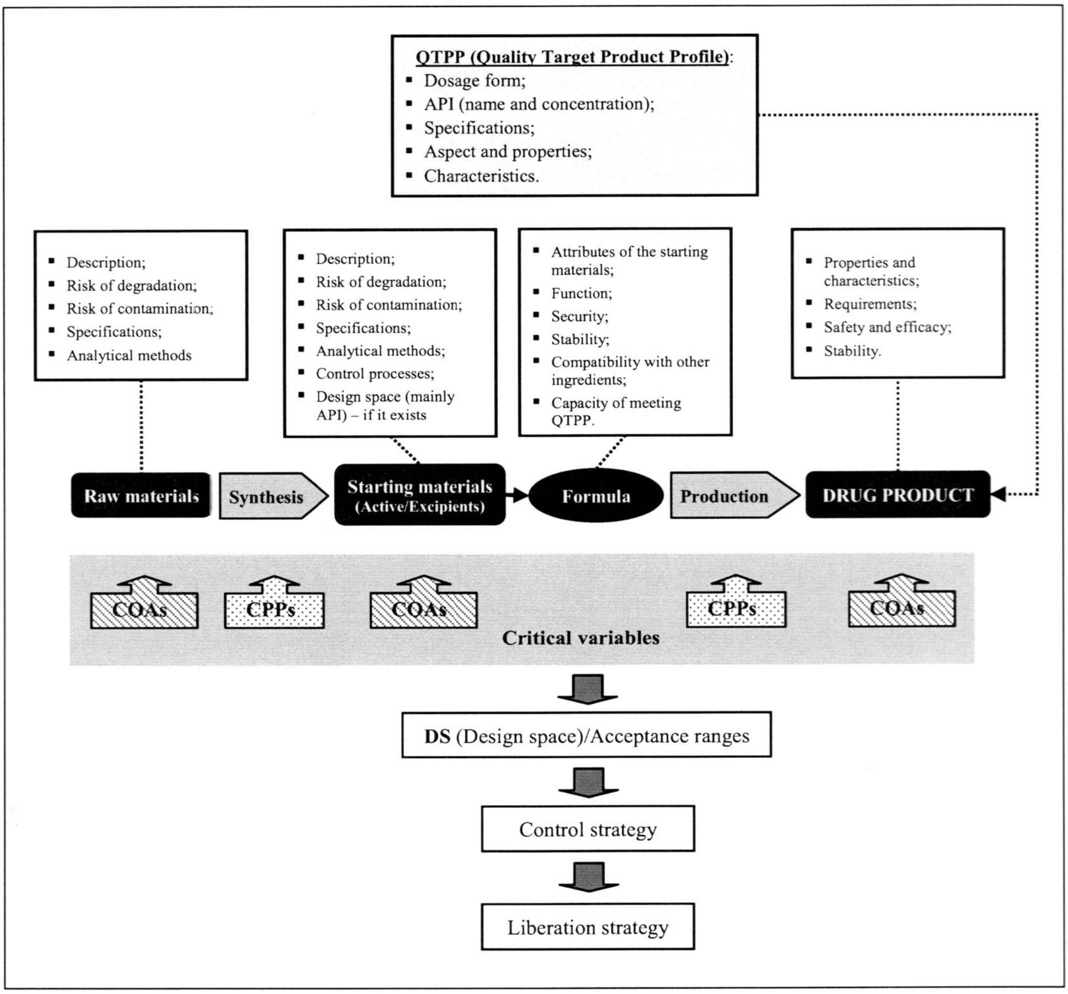

Fig. (4). Quality by design.

Determining the relation that exists between starting materials, manufacturing process and finished product allows for the knowledge of its behavior before variations (regarding physico-chemical conditions, characteristics of the starting materials, relative proportions of excipients and active ingredients in the formula, *etc.*).

Raw materials which are used for the preparation of the starting materials, these starting materials themselves and the finished pharmaceutical itself all possess "Critical Quality Attributes" (CQAs).

A CQA *is a physical, chemical, biological or microbiological property or characteristic that should be within an appropriate limit, range, or distribution to ensure the desired product quality* [10].

The adequacy of a product is determined by the CQAs. Whereas the "Critical Process Parameters" (CPPs) can be used for the monitoring of processes.

A CPP *is a process parameter whose variability has an impact on a critical quality attribute and therefore should be monitored or controlled to ensure the process produces the desired quality* [11].

The ensemble of CQAs and CPPs can be defined as the "critical variables", which can be identified and their criticality evaluated by performing risk analysis. This allows for the distinction between critical and non-critical parameters. The former should be monitored, unless that a process modification turn them into non-critical. These non-critical parameters are not necessarily monitored. Monitoring a variable requires knowing its operating and acceptable ranges (Fig. **5**).

A "Proven Acceptable Range" can be defined as *a characterized range of a process parameter for which operation within this range, while keeping other parameters constant, will result in producing a material meeting relevant quality criteria* [12].

Apart from determining individually the acceptable ranges for each one of the variables it is possible to combine all data (input variables, process parameters and finished product specifications) in a "space" where all CQAs will be fulfilled and, consequently, where the quality of the product will be guaranteed. This space, known as "design space" (DS), is determined by applying statistical methods of "design of experiments" (DoE), in order to reduce the number of essays which are necessary for establishing the multifactorial influences of the variables among them. Despite the fact that it is possible to represent graphically the design space, the aim is to be able to set up a predictive mathematical model.

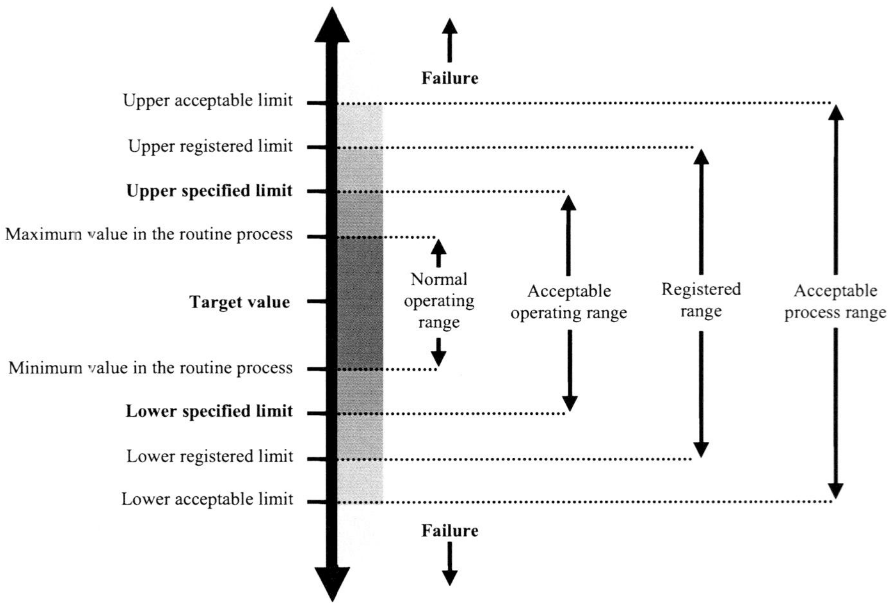

Fig. (5). Operational and acceptable ranges.

A "Design Space" can be defined as *the multidimensional combination and interaction of input variables (e.g., material attributes) and process parameters that have been demonstrated to provide assurance of quality. Working within the design space is not considered as a change. Movement out of the design space is considered to be a change and would normally initiate a regulatory post approval change process. Design space is proposed by the applicant and is subject to regulatory assessment and approval* [13].

Both options, either determining the individualized ranges of critical variables or establishing a design space are acceptable. Although it is evident that better product knowledge means easier quality assurance, it is not less certain that establishing a design space requires an important amount of laboratory work and consequently it is expensive. This is why there have been raised doubts about its utility. Companies which have established design spaces point out the following advantages:

- Process is more robust;
- Product is better known and this represents an improved final control;

- Deviations and rejects diminish;

- Greater flexibility in manufacturing, because many modifications can be managed without regulatory approval (movements within the space of design are not considered modifications requiring approval and can be handled within the change management system);

- Increases confidence on the quality of the product by the authorities and by other companies;

- Resources used for the definition and registration of the design space are compensated by the advantages in terms of time and means saving, and because of the flexibility that it supposes.

Once that critical variables are known and their behavior has been analyzed it is possible to define a control strategy intended to ensure consistent product quality, according to the QTPP. A "control strategy" can be defined as *a planned set of controls, derived from current product and process understanding that ensures process performance and product quality. The controls can include parameters and attributes related to drug substance and drug product materials and components, facility and equipment operating conditions, in-process controls, finished product specifications, and the associated methods and frequency of monitoring and control* [14].

Process can be monitored by means of critical variables. This can be done by out of line traditional sampling and analysis or by real-time monitoring using "process analytical technology" (PAT) [15], which can be defined as *a system for designing, analyzing, and controlling manufacturing through timely measurements (i.e., during processing) of critical quality and performance attributes of raw and in-process materials and processes with the goal of ensuring final product quality* [16]. This latter approach makes unnecessary sampling (an operation subjected to inevitable bias).

A good knowledge of the process and the application of a risk management approach determine the control strategy. The objective of this strategy is ensuring a steady level of product quality, as defined by the quality profile (QTPP).

Complementarily to the control strategy a liberation strategy should be defined. According to the traditional approach the finished product is analyzed, but when there is monitoring by real-time (or almost) testing, it can be used "real time release testing" (RTRT), that is *the ability to evaluate and ensure the quality of in-process and/or final product based on process data, which typically include a valid combination of measured material attributes and process controls* [17].

The use of automated systems (PAT) permits real time liberation of products. This liberation offers equal assurance and even more than traditional methods, because:

- the parameters which are monitored are related to analytical results;
- testing is realized automatically during the operation itself;
- the critical variables are kept under control;
- every batch can be deemed "validated".

Exactly like final analysis in traditional manufacturing, control strategy is just one of the items which should be considered when liberating a batch (*i.e.* any other element related to production like environmental and personnel monitoring, in-process sampling, analysis of deviations – if they exist, *etc.*). It also has to be reminded that RTRT, like design space, is just an option, not a requirement.

Anyway, this approach is not new, as GMP had recognized "parametric release", *a system of release that gives the assurance that the product is of the intended quality based on information collected during the manufacturing process and on the compliance with specific GMP requirements related to Parametric Release.*

It is recognized that a comprehensive set of in-process tests and controls may provide greater assurance of the finished product meeting specification than finished product testing [18].

Although parametric release may be authorized by the regulatory authorities for definite specific parameters as a substitute for the routine analysis of the finished product, in practice it was mainly thought for sterile products, because the final sterility testing offers less assurance than a tight control of critical process parameters [19].

Sterility tests are limited in their ability to detect contamination because of the small sample size typically used. ... To further illustrate, if a 10,000-unit lot with a 0.1 percent contamination level was sterility tested using 20 units, there is a 98 percent chance that the batch would pass the test [20].

Technological Transfer

The goal of technology transfer activities is to move product and process knowledge from development to manufacturing, and within or between manufacturing sites, in order to achieve product realization. This knowledge forms the basis for the manufacturing process, control strategy, process validation approach and ongoing continual improvement [21].

This is a very important stage even if it tends to be somewhat obscured because it is "squeezed" between the two great phases of development and commercial manufacturing and it lasts not long, at least in comparison with the two other phases. Transfer means starting the process in new conditions and verifying and ensuring that its performance is maintained. This transfer can refer to a new process (from the development center to a manufacturing plant) or to an old process with well proven performances (from a facility to another one).

Transfer supposes:

- keep increasing product knowledge under different circumstances;
- verifying that change in scale (development → production) does not affect product quality;
- verifying that change in production site does not have an effect on the product either;
- writing the necessary procedures (SOPs);
- personnel training;
- facility qualification;
- process validation.

Commercial Manufacturing

This is the life cycle phase which has received traditionally primary attention and to which most of the information contained in this book refers. It is true, however, that current manufacturing is not simply understood as the meticulous repetition of the same operations, but as a continuous process of improvement thanks to an steady increase of knowledge on the product.

The goals of manufacturing activities include achieving product realization, establishing and maintaining a state of control and facilitating continual improvement. The pharmaceutical quality system should assure that the desired product quality is routinely met, suitable process performance is achieved, the set of controls are appropriate, improvement opportunities are identified and evaluated, and the body of knowledge is continually expanded [22].

Product Discontinuation

Although this, properly speaking, is not an "operational" stage like the others because there are no preparation operations, it plays an important role in the life cycle, concluding it.

The goal of product discontinuation activities is to manage the terminal stage of the product lifecycle effectively. For product discontinuation, a pre-defined approach should be used to manage activities such as retention of documentation and samples and continued product assessment (e.g. complaint handling and stability) and reporting in accordance with regulatory requirements [23].

Discontinuation means that the product will not be manufactured anymore. From the point of view of facilities it is just a logistical problem (they keep going with other products, they are adapted or transferred for other uses or are disassembled), but the product will be distributed and used by patients until the end of its shelf-life. In other words, from the closing of its production to its disappearance from the market there is a period of time corresponding to its shelf-life. Authorities require that during this period of time the drug product should provide the same level of assurance that it offered when it was manufactured (keeping documentation, attention to complaints, pharmacovigilance, stability control, maintenance of samples, recall system, *etc.*).

PROCESS VALIDATION

The validation approach of the organization is described in a Validation Master Plan (VMP). Before starting any validation, all intervening equipment/systems should have been qualified.

Preparation of a VMP

The contents of a VMP vary according to the particular circumstances of each organization, but we could propose this general one:

1. Objective: This VMP has the following objectives:

- Define how validation will be organized and performed.
- Ensure the adequate planning of the validation activities and the allocation of the necessary resources.
- Ensure that the validation activities will be appropriately documented.
- Provide easy-access information on validation.

2. Scope: Identify and describe the situation of the plant or unit. Provide information on the processes to be validated.

3. Responsibilities: There will be a validation team (Table **1**) usually headed by a technician belonging to the QA department and composed basically by technicians of production, of QC and of the engineering department.

Table 1. Example of responsibilities regarding validation documentation.

Task	**Personnel**			
	Plant Director	QA Head	Validation Team Head	Validation technician
VMP	Approves	Reviews	Writes	---
Validation protocols	---	Approves	Reviews	Writes
Validation reports	---	Approves	Reviews	Writes

The exact composition of the validation team, in quantity and quality, is dictated by each practical case.

4. Definitions: Introduce the GMP definitions for the main terms (*e.g.* validation, protocol, report, *etc.*) and for other words or expressions, as necessary.

5. Summary of processes to be validated: Brief description of the types of products which are manufactured in the plant. The processes which are validated belong to three types: production, cleaning and computerized systems (analytical procedures are usually treated separately by the QC laboratory).

6. Organizational structure of validation activities: This VMP identifies and lists the processes to be validated. Following the same pattern described for the qualification, are prepared validation protocols, which should be reviewed and approved. The approved protocols will be realized by the validation team. When

completed, the corresponding reports will be prepared (Fig. **6**). The approval of a report amounts to the liberation of the process as successfully validated.

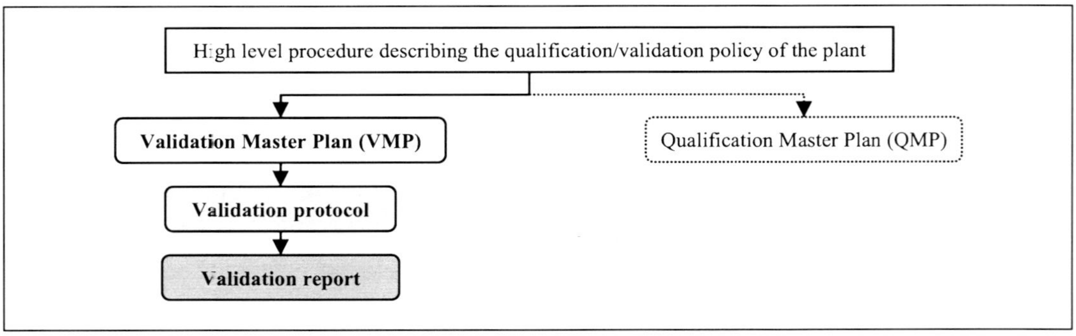

Fig. (6). Validation documentation.

7. Documentation format: Each protocol has a front page identifying the document and providing the adequate spaces for approval, review and writing (name, post, signature and date). Then the protocol describes briefly its object and scope and details the tests to perform. A tentative content of a validation protocol can be as follows:

- Objective: Demonstrate that the process can perform as purported.
- Scope: Process NNN.
- Brief description of the characteristics of the process to be validated.
- Validation approach: Describe the number of batches to be used for validation and how this validation will be performed. See below for more details.
- Prerequisites: Verify that equipment is qualified, that measuring instruments are calibrated, that personnel are trained, and that analytical methods are validated.
- Validation operations: Prepare a batch processing record to gather all information relating to each one of the validating batches. It should contain acceptance ranges for each one of the critical variables (the intention is showing that following these instructions it is possible obtaining a product meeting its requirements and that critical variables remain within their pre-established acceptance ranges).

Reports can follow the same pattern described for qualification.

8. Codification of the qualification documentation: The above mentioned documents will be identified by a code composed of three letters (identifying the type of document) and three numbers (for successive numbering). See Table **2**.

Table 2. Example of codification of the validation documents.

Type of document		Identification
Validation Master Plan		VMP
Validation protocol	Production process	PVP
	Cleaning Method	CVP
	Computerized system	SVP
Validation report	Production process	PVR
	Cleaning Method	CVR
	Computerized system	SVR
Note: Revalidation protocols/reports keep the initial code, but changing the version number.		

9. Planning: The documents comprising the validation program are listed (Table **3**).

Table 3. Example of planning of validation tasks.

Process		#	Protocols/Reports
Production	AAAA	001	PVP-001/PVR-001
	BBBB	002	PVP-002/PVR-002
	CCCC	003	PVP-003/PVR-003
Cleaning	DDDD	004	PVP-004/PVR-004
Computerized system	EEEE	005	PVP-005/PVR-005

10. Scheduling: See Table **4**.

Table 4. Validation chronogram.

Qualification	**Period (year: ....)**					
	January-February	**March-April**	**May-June**	**July-August**	**September-October**	**November-December**
Process #1	X					
Process #2			X			
Process #3			X			
Process #4					X	
Process #5						X

11. Change control: Any change will be handled following the approved procedure (SOP-nnn).

12. Filing: Validation documentation will be archived by the QA department.

13. Training: All personnel taking part in validation tasks will be provided with the adequate training.

14. Calibration: All instruments used in validation should be in state of calibration.

15. Analytical methods: The analytical methods used in validation should be validated.

16. Revalidation: See below.

Approaches to Validation

Here are compared the two existing approaches to validation. On one side, the traditional one focused on prospective validation, and on the other, the new one which relies basically on concurrent validation.

Traditional Approach

Usually validation *is completed prior to the manufacture of the finished product that is intended for sale* [24]. This is known as "prospective validation" and it supposes that several batches are prepared to verify that the manufacturing process as described in the registering file of the product allows for the preparation of a product with the required quality. The number of batches has to be sufficient for ensuring that the process operates as intended. In practice it is often considered that three batches meet this requirement.

For legacy products which possess a long history of satisfactory manufacturing, GMP accepts "retrospective validation" which can be defined as the *validation of a process for a product which has been marketed based upon accumulated manufacturing, testing and control batch data* [25]. In this case validation is realized analyzing the batch manufacturing records of all the manufactured batches of a given period with the aim of getting the assurance that the process performs as required. The number of batches to evaluate should be determined case by case, but in general it is considered that at least ten batches should be scrutinized. The main obstacle for this type of validation is the lack of homogeneity in the batches being analyzed. It is evident that retrospective validation has only meaning if the batches which are analyzed are completely similar (in procedure, equipment, utilities, materials, *etc.*).

The "state of validation" obtained after a successful validation can be modified as a result of the inherent variability of operations (worn-out equipment, new personnel, tiny variations in the characteristics of materials, *etc.*). The change management system plays an important role, but has to be complemented with a periodic evaluation system. Both determine the need of revalidation (Fig. **7**).

This is, however, an unacceptable approach for critical processes like manufacturing of sterile pharmaceuticals which require periodical revalidation, at least performing "media fills".

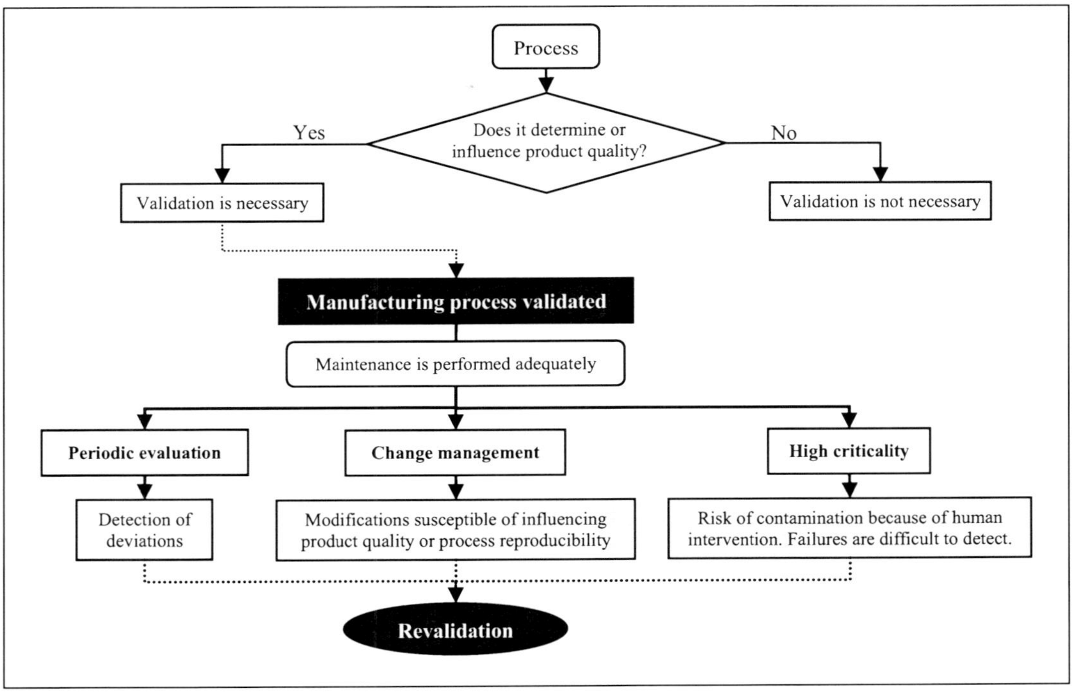

Fig. (7). Revalidation.

The approach used by the company should be described and explained in the Validation Master Plan (VMP) or in the general procedure dealing on Qualification/Validation policy.

New Approach

Although there is no need to discuss about the utility of validation, its practical implementation has always raised many doubts. Just to mention a few: how many batches should be considered sufficient? Which testing should be performed? How should validation be performed, either prospectively or retrospectively? For how long a validated process remains as such?

These common questions suggest that the problem was not validation itself but how it was approached. Manufacturing is a continuous process, whereas traditional validation is a very limited process performed during a short time. How can a limited process ensure the quality of a continuous one?

To answer these questions a new approach on validation was necessary and it should be based on two main points: First, validation should accompany the manufacturing process and be a never ending process too. Second, validation should take into account the product life cycle.

After technological transfer three lots of the product are prospectively validated. The intention of this validation is showing that the manufacturing documentation is correct and that the process can be appropriately monitored. In other words these batches are used to show that the product is ready for the subsequent "concurrent validation", that is, a *validation carried out during routine production of products intended for sale* [26]. Then all manufactured batches are validated.

The validation guarantees that the manufacturing process can produce in a reliable manner a product consistent with the QTPP.

Aseptic Process Simulation with Media Fills

In aseptic processes sterility can be compromised at any moment because of microbiological contamination. This contamination can be the consequence of sterilization failure (regarding materials, products, containers, closures, tools, *etc.*) but also of a human error (contact of sterile items with non sterile ones). Thus the validation of aseptic processes requires showing that they perform as purported in terms of critical variables, but also of asepsis. The process simulation by using culture media, known in a simplified way as "media fill", reveals easily the presence of contamination by microorganisms because of the growth of colonies after incubation of the closed containers filled with media (Fig. **8**).

Risk Analysis of the Process

A media fill has only sense if it reproduces exactly the conditions of the real manufacturing process. This requires a previous risk analysis in order to ascertain all operations likely of contaminating the product (*e.g.* different operators, equipment assembly, product loading, equipment adjustment, interventions on equipment, line speed, sampling, logistic starts and stops, closure and container loading, filling, stoppering, crimping, *etc.*).

This can be done by preparing a process flowchart and analyzing carefully its steps in terms of personnel, equipment, products and closures and containers. It should be followed a worst case approach by considering in each step not only the routine situation, but the most complex one in terms of people, equipment problems, *etc.*

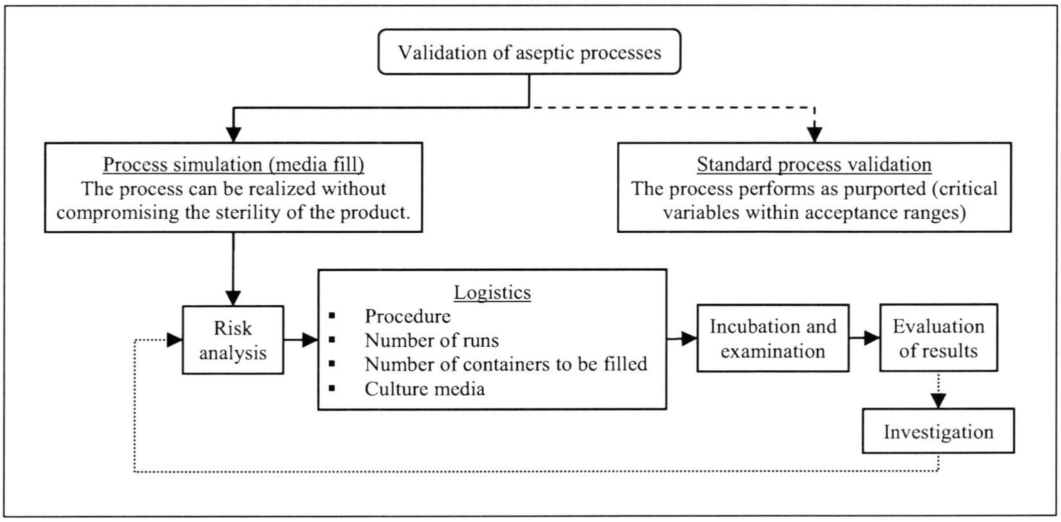

Fig. (8). Rationale for the validation of aseptic processes.

FDA recommends that the media fill program address applicable issues such as:

- *Factors associated with the longest permitted run on the processing line that can pose contamination risk (e.g. operator fatigue);*
- *Representative number, type, and complexity of normal interventions that occur with each run, as well as non-routine interventions and events (e.g. maintenance, stoppages, equipment adjustments);*

- *Lyophilization, when applicable;*
- *Aseptic assembly of equipment (e.g. at start-up, during processing);*
- *Number of personnel and their activities;*
- *Representative number of aseptic additions (e.g. charging containers and closures as well as sterile ingredients) or transfers;*
- *Shift changes, breaks, and gown changes (when applicable):*
- *Type of aseptic equipment disconnections/connections;*
- *Aseptic sample collections;*
- *Line speed and configuration;*
- *Weight checks;*
- *Container closure systems (e.g. sizes, type, compatibility with equipment);*
- *Specific provisions in written procedures relating to aseptic processing (e.g. conditions permitted before line clearance is mandated)* [27].

Logistics

Procedure

Media fills should be performed by following a special version of the batch master record gathering all the worst case considerations of the risk analysis and where instead of product is used culture medium.

In the media fills should take part, at least one a year, all persons (either operators or personnel of maintenance) who are allowed to enter the clean room where the aseptic process is performed. Each person should play during the media fill the same role they play during routine production. Although the simulation should mimic the true process, often the main objective is less reproducing exactly its duration than performing all the operations that might produce contamination.

For lyophilization operations, FDA recommends that unsealed containers be exposed to partial evacuation of the chamber in a manner that simulates the process. Vials should not be frozen, and precautions should be taken that ensure that the medium remains in an aerobic state to avoid potentially inhibiting the growth of microorganisms [28].

Number of Runs

The initial qualification of the line should comprise a minimum of three consecutive and separate runs performed successfully. Afterwards, media fills should be performed twice a year for every shift and process.

Number of Containers to be Filled

The number of containers which are filled should be sufficient for ensuring that it is representative of the routine process. When the standard batch is composed of a reduced number of containers, the process simulation should use at least this same number. In general it is considered that 5,000 – 10,000 is an acceptable range for starting the process simulations.

Culture Media

Soybean casein digest medium is typically used. In particular cases it can be justified to use anaerobic growth media, such as fluid thioglycollate medium. Any growth medium which is used should show its ability to promote growth of gram-negative and gram-positive bacteria and of yeasts and moulds with a <100 cfu challenge (of indicator microorganisms and/or microorganisms isolated from the environment). In case of failure of the growth promotion tests the media fill should be repeated. Notwithstanding that, if it was found any contamination during the assay, its origin has to be investigated.

The quantity of medium filled per container should suffice for contacting the inner surfaces of container and closure and allow for the visual detection of microbial growth. In order to ensure contact of the medium with all the surfaces the units are either inverted or methodically swirled.

Once the media fill run is completed the filling line has to be promptly cleaned, sanitized and sterilized, as necessary, in order to discard any risk of contamination.

Incubation and Container Examination

Temperature: The units filled during the media fill should be incubated at a temperature suitable for the recovery of microorganisms.

The incubation temperature should be kept within the range of 20-35°C and it should be maintained within ±2.5°C of the target temperature.

Time: The units should be incubated at least during 14 days. In case of using two temperatures for the incubation, the units should be incubated for at least 7 days at each temperature, starting with the lower temperature.

Examination: All the units should be examined by expert personnel in search of microbiological contamination. According to FDA it is advised to use amber or opaque containers for a better detection of microbial contamination. When the authorized product is filled in clear containers, they can be substituted in the media fill by amber ones, provided that they have the same physical properties.

Faulty units: All integral units should be incubated. Units possessing cosmetic defects but maintaining their integrity should be incubated too. Only units which lack integrity should be rejected. Units which were erroneously rejected should be immediately returned to incubation.

Once that incubation is underway, units found defective should be considered accounted in the media fill results, because they might represent a real case (*e.g.* a defective unit which was not detected and thus might have been released to the market). Any unit lacking integrity excluded from the incubated units should be fully justified in the final media fill report. Any correlation between faulty units difficult to detect and microbial contamination should be investigated and corrected.

Although the intent of process simulation is showing that the conditions under which the routine process is performed allow asepsis, it can also be used for increasing knowledge on the process. Thus, by incubating defective units, media remainders in pipes or in receptacles, which in routine production would be discarded, it is possible to acquire more information on the quality of the process. These supplementary samples should be incubated separately and not being taken into account in the evaluation of the media fill.

Evaluation of Results

The objective of a media fill is showing asepsis (*i.e.* not a single contaminated container in the batch). Thus it is evident that a process simulation process is considered “passed” when there is not a single container showing growth. Conversely, a simulation process is deemed “failed”, when there is growth in several containers. A more complex issue appears when there is “just” one container showing growth. See Fig. (**9**).

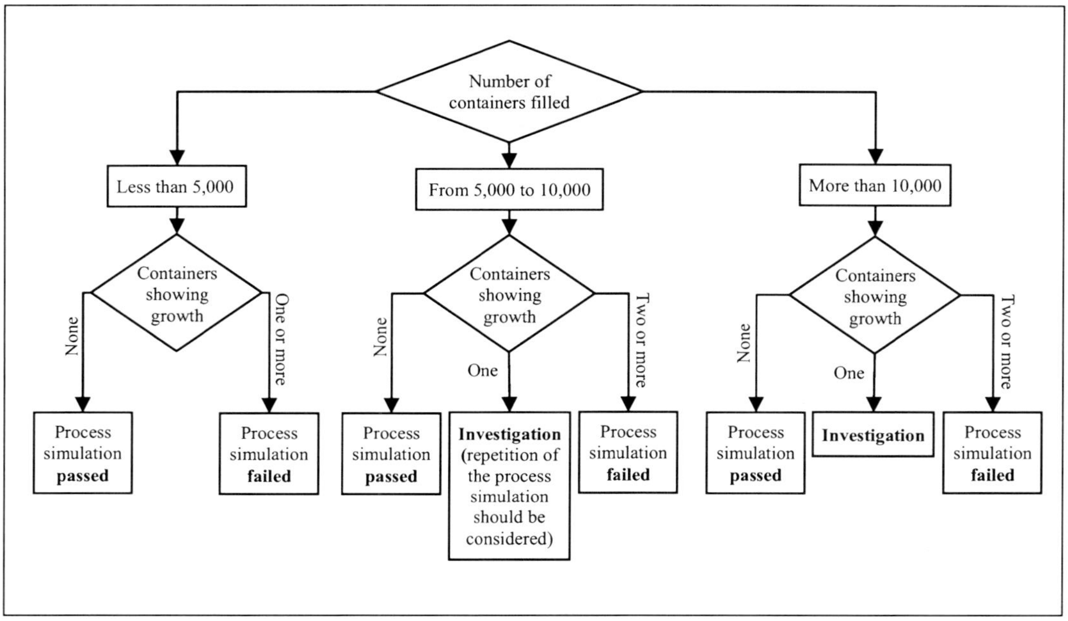

Fig. (9). GMP approach to the evaluation of the results of a process simulation with media fill.

Investigation

A failed media fill should be followed by an accurate investigation in order to determine the causes and extent of the problem and the origin of the contamination. This would be followed by the application of the CAPA system. As soon as the adequate corrective and preventive measures have been implemented, the media fill can be repeated. The aim of this repetition is verifying that the process performs as specified. If it appears impossible to detect the causes of the media fill failure it is considered acceptable performing three consecutive successful runs in tandem with more intensive monitoring of the production process.

Contaminated units should be investigated and the species of the contaminating microorganisms should be identified. The origin of the contamination should be established. In case of media fill failure the investigation should include an assessment of the batches produced since the previous media fill to determine if there might be contaminated units.

ANALYTICAL VALIDATION

Analytical methods should be validated to show that they are adequate for providing reliable results [29, 30]. See Table **5**.

Analytical validation follows the same general pattern that has been previously described for qualification (chapter 2) and validation (chapter 10).

Table 5. The most common types of analytical procedures.

Identification tests	The aim of these tests is ensuring the identity an analyte in a sample.
Testing for impurities	Testing for impurities is performed to verify the characteristics of purity of a sample. This can be a limit test for impurities in a sample or a quantitative test.
Assay tests	Here are considered two types of test regarding the analyte present in a determinate sample: measurement of dissolution and content/potency.

Pharmacopoeial methods or methods approved by regulatory authorities need not be validated as such, but they have to be verified in the laboratory to show that they are suitable and that do not show interference with substances in the product which is actually assayed.

Analytical validation is based on the verification of characteristics of the procedure, which are defined here:

<u>Accuracy (or trueness)</u> is the closeness of agreement of the results obtained by the procedure with the true value or an accepted reference value.

<u>Precision</u> is the degree of agreement among individual results. It may be considered at three levels: repeatability, intermediate precision and reproducibility.

- Repeatability (or intra-assay precision) expresses the precision under the same operating conditions over a short interval of time.

- Intermediate precision expresses within-laboratory variations (usually on different days, different analysts, different equipment, *etc.*).

- Reproducibility expresses the precision between laboratories (collaborative studies, usually applied to standardization of methodology).

Specificity (selectivity) is the ability to measure unequivocally the analyte in the presence of other substances which may be expected to be present (excipients, degradation products, impurities, *etc.*).

Detection limit is the smallest quantity of analyte which can be detected but not necessarily quantified.

Quantitation limit is the lowest amount of analyte in a sample which can be quantitatively determined with acceptable precision and accuracy.

Linearity is the ability (within a given range) to produce results which are directly proportional to the concentration of analyte in the samples.

Range is the interval between the upper and lower concentration (amounts) of analyte in the sample (including these concentrations) for which it has been demonstrated that the analytical procedure has a suitable level of precision, accuracy and linearity.

Table 6. Characteristics that should be verified for the validation of an analytical procedure.

Characteristics		**Type of analytical procedure**			
		Identification	**Testing for impurities**		**Assay**
			Quantitative test	**Limit test**	
Accuracy (trueness)		-	+	-	+
Precision	Repeatability	-	+	-	+
	Intermediate precision	-	+[1]	-	+[1]
Specificity (selectivity)[2]		+	+	+	+
Detection limit		-	-[3]	+	-
Quantitation limit		-	+	-	-
Linearity		-	+	-	+
Range		-	+	-	+

[1] in cases where reproducibility has been performed, intermediate precision is not needed.

[2] Lack of specificity of one analytical procedure could be compensated by other supporting analytical procedure/s.

[3] It may be needed in some cases.

Table **6** shows the characteristics which should be verified for the validation of an analytical procedure. As requirements depend on the type of test, (-) means that the characteristic is not normally evaluated, whereas, (+) signifies that this characteristic is normally evaluated. The revalidation of an analytical procedure is necessary when there are significant changes, such as those regarding the laboratory (*e.g.* different equipment, modification of the analytical procedure, *etc.*), the APIs (*e.g.* changes in their synthesis) or in the product (*e.g.* different composition). The extension of this revalidation depends on the nature of the changes and should be evaluated in each case.

VALIDATION OF COMPUTERIZED SYSTEMS

Computerized systems should be validated at the level appropriate for their use and applications [31, 32].

The lifecycle model approach is also useful for computerized systems and the four well-known stages (see chapter 2) should be considered here too:

(1) Planning, specification and programming.

(2) Testing on site.

(3) Service life with monitoring, change management and revalidation (as necessary).

(4) Discontinuation (ensuring that data will be maintained).

The security of computerized systems is a very important point to be taken into account (see chapter 10).

Computer systems have two quite different components: Hardware and software.

Hardware is constituted by the equipment (input/output devices, signal converters, central processing units - CPUs, distribution systems and peripheral devices). Its elements should be identified, characterized and verified. It is important ensuring that these elements are protected from conditions which might jeopardize their adequate operation (*e.g.* interferences, dust, stress conditions, *etc.*).

Software is composed by the programs which are used by the system. They should be identified and provide assurance that they will consistently perform as expected. It is tested that the system functions according to expectations under normal and worst case conditions. The necessary degree of validation depends on the type of program [33].

Those which have been tailor-made require thorough validation, whereas standard programs in principle can be considered as validated. Between these two situations the necessary amount of validation is linked to the amount of changes made to an existing program to meet particular requirements.

The common approach for the validation of computerized systems is the same that was described in chapter 2 regarding qualification in general. Validation requires describing what the system is expected to perform and then preparing tests in order to proof that the system is actually capable of doing this.

Validation should go on with permanent monitoring to ensure that the system continues to perform as expected during the service life and by revalidation whenever significant changes are introduced.

APPLICATION OF THE LIFECYCLE MODEL TO LEGACY PRODUCTS

The Pharmaceutical Quality System (PQS) applied to the product lifecycle model allows for a successful GMP implementation and provides a good frame for ensuring quality. Unfortunately most of the existing pharmaceutical products were developed before this model had been devised. Consequently, it might seem that their quality should remain tied to 20th century approaches, which ignored quality by design. Yes, of course, this is a possibility. Another one could be a redevelopment of these products following the 21st century approach, like any new product. Yes, this is an option too, but not a very realistic one. There is however, a third, intermediate option, because the application of concepts of the present century to products created in the last century offers a great prospect for improvement. In fact, the expenses related to this task can be compensated by the increase and updating of the existing knowledge on the products and also by the diminution of the costs associated with validation, quality assurance and quality control.

Although the "redevelopment" of old products following current approaches is normally inapplicable, we should not forget that the backbone of these approaches is constituted by science-based and risk-assessed decisions and that the motor which impulses everything is continual improvement. Thus, it is possible, little by little, transforming legacy products into products which somewhat approach the current model of quality insurance.

New products are well understood because of the knowledge acquired during their development, transfer and commercial manufacturing and as a consequence they can be closely monitored. Although this is not the case for legacy products, it is possible to follow with them a reverse procedure (*i.e.* gather the currently existing manufacturing information in order to reconstruct, as far as possible, a quality by design approach). Whereas for new products the lifecycle steps allow for building a structured knowledge and this is translated into better quality insurance, for legacy products it is necessary gathering the existing unstructured knowledge for turning it into structured knowledge.

The life-cycle strategy that is described here might be called "DAME", an acronym derived from the names of its four steps (Definition, Approval, Monitoring and Evaluation). The application of DAME requires the previous implementation of the PQS as it has been described in chapter 5, but as the strategy that is here proposed is a progressive one, implemented step by step, it is also possible to start by developing and implementing the PQS at the same time than this strategy. In this case it is advisable to start with structures as simpler as possible and with clearly defined and outlined responsibilities.

The DAME strategy, intended to ensure the quality of the products runs parallel to the life-cycle of the product (Fig. **10**).

The purpose of DAME is to compile information. It does not intend to duplicate work which was performed by the departments in charge of the different stages of the life-cycle of a product, because it is evident that even if the life-cycle model did not exist as such, these stages may have been, more or less, followed. DAME ensures that critical data are known and then used in an appropriate way.

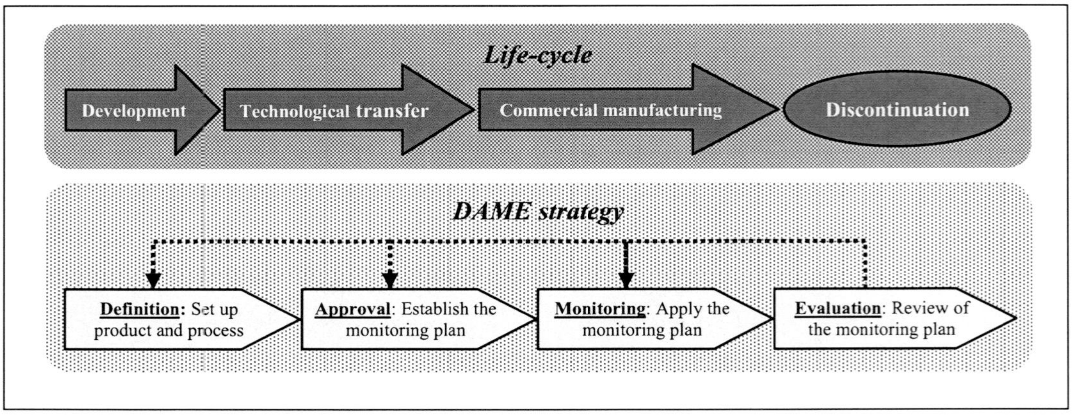

Fig. (10). DAME strategy.

When applying the DAME strategy to legacy products it has to be born in mind that there are matters which might require a modification of the manufacturing authorization prior to its implementation. This is why, in many cases, it is convenient to start DAME by applying it to assay batches or informally in parallel to the current procedure approved for production. The new approach can only be implemented once that it has been well proven and the request for modification has been approved by the regulatory authorities

Whenever applying the four stages of the DAME strategy it will be necessary to take into account the following facts:

1st The review of the existing knowledge about legacy products is not a loss of time, but a way of enhancing their quality.

2nd Improving the diffusion of information among the different departments and posts of a company is very important and it should be done in both directions: forwards (from generator to receiver) and backwards (from receiver to generator). The gaps or shade areas between departments suppose a loss of time and money. This is why it is important to detect and correct them as far as possible.

3rd The application of new concepts, such as process analytical technology (PAT), design space or real time release testing (RTRT), can start in a modest way and progress according to the possibilities. Processes can be controlled by using the existing technology and quality control testing or by using PAT and RTRT. Both options are acceptable.

4th The introduction of concepts such as continual monitoring or improvement are essential for ensuring the quality of the products and the state of control on the processes.

5th The selection of the first product to which the DAME strategy will be applied is very important. In general it can be said that it is advantageous to choose the biggest seller, the most "strategic", or the product which shows lesser state of control. This first product will open the way for the others.

1st Step: Definition of a Product Profile

DAME should be started by defining the "Quality Target Product Profile" (QTPP) of the product (Fig. **11**).

The outcome of development is the formula and the manufacturing procedure of a product, but also the definition of the specifications for the starting and packaging materials and for the products (intermediate and finished).

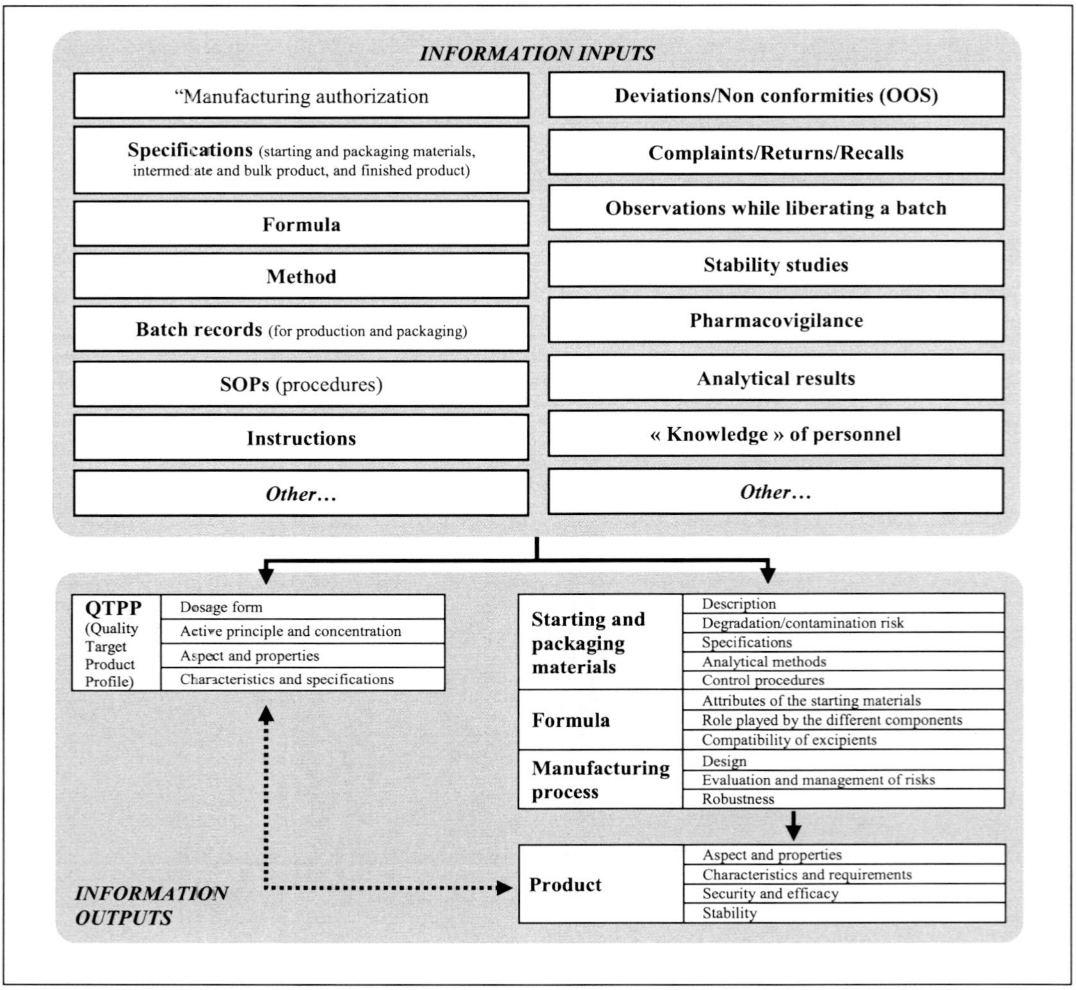

Fig. (11). Definition of the product profile.

It can be said that the manufacturing process links the starting materials with the finished product. The characteristics of the product depend on the properties of the materials and on the parameters of the process. This is why it is possible to determine these relations and to establish their behavior as regards variations (in physico-chemical conditions, in relative proportions, in processing times, *etc.*).

Legacy products are already "defined" and consequently the necessary information to apply a new quality approach is already available. In any case, it is always possible to realize additional testing and to describe QTPP in a retrospective way (if this baseline definition does not exist yet). See Fig. (**12**).

2nd Step: Approval

Study of Critical Variables

Even if the possibility of performing multivariable studies in order to establish a design space remains always open, in most of cases it will suffice with the determination of critical parameters and with the establishment of their acceptation ranges, defined by their alert and action limits.

The critical variables are made up of the set of CQAs and CPPs. This involves, firstly the identification of all the existing variables, and secondly the assessment of their criticality by means of risk analysis. As usual, the method which is chosen to perform this analysis is less important than the characteristics of the existing information. Critical variables should be submitted to monitoring, unless that a change in the process might transform them into non critical.

From the three factors determining the level of risk of a hazard (severity, probability and detection), in most of cases it is only possible to act on the last two. Probability can be diminished by improving technologically the process. The capacity of detecting deviations of the critical variables can be increased by introducing new instrumentation. And both can be improved by better personnel training and experience.

Although in the case of legacy products there will likely be sufficient information to perform risk analysis directly in one stage, using, for instance, FMECA, it will often be convenient to develop this analysis in three phases, in relation with the existing level of knowledge:

- A preliminary analysis, using, for instance, PHA (primary hazard analysis), in order to identify the CQAs and HACCP (hazard analysis and critical control points) to determine the CPPs.

- Afterwards, as more information has been gathered, it is possible to use other methods such as FMECA (Failure Mode, Effects & Criticality Analysis), in order to assess the level of risk of the process.

- Finally, the analysis performed will be revised in order to verify that the implemented monitoring procedures allow for the reduction of residual risk to acceptable levels.

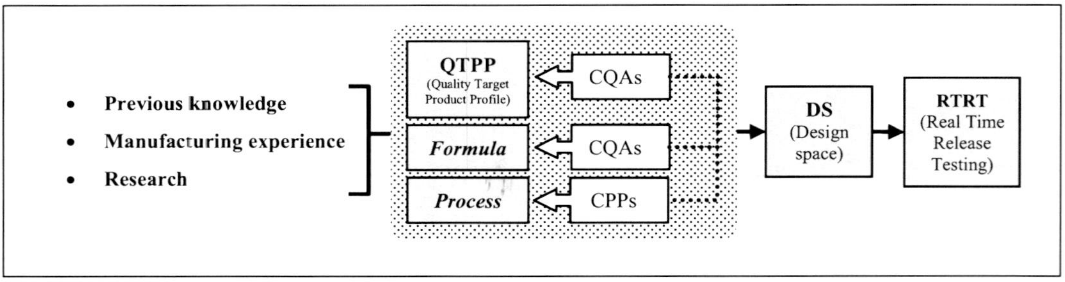

Fig. (12. Global strategy of Quality by Design (QbD).

Control

When critical variables have been identified (materials/product attributes or process parameters) it is necessary to know which are their acceptable ranges. As it was said, if CPPs within acceptation range ensure the adequacy of CQAs, the monitoring/measure of CPPs is a way for assessing the quality of the product.

Once critical variables are well established it will be necessary to choose the adequate monitoring system. This will also require the implementation of a written procedure describing how to act in case of excursion from the defined limits.

Then, control of products can move from the traditional off-line analysis to real time monitoring by using process analytical technology (PAT). This last approach has the advantage of not requiring sampling and of providing real-time data.

Liberation

The strategy to be followed for the liberation of the product should follow in parallel the strategy of control. It is possible to choose the traditional approach of liberation after analysis of the finished product or, when there is monitoring/measuring in real time (or almost), to liberate it also in reduced time.

If it is decided to perform real time release testing (RTRT) it should be defined the procedure to be followed in case of failure of the monitoring equipment (for instance, traditional liberation after analysis, use of reserve equipment, *etc.*; the chosen option should be justified in a scientific way and to be based on risk assessment).

Validation

Validation provides confidence in the product and in the manufacturing process. Thus, it consists in showing that the manufacturing process is capable of yielding a product which corresponds to the QTPP.

Current validation strategy is based on:

- Knowledge acquired during the development (and enhanced afterwards),
- Risk assessment,
- Data derived from process monitoring,
- Statistical studies of "process capability".

It is necessary to point out that the qualification of equipment, as it has been performed until now, is not modified. It is necessary, however, to link qualification with risk assessment and, consequently, concentrate on the critical aspects. See Table **7**.

Table 7. General process validation checklist.

	Topic	Action
1	Qualification of equipment	Verify that all the items of equipment involved in the manufacturing process have been qualified.
2	Qualification of utilities	Verify that all utility systems intervening in the manufacturing process have been qualified: - HVAC (see clean rooms); - Dust exhaust; - Water for pharmaceutical use; - Compressed air.
3	Qualification of clean rooms	Verify that all the clean rooms intervening in the process have been qualified and particularly: - particle counting for classification; - class recovery time; - cascade of pressures.
4	Calibration of critical instruments	Verify that all critical instruments are in state of calibration (both in manufacturing equipment and in apparatus used during validation).
5	Operating procedures/instructions	- Verify that there are approved documents regarding assembly, use, cleaning and maintenance of equipment/tools. - Verify that there are approved documents describing how to perform operations related to the process which is validated.
6	Manufacturing documentation	- Verify that there are approved batch formula, batch manufacturing instructions and batch manufacturing record.

Table 7: contd...

7	Personnel training	Verify that personnel has been trained: - Regarding validation (for those who are in charge of the validation); - Regarding the product manufacturing process and its related operations.
8	Validation of the cleaning procedures	Verify that the cleaning procedures of equipment/tools intervening in the manufacturing process have been validated.
9	Validation of the analytical procedures	Verify that analytical procedures related to the process have been validated: - Starting and packaging materials; - In process controls; - Intermediates; - Bulk product; - Finished product.
10	Validation of computerized systems	Verify that the computerized systems intervening in the process have been validated.
11	Product specification (QTPP)	Verify that there are approved specifications for the product and that its QTPP has been defined.
12	Starting/packaging materials specification (CQAs)	Verify that there are approved specifications for the starting and packaging materials. Verify that their CQAs have been determined and acceptable ranges established.
13	Risk analysis of the manufacturing process (CPPs)	Verify that the risk analysis of the process has been performed and that its CPPs have been identified and for them acceptable ranges have been established.
14	Intermediates and bulk product specifications (CQAs)	Verify that there are approved specifications for the intermediates (if they exist) and for bulk product. Verify that their CQAs have been determined and acceptable ranges established.
15	Finished product specification (CQAs)	Verify that there are approved specifications for the finished product. Verify that their CQAs have been determined and acceptable ranges established.
16	Incidents/deviations	Verify that there is a procedure for handling incidents/deviations during manufacturing. In case of having detected incidents/deviations they have been adequately managed.
17	Results obtained in the validation of batch #1	Verify the batch manufacturing record of batch #1 and the associated monitoring and control operations to confirm that everything is correct.
18	Results obtained in the validation of batch #2	Verify the batch manufacturing record of batch #2 and the associated monitoring and control operations to confirm that everything is correct.
19	Results obtained in the validation of batch #3	Verify the batch manufacturing record of batch #3 and the associated monitoring and control operations to confirm that everything is correct.
20	Validation report	Write a validation report summarizing all the previous verifications

In case of aseptic processing it is necessary to add a particularized control of sterilization which is an extremely critical point and a media fill assay to verify that the process as it is performed ensures product sterility. See Table **8**.

Table 8. Sterile process validation checklist.

	Topic	Action
1	Qualification of equipment	Verify that all the sterilization processes have been adequately performed: - There are approved procedures for sterilization; - Sterilization processes are validated; - The CPPs of sterilization are correct; - The bioindicators show no growth when incubated.
2	Media fill	A mock process with culture medium yields containers that when are incubated show no growth.

3rd Step: Monitoring

Routine production can be adequately overseen by monitoring the parameters of the manufacturing process and the CQAs and the CPPs. This can be performed by using automatic methods providing information in real time (PAT). Although this is the best solution, in most cases this would only be applied after having reached some degree of "maturity". In most cases, it is preferable to start in a humble way, by identifying the critical variables and defining methods to supervise them, both "on line" and "off line". Afterwards experience and assay will indicate the better approach to automation. See Fig. (**13**).

Obviously, the application of the DAME strategy does not modify the situation of the quality unit (QA/QC), although it may allow for a certain degree of simplification as a consequence of a sharper distinction between "analytical" and "monitoring/supervision" tasks.

Monitoring should be extended to the gathering of analytical data of commercial batches in order to confirm or, if necessary, correct the predictive model (does the commercialized product during all his life correspond to the product which has been developed, clinically tested and authorized in all its critical aspects? Is it stable?).

A written procedure should describe the method followed to oversee the critical variables (what, how, when, by whom).

4th Step: Evaluation

As indicated previously, it is necessary to implement a system of periodical evaluation of the existing data. Even in "mature" processes (*i.e.* well known and under control) deviations, imperceptible for those who take part in routine manufacturing, may appear. Therefore, it is necessary a close data follow-up regarding:

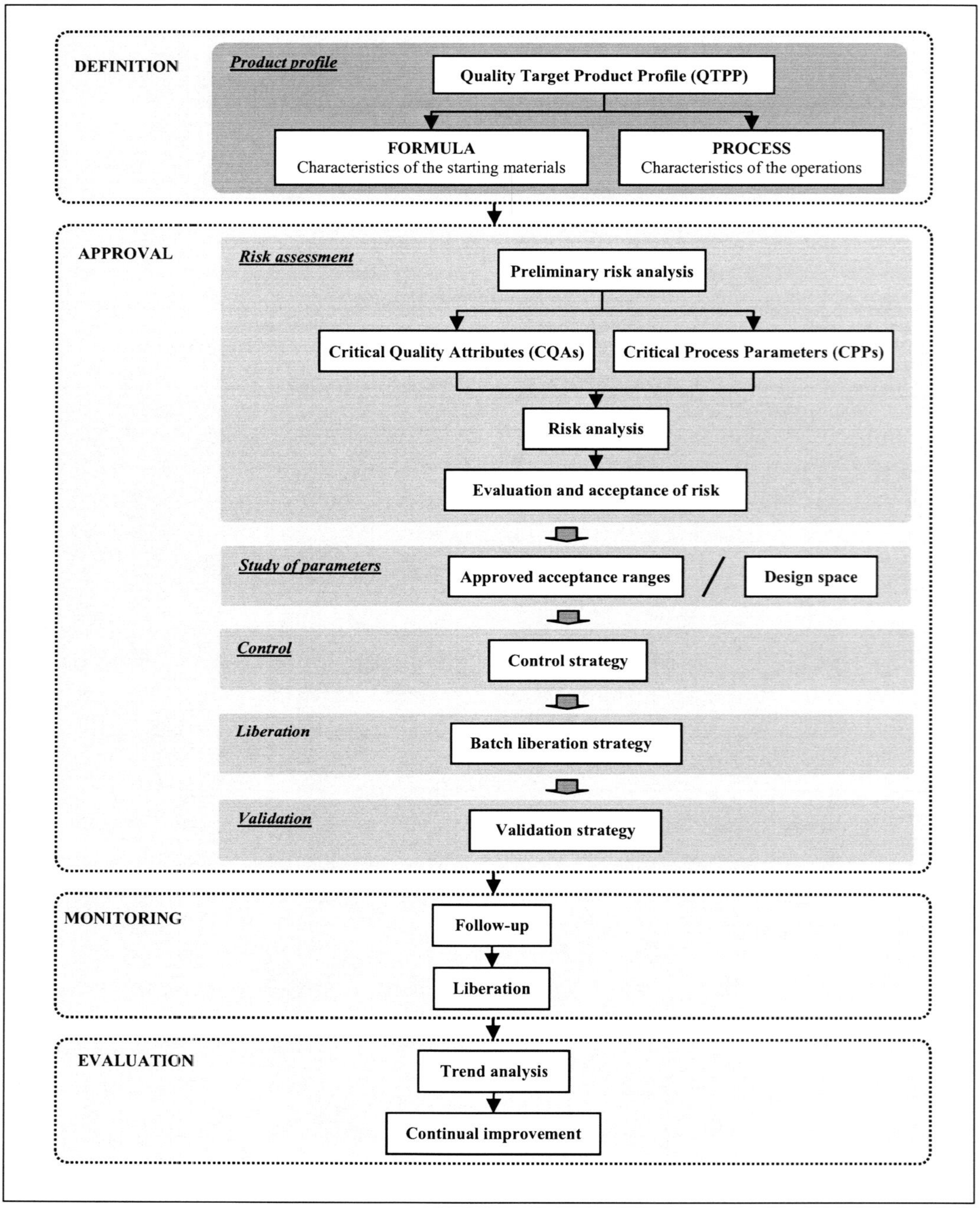

Fig. (13). DAME strategy step by step.

- deviations (CAPA system);

- variations;
- manufacturing experience;
- complaints;
- trend analysis of monitoring and testing data;
- product quality reviews and management reviews;
- liberation of batches.

Continual improvement will be a consequence of this evaluation, with the objective of reducing variability.

DAME strategy is based on the life-cycle and thus it is also submitted to continual improvement by a double process of increase of information ("feed forward") and of modification of existing premises ("feedback"), so that process parameters may be adjusted during the life-cycle. See Fig. (**14**).

As it has been mentioned before, DAME is a strategy for "updating" legacy products and as such it has to be born in mind that the objective is improving as much as possible the control strategy of those products, but always taking into account the existing resources and possibilities. In between the two extreme situations (*i.e.* quality by design and purely empirical design) there may always be different possibilities and the aim is advancing as much as possible towards the top situation. It is better a partial improvement than no improvement at all.

CONCLUDING REMARKS

The quality of pharmaceutical products is the result of a number of activities realized concurrently. First of all, a product should not be simply seen as a formula, a manufacturing procedure and some specifications, but as the global result of a whole life-cycle, where the product is scientifically developed and analyzed in order to gain sufficient knowledge for understanding its behavior (in terms of attributes and parameters). Only a product that has quality by design can be manufactured with quality, because only if the factors from which depends its quality are known, can this quality be ensured. Knowledge is far from being information that can be acquired once and for all during the development. This is why it is spoken of risk and knowledge management and of continual improvement. Since development to discontinuation knowledge of a product is improved and this insures that it will always remain valid, because slight drifts will be detected, analyzed and corrected as necessary.

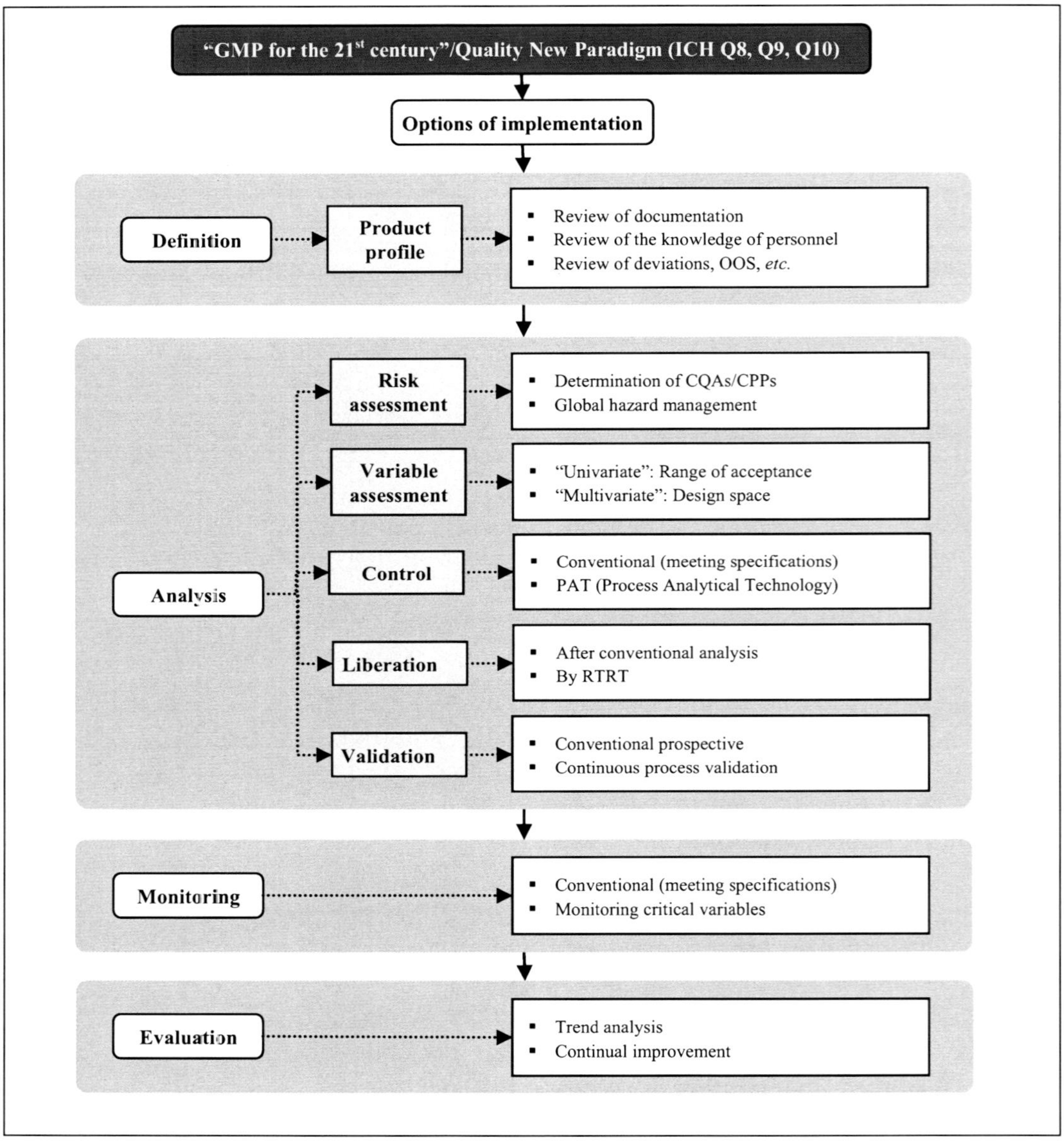

Fig. (14). DAME strategy: Options for its implementation.

CONFLICT OF INTEREST

The author confirms that this chapter contents have no conflict of interest.

ACKNOWLEDGEMENT

Declared None.

REFERENCES

[1] ICH (International Conference on Harmonisation of Technical Requirements for registration of Pharmaceuticals for Human Use). Pharmaceutical development. Harmonised Tripartite Guideline. Q8(R2). ICH, Geneva, Switzerland, 2009. 2.

[2] U.S. Department of Health and Human Services Food and Drug Administration Center for Drug Evaluation and Research (CDER) Center for Biologics Evaluation and Research (CBER) Office of Regulatory Affairs (ORA). CGMP for Phase 1 Investigational Drugs. Guidance for Industry. CGMP. FDA, Rockville, MD, USA, 2008.

[3] European Commission. Enterprise and Industry Directorate-General. Investigational Medicinal Products. In: EudraLex. The Rules Governing Medicinal Products in the European Union. Volume 4. EU Guidelines to Good Manufacturing Practice. Medicinal Products for Human and Veterinary Use. European Commission, Brussels, Belgium, 2010. Annex 13.

[4] WHO (World Health Organisation). Handbook for Good Clinical Research Practice (GCP). Guidance for implementation. WHO, Geneva, Switzerland, 2002.

[5] ICH (International Conference on Harmonisation of Technical Requirements for registration of Pharmaceuticals for Human Use). Guideline for Good Clinical Practice. Harmonised Tripartite Guideline. E6(R1). ICH, Geneva, Switzerland, 1996.

[6] Commission of the European Communities. Directive 2005/28/EC of 8 April 2005 laying down principles and detailed guidelines for good clinical practice as regards investigational medicinal products for human use, as well as the requirements for authorisation of the manufacturing or importation of such products. Official Journal of the European Union. L 91/13, 9.4.2005.

[7] Schmitt S. Quality by design: Putting theory into practice. PDA Bethesda, MD, USA, 2011.

[8] ICH (International Conference on Harmonisation of Technical Requirements for registration of Pharmaceuticals for Human Use). Pharmaceutical development. Harmonised Tripartite Guideline. Q8(R2). ICH, Geneva, Switzerland, 2009. Glossary (part 2).

[9] Ibid.

[10] Ibid.

[11] Ibid.

[12] Ibid.

[13] Ibid.

[14] ICH (International Conference on Harmonisation of Technical Requirements for registration of Pharmaceuticals for Human Use). Pharmaceutical Quality System. Harmonised Tripartite Guideline. Q10. ICH, Geneva, Switzerland, 2008. Glossary.

[15] U.S. Department of Health and Human Services. Food and Drug Administration. Center for Drug Evaluation and Research (CDER). Center for Veterinary Medicine (CVM). Office of Regulatory Affairs (ORA). PAT – A Framework for Innovative Pharmaceutical Development, Manufacturing, and Quality Assurance. Guidance for industry, FDA, Rockville, MD, USA, 2004.

[16] ICH (International Conference on Harmonisation of Technical Requirements for registration of Pharmaceuticals for Human Use). Pharmaceutical development. Harmonised Tripartite Guideline. Q8(R2). ICH, Geneva, Switzerland, 2009. Glossary.

[17] Ibid.

[18] European Commission. Enterprise Directorate-General. Parametric Release. In: EudraLex. The Rules Governing Medicinal Products in the European Union. Volume 4. EU Guidelines to Good Manufacturing Practice. Medicinal Products for Human and Veterinary Use. European Commission, Brussels, Belgium, 2001. Annex 17.

[19] PIC/S (Pharmaceutical Inspection Convention/Pharmaceutical Inspection Co-Operation Scheme). Guidance on Parametric Release. Recommendation PI 005-3. PIC/S, Geneva, Switzerland, 2007.

[20] U.S. Department of Health and Human Services. Food and Drug Administration. Center for Drug Evaluation and Research (CDER). Center for Biologics Evaluation and Research (CBER). Office of Regulatory Affairs (ORA). Sterile drug products produced by aseptic processing – Current Good Manufacturing Practice. Guidance for Industry. FDA, Rockville, MD, USA, 2004. B.

[21] ICH (International Conference on Harmonisation of Technical Requirements for registration of Pharmaceuticals for Human Use). Pharmaceutical Quality System. Harmonised Tripartite Guideline. Q10. ICH, Geneva, Switzerland, 2008. 3.1.2.

[22] Ibid. 3.1.3.

[23] Ibid. 3.1.4.

[24] PIC/S (Pharmaceutical Inspection Convention/Pharmaceutical Inspection Co-Operation Scheme). Validation Master Plan, Installation and Operational Qualification, Non-sterile Process Validation, Cleaning Validation. Recommendations PI 006-3. PIC/S, Geneva, Switzerland, 2007.

[25] Ibid.

[26] Ibid.

[27] U.S. Department of Health and Human Services. Food and Drug Administration. Center for Drug Evaluation and Research (CDER). Center for Biologics Evaluation and Research (CBER). Office of Regulatory Affairs (ORA). Sterile drug products produced by aseptic processing – Current Good Manufacturing Practice. Guidance for Industry. FDA, Rockville, MD, USA, 2004.

[28] Ibid.

[29] WHO (World Health Organisation). Supplementary guidelines on good manufacturing practices: validation. In: WHO Expert Committee on Specifications for Pharmaceutical Preparations. Fortieth report (WHO Technical Report Series, No. 937). WHO, Geneva, Switzerland, 2006. Annex 4 (Appendix 4: Analytical method validation).

[30] ICH (International Conference on Harmonisation of Technical Requirements for registration of Pharmaceuticals for Human Use). Validation of Analytical Procedures: Text and Methodology. Harmonised Tripartite Guideline. Q2(R1). ICH, Geneva, Switzerland, 2005.

[31] WHO (World Health Organisation). Supplementary guidelines on good manufacturing practices: validation. In: WHO Expert Committee on Specifications for Pharmaceutical Preparations. Fortieth report (WHO Technical Report Series, No. 937). WHO, Geneva, Switzerland, 2006. Annex 4 (Appendix 5: Validation of computerized systems).

[32] ISPE (International Society of Pharmaceutical Engineering). GAMP: A risk-based approach to GXP process control systems. Second edition. ISPE, Tampa, Florida, USA 2011.

[33] Gough J, Nettleton D. Risk-based software validation. PDA Bethesda, MD, USA 2006.

CHAPTER 12

Global Quality

Abstract: Current pharmaceutical quality requires a global approach based on a quality system established on GMP and on risk analysis. Quality can be only ensured if hazards are identified and controlled to be kept at an acceptable risk level. Consequently, nowadays quality audits are not seen anymore as a simple compilation of checklist questions (yes/no/n. a.), but as an investigation to see if existing problems are detected and solved/controlled satisfactorily. This requires good knowledge and deep analysis on processes and products. As for the rest, it is also necessary to ensure that those pharmaceutical products which are dispatched from the warehouse, after being certified and released, maintain their quality when they reach their final consumers. Thus, it has been paid progressively attention to the hazards that waylay them in the often very complex distribution chain, including the risk of theft and counterfeiting. Taking into account the successful experience of GMP equivalent GDPs (good distribution practices) have been developed. It is also necessary to ensure the soundness of studies on drug products which are performed in different laboratories. And this requires a homogeneous quality approach. This is why, following again the same track, GLP (good laboratory practice) was prepared. And, finally, it is necessary to bear in mind that once a drug product has been licensed it is used by much more people than when it was tested during development, and this opens the door to unexpected reactions. Thus a pharmacovigilance system is necessary to keep updated its benefit-risk safety profile.

Keywords: ADR, counterfeiting, dispatch, GCP, GDPs, GLP, GVP, FEFO, pharmacovigilance, pharmacovigilance centre, PQS, sponsor, study, study director, study plan, supply chain, test substance, reference substance, transportation, warehousing.

CONCEPT

The different elements which make possible manufacturing quality pharmaceuticals have been analyzed in previous chapters. These elements are so varied (documentation, premises, equipment, personnel, *etc.*) that they require to be studied separately. Notwithstanding that, all these elements have to be designed for building together a precise system of global quality.

Although each case is different, in a general way it is possible to say that pharmaceutical plants can belong to two categories. In the first one appear those which do possess quality and in the second one those which do lack it. This way of putting things might seem surprising and too reductionist, but using current quality thinking it is rather correct, because possessing quality does not mean that everything is done faultless and there are no problems. It means, on the contrary,

Jordi Botet

that hazards linked to processes are known and understood, that a system is in place to monitor them and, most important of all, when problems arise this system can provide the adequate response to keep processes going under control. This is what makes the big difference; only pharmaceutical plants that know how to handle adequately problems have quality. A company managing satisfactorily several problems can be relied upon, whereas a firm just having a couple of problems, but not conducting them appropriately is very dangerous. This is why it has been said that having problems is not the problem; the problem is having problems and being unable of reacting adequately.

Thus, global quality means possessing a quality system capable of preventing most of problems, handling them satisfactorily and, thanks to continual improvement, reducing progressively their occurrence. Unfortunately the alternative to global quality is simply lack of quality. Let's suppose a plant manufacturing hundreds of batches and all of them meeting requirements, but where every now and then a batch happens to be out-of-specifications and nobody knows why or detects it. Would it be possible to say that this plant has global quality?

Nowadays a global quality system should be capable of detecting and handling all problems and then finding out the root causes of these problems and implementing actions which improve the system in order to impede relapsing.

GLOBAL QUALITY ORGANIZATION REVIEW

The global review of the organization of a pharmaceutical plant from the quality point of view requires a grouping of the intervening topics in logical areas:

- Quality Assurance (QA);
- Supply chain (manufacturing processes);
- Personnel;
- Premises, Facilities & Equipment;
- Quality control (QC);
- Hygiene, security and environment.

Although this does not intend to be an audit guide it is recognized that can be used as such. In fact it means to be used as an "aide-memoire" to analyze a pharmaceutical plant in terms of quality assurance compliance. Topics which have to be considered are numerous, varied and difficult to group in a coherent way, but some degree of systematization is indispensable not to get lost and in a maze of matters (Table **1**).

Table 1. Global quality organization aide-memoire.

Area	Topic
(1) **Quality Assurance** (QA)	▪ Organization of the Pharmaceutical Quality System (PQS); ▪ Administration of the Pharmaceutical Quality System (PQS); ▪ Batch certification.
(2) **Supply chain**	▪ Supplier qualification and purchase; ▪ Warehousing of starting & packaging materials; ▪ Weighing of starting materials; ▪ Preparation of packaging materials; ▪ Production; ▪ Process validation; ▪ Cleaning validation; ▪ Warehousing of intermediate, bulk & finished products; ▪ Shipping & distribution of finished products ▪ Outsourcing (vendor/contractor management)
(3) **Personnel**	▪ Organization; ▪ Management; ▪ Training.
(4) **Premises, Facilities & Equipment**	▪ Area classification; ▪ Management; ▪ Qualification; ▪ Maintenance; ▪ Calibration.
(5) **Quality control** (QC)	▪ Sampling; ▪ Testing; ▪ Environmental monitoring; ▪ Water, steam and compressed air monitoring; ▪ Approval/rejection; ▪ Cross-contamination & mix-up control; ▪ Retain & reference samples; ▪ Stability management; ▪ Pharmacovigilance.
(6) **HSE** (hygiene, security, environment)	▪ Hazard detection and security measures ▪ Waste and effluent disposal ▪ Outdated product disposal ▪ Vermin control

(1) Quality Assurance (QA)

Organization of the PQS

- There is a Quality Manual approved by the Senior Direction;
- There is a Declaration of the quality policy of the company approved by the Senior Direction;
- There is a Manual of Processes;
- There is a Site Master File;
- There is a procedure detailing how documentation should be managed. There is a list of existing procedures.

Administration of the PQS

- There is a Corrective Action/Preventive Action (CAPA) system in place;
- There is a Change management system in place;
- There is a Process Performance and Product Quality Monitoring system in place;
- There is a procedure describing how Management reviews have to be planned. Management reviews are realized;
- There is a procedure describing how Product Quality Reviews have to be performed. Product Quality Reviews are realized;
- There is a procedure describing how Audits have to be planned. There is an annual plan regarding internal audits and it is implemented. There are corrective/preventive plans for the deviations detected during the audits and the corresponding follow-up;
- There is a procedure describing the approach on Risk management and it is implemented;
- There is a procedure describing the approach on Knowledge management and it is implemented;

- There are procedures describing how quality issues (incidents, deviations, out-of-specifications, out-of-trends, complaints, recalls, returns, out-of-temperature excursions, counterfeiting) have to be handled and they are implemented;

- Procedures are available to the personnel where they are needed. All procedures are within their period of validity. There are no unidentified supplementary documents besides the procedures of the PQS in the premises;

- Entries of data in records are made at the time each action is performed. Alterations or corrections are dated and signed and allow to read the original information. There are no blank spaces left (lines are drawn or "n. a." is written).

Batch Certification

- Batch Manufacturing records are revised. A check-list is very useful to ensure that nothing is forgotten;

- Batches of finished product are released after certification by the Qualified Person.

(2) Supply Chain

Supplier Qualification and Purchase

- There is a procedure on assessment of suppliers and their classification according to auditing, experience and confidence level;

- Suppliers are audited and approved. There is a list of approved suppliers;

- There is a procedure describing how purchases are made.

Warehousing of Starting & Packaging Materials

- There is a procedure on reception, identification, cleaning (if necessary), labeling and quarantine of materials;

- There is a procedure on internal lot numbering of materials;

- There is a procedure on storage (organization and temperature control) of materials;
- There is a procedure on weighing of starting materials;
- There is a procedure on inventory of materials;
- There is a procedure on handling of outdated materials;
- There is a procedure on handling of spillages;
- The receiving and dispatch bays are separated;
- The receiving and dispatch bays act as airlocks for the storage areas;
- The receiving and dispatch bays shelter materials and products from the weather;
- The receiving bays are prepared to clean the containers of incoming materials before storage, if this is necessary;
- There is adequate segregation for rejected materials and it is ensured that they cannot be used by mistake;
- There is adequate control of stocks (FEFO). There is assurance that only approved and within their shelf-life lots will be used;
- Appropriate temperature conditions are maintained in the storage areas (thermal mapping to detect worst-case points, temperature probes and data recording) both for materials kept at room temperature and for materials requiring particular temperatures (freezer, refrigerator). There is an effective alarm system and there is a procedure describing how to handle excursions of temperature;
- There are specialized areas for inflammables, pressurized gases, highly active substances, hazardous materials and for substances subjected to particular regulations. Materials are safely stored in these areas;
- There is a closed area for the storage of printed packaging materials;
- There is a separated area for the sampling of packaging materials;

- There is a separated area for the sampling of starting materials where they are protected from cross-contamination and mix-up;
- Outdated materials are separated and stored in an specific area to be disposed of, so that there is no risk of mistake;
- Storage areas are clean and orderly;
- Materials are stored on pallets to avoid contacting the floor and adequately spaced to allow cleaning and checking;
- Pallets are clean and in good state of repair;
- Containers of materials bear adequate information (either on the label or by a computerized system): name, code reference, supplier batch number, internal batch number (if it exists), status (released, quarantine, rejected) and expiry/retest date;
- Access to warehouse is controlled and limited to authorized personnel.

Weighing of Starting Materials

- There is a procedure on weighing. The handling of rests of batches is described in it;
- There is a separated area for the weighing of starting materials where they are protected from cross-contamination and mix-up;
- Before starting the operations it is verified that the working area is free from any element of a preceding batch;
- The adequate operation of the weighing booth is verified. There is an alarm to signal malfunction;
- Weighing reports are printed and verified;
- Weighed materials are adequately protected (in bags, drums, *etc.*) and labeled;
- Weighed materials are transferred to production on pallets adequate for clean areas (non shedding particles: aluminum, stainless steel, polymeric) grouped by batches and clearly identified.

Preparation of Packaging Materials

- There is a procedure on preparation of packaging materials;

Production

- Each product has the necessary documentation (specifications, master formulae, processing and packaging instructions, batch master records);
- There are procedures describing how to assemble, use and clean each item of equipment;
- There are procedures describing how to perform operations and they are available for the operators;
- There is a procedure on batch numbering;
- There is a procedure indicating how to act in case of incident or deviation and personnel have been trained;
- There is a procedure on handling of spillages;
- There is a procedure describing how and where to use gloves, masks and other personal protection equipment (PPE). Personnel know and follow these instructions;
- Rooms and equipment have associated log-books and they are filled in;
- Rooms and equipment are identified (code number/name) and adequately labeled (status, product, batch). The status of pieces/utensils is identified. Clean items are protected from dust (plastic bag/film) and labeled as such;
- Critical environmental parameters (ΔP, T, RH) are monitored and recorded;
- Are there light-sensitive materials? Are they adequately protected?
- Rooms are clean and orderly;
- Personnel wear adequate and clean clothing appropriate for each clean area level;
- Intermediate and bulk products are adequately stored (protected in their containers, labeled and kept at the right temperature range);

- Before starting the operations it is verified that the working area is free from any element of a preceding batch;
- Access to the production areas is controlled and limited to authorized personnel;
- There is an adequate control on labels and packaging materials (reconciliation);
- Yields are controlled;
- The quality of the water used for production is adequate for the products which are prepared;
- Service pallets in the production areas (and particularly in the packaging areas) are orderly placed (spaces marked on the floor/labels on the wall or partition indicating which pallets can be placed there);
- Waste bins are adequately identified, placed and used;
- Packaging lines are sufficiently separated for ensuring that there is no risk of cross-contamination;
- Samples taken from the production equipment/line are not sent back to it;
- In the areas where utensils/equipment are washed there is clear identification and separation between items to be cleaned and items already clean;
- There are no unidentified containers or flasks in the premises;
- There are no pipes or other items left with water or other liquids inside after finishing the operations of the working shift;
- There are no unidentified/left over items in the lockers or drawers.

Process Validation

- There is a Validation Master Plan (VMP);
- Production processes are controlled by critical variables;

- The quality product profile is defined for each product;
- Critical variables for starting and packaging materials and for intermediates and products are defined and their proven acceptable ranges determined;
- Process parameters and their acceptable proven ranges are established;
- Production processes are validated taking into account the above mentioned variables. Firstly by verifying with three batches that by controlling these variables the process can be adequately controlled (prospective validation) and secondly by monitoring these variables for each manufactured batch (concurrent validation).

Cleaning Validation

- There are cleaning procedures for equipment and tools coming in contact with materials and products;
- These cleaning procedures have been validated to discard any risk of cross-contamination;
- Cleaning validation also determines the expiry date of cleaning and the maximum acceptable period between equipment utilization and cleaning;
- In case of campaign working the number of consecutive lots that can be produced without cleaning is validated;
- New equipment is analyzed to determine if further validation is necessary;
- The effectiveness of cleaning is periodically assessed and if necessary revalidation is performed.

Warehousing of Products

- There is a procedure on storage (organization and temperature control);
- There is a procedure on inventory of products;

- There is a procedure on handling of outdated products;
- There is an adequate control of stocks (FEFO);
- Appropriate temperature conditions are maintained in the storage areas (thermal mapping to detect worst-case points, temperature probes and data recording) both for products kept at room temperature and for products requiring particular temperatures (freezer, refrigerator). There is an effective alarm system and there is a procedure describing how to handle excursions of temperature;
- Products are adequately labeled: name, presentation, code reference, batch number, expiry date;
- There is an area for rejected products and it is ensured that they cannot be shipped by mistake;
- There are areas for returned and recalled products and it is ensured that they cannot be shipped by mistake;
- There is an area for products subjected to particular regulations and they are safely stored in these areas;
- Outdated products are separated and stored in an specific area to be disposed of, so that there is no risk of mistake;
- Storage areas are clean and orderly;
- Products are stored on pallets to avoid contacting the floor and adequately spaced to allow cleaning and checking;
- Pallets are clean and in good state of repair;
- Access to warehouse is controlled and limited to authorized personnel.

Dispatch and Distribution of Finished Products

- There are procedures describing how products are to be selected and prepared for shipping;
- It is ensured that only approved and within their shelf-life batches are shipped. However, batches which expiry date is so close that it is

unlikely that they will reach the consumer before expiration are not dispatched;

- There is a procedure on transportation (conditions, cold chain management, vehicles);
- There is an adequate area for the preparation of products to be shipped;
- Shipped products are adequately protected and labeled;
- There is adequate traceability on shipments for ensuring that in case of recall the destination of all the units of a batch of product is known and only approved distributors can receive products.

Outsourcing (Vendor/Contractor Management)

- There is a procedure on vendor/contractor management, indicating that a contract describing in detail the responsibilities of the intervening parts will be signed;
- There are contracts in force for the outsourced operations and the respective responsibilities are fulfilled.

(3) Personnel

Organization

- There is an organizational chart;
- The responsibilities of key persons are described and meet GMP requirements;
- There are CVs and job descriptions.

Management

- There are procedures describing the qualification and employment policy;
- Personnel knowledge and competence is adequately managed (training matrix). Only trained personnel can perform operations;

- Substituting personnel in case of absence (illness, vacation, *etc.*) has the necessary qualification, experience and training for the work they perform.

Training

- New employees receive general reception training;
- All employees receive specialized training related to their post;
- There is a training program, which is implemented and there are records;
- Personnel is trained on the procedures and other relevant documents;
- Training is assessed.

Behavior

- Personnel neither smoke, eat, drink or chew in the QC laboratory nor in the storage and production areas;
- Personal medicines, smoking material, plants, food and drinks are not allowed in the QC laboratory and in the storage and production areas;
- Personnel do not wear jewels or wrist-watches in the clean areas. They neither use cosmetics shedding particles in these areas.

(4) Premises, Facilities & Equipment

Organization

- There are updated plans of the premises and facilities;
- Personnel, materials, product and waste flows are adequate;
- Production areas are classified according to the operations which are carried out in them;
- Clean rooms possess the necessary measuring elements for controlling their environmental parameters (pressure, temperature, humidity);

- There are adequate changing rooms for each clean area grades (D, C and A/B).
- Outdoor clothing is not brought into changing rooms leading to grade C and B clean rooms. Changing rooms giving access to grade D clean areas are provided with lockers to leave personal outdoor clothes;
- Changing rooms are provided with instructions reminding people that they have to wash (and disinfect, as necessary) hands before donning clothes. There are instructions about clothing and a mirror to verify the adequate donning of clothing. The part of a changing room near to the entrance is where are located the washbasins;
- Both changing room and airlock doors are interlocked and cannot be opened simultaneously;
- Canteens and relaxing rooms for personnel are separated from the production and QC areas. Toilets are not connected directly with production, storage or QC areas;
- Maintenance workshops are separated from production or QC areas to avoid any risk of contamination. Parts and tools stored in the production areas are kept in rooms or lockers kept for that particular purpose;
- Pressure gauges (indicating the ΔP of rooms and HEPA filters) bear a label showing their acceptable ranges;
- Thermometers and hygrometers (as necessary) bear a label showing their acceptable ranges.

Qualification

- There is a Qualification Master Plan;
- Clean areas are periodically requalified;
- Utility systems are qualified;
- Equipment is qualified;

- Critical utility systems and equipment are periodically requalified.

Maintenance

- There are procedures on maintenance of premises, utility systems and equipment. They take into account the conditions to be fulfilled by equipment before being restarted after maintenance (cleaning, sanitization, authorization);
- There is a maintenance plan and it is implemented.

Calibration/Verification

- There is a procedure on calibration management;
- There is a list of critical instrumentation to be calibrated periodically;
- There is a calibration plan and it is implemented. Instruments bear the calibration labels;
- Weighing equipment is frequently checked for leveling and tested with standard weights;
- There is a procedure describing how to take action when an instrument is discovered to be out of calibration.

Computerized Systems

- There is a procedure for ensuring restricted and personalized access to these systems;
- There is a procedure describing how to act in case of breakdown of these systems;
- There is a procedure on data back-up;
- Access passcodes are adequately managed;
- Back-up is regularly realized and the effectiveness of data recovery is verified;
- When modifications of data are made the author, the data and the previously existing data are recorded (audit trail).

(5) Quality Control (QC)

Sampling

- There are procedures indicating how to sample starting materials, packaging materials, intermediates, bulk products and finished products;
- There are people trained for sampling;
- There is a procedure indicating how samples should be received, recorded (log-book), stored and assigned for testing;
- There is a place for the appropriate reception and storage of samples in the laboratory (pending testing).

Testing

- There are specifications for starting materials, packaging materials, intermediates, bulk products and finished products;
- There are procedures regarding the utilization of instrumentation and equipment;
- Analytical equipment is qualified;
- Analytical equipment is maintained and calibrated;
- Pieces of analytical equipment have their associated log-books and operations are adequately recorded;
- There are procedures describing how to perform testing and associated operations;
- There is a procedure on handling of spillages;
- Analytical methods are validated;
- There are procedures describing the handling of reagents, solutions and reference standards;
- Reagents, solutions and standards are adequately stored (label identifies the substance, the date of reception, the expiry date and the storage conditions);

- Adequate handling procedures and safe storage is provided for flammable, explosive, toxic, irritant, *etc.* substances;
- Reagents and solutions for use are adequately labeled (signatures of the persons who prepared them, dates of preparation, expiry dates, specific storage conditions, standardization factors);
- Raw data are recorded and maintained (laboratory workbooks ensure full traceability and indelibility of data);
- Calculations are critically examined;
- There is a procedure on handling of out-of-specifications;
- The accuracy of volumetric glassware is ensured;
- The adequacy of the cleaning procedures for glassware is verified;
- Analytical scales are checked for leveling and tested with standard weights before being used for critical weighing;
- There is a procedure on reanalysis of materials as necessary;
- In the washing rooms for utensils, glassware and equipment there is clear identification and separation between dirty items and items already clean;
- There are no unidentified containers or flasks;
- There are no pipes or other items left with water or other liquids inside after finishing the operations of the working shift;
- There are no unidentified/left over items in the lockers or drawers;
- The microbiological laboratory is separated and has an adequate particulate environmental classification;
- There is an adequate air supply to the physico-chemical areas to hinder contamination. Operations liberating fumes are performed within safety hoods ensuring adequate exhaust;

- There is adequate separation of operations in the laboratory for ensuring that there is neither mix-up nor cross-contamination;
- Access to the laboratories is controlled and restricted to authorized personnel;
- There are separated laboratories devoted to the control of biologicals and radioisotopes;
- Waste is adequately collected;
- Sensitive instruments are adequately protected from inadequate conditions such as humidity, vibration, electrical interference, *etc.*

Environmental Monitoring

- Airborne contamination of clean areas of grade A is permanently monitored during operations;
- Clean areas are monitored during operations as recommended by GMP (plates, active sampling);
- Monitoring results are analyzed for verifying that they meet requirements but also to detect negative trends;
- In case of deviation appropriate measures are foreseen and implemented.

Water, Steam and Compressed Air Monitoring

- There is supply of potable water. There is a sampling and testing program. Testing shows the adequacy of the supply;
- Water for pharmaceutical use is produced. There is a sampling and testing program which shows that the supply of pharmaceutical water is adequate;
- There is production of pharmaceutical steam. There is a sampling and testing program. Testing shows the adequacy of the pharmaceutical steam;

- There is production of pharmaceutical compressed air. There is a sampling and testing program. Testing shows the adequacy of the supply of pharmaceutical compressed air.

Cross-Contamination & Mix-Up Control

- There is a procedure describing how cross-contamination and mix-up are controlled;
- There is permanent monitoring to keep low risk of cross-contamination and mix-up.

Retain & Reference Samples

- There is a log-book recording sample movement (in or out from the room);
- There is a procedure describing how retain and reference samples are taken, maintained for the prescribed time and finally discarded;
- Retain and reference samples are kept in adequate environmental conditions in a room with controlled access.

Stability Management

- There is a procedure describing the ongoing product stability program;
- Samples of product are kept for study in the ongoing stability program and data are controlled;
- There is a log-book recording samples in and out from the program.

Pharmacovigilance

- There is a procedure on pharmacovigilance;
- Reports on product reactions are studied and communicated as necessary.

(6) HSE (Hygiene, Security and Environment)

- There is a study of potential hazards to personnel (*e.g.* fire, earthquake, flood, electrocution, crushing, contusion, fall, *etc.*). The corresponding preventive measures are implemented. There are MSDS (Material Safety Data Sheets);

- The disposal of waste and effluent is safely organized and performed;
- The disposal of outdated product is safely realized;
- There is a program for the control of vermin. Baits and traps are identified, placed and maintained. There are diagrams of the plant showing the position of these baits and traps in the plant;
- The QC laboratory has adequate protective measures (showers, eye-washers, safety goggles).

GOOD DISTRIBUTION PRACTICES

As discussed previously, the aim of pharmaceutical industry is providing the patients with suitable drug products. On the one hand this means that these products have to be well designed (and this is the object of the two first stages of life cycle: development and technological transfer) and supervised by the competent authorities. On the other this quality designed product has to be commercially manufactured and delivered to the patients. This means reproducing faithfully and safely the approved product and distributing it or, put in other words, ensuring a reliable supply-chain management. In previous chapters we have basically considered the first part of this chain which starts with the purchase of starting and packaging materials and finishes with the storage of the finished pharmaceutical products in the warehouse of the manufacturing plant. Even if these products have been produced accordingly to GMP and within a well designed and managed quality system, they still have to reach the patients who need them. This second part of the supply chain is called "distribution" and is defined as *the procuring, purchasing, holding, storing, selling, supplying, importing, exporting, or movement of pharmaceutical products, with the exception of the dispensing or providing pharmaceutical products directly to a patient or his or her agent* [1].

In practice, however, for a pharmaceutical manufacturer distribution is the division and conveyance of drug products from its premises, or from another point (*e.g.* a logistic distribution center), to the end user, through one or more intermediates (storage/health establishments) by means of various transport methods.

Thus, following the GMP model, "good distribution practices for pharmaceutical products" (GDPs) have been developed. GDPs can be defined as *that part of quality assurance which ensures that the quality of medicinal products is maintained throughout all stages of the supply chain from the site of manufacturer to the pharmacy or person authorized or entitled to supply medicinal products to the public* [2].

Their aim is ensuring that medicinal products while being shipped and carried to their final users are adequately protected and thus their quality is maintained. Putting it in other words, GDPs make sure that patients receive pharmaceuticals possessing exactly the same level of quality that they had when they had been dispatched by the manufacturing laboratory, even if in the meantime different actors in different places have intervened [3].

As GDPs closely follow the GMP pattern it is not necessary to repeat what has already been said, but just comment on some points which are not dealt in GMP (*e.g.* vehicles or shipment containers). In fact what GDPs intend is "extending" GMP from the warehouse of the pharmaceutical plant to the patients themselves. Let us then consider the different aspects covered by GDPs

Organization and Management

Authorization: All actors taking part in the distribution of pharmaceutical products should have been authorized by the relevant authorities.

Quality system: Products have to be at all times managed under a quality system which states how things should be done, by whom and under which supervision. Each distribution point should have a designated person with the authority and responsibility to ensure the implementation and maintenance of the system.

Quality management: There should be adequate documents describing how operations have to be performed. Products should be handled as stated in the procedures. Operations should be registered to ensure traceability and monitored to ensure that they are done as intended. Any discrepancy in stock, deviation or OOS should be handled within the CAPA system (investigated and the necessary corrective/preventive actions implemented). Computerized systems should meet the requirements already described in previous chapters.

Procedures defining how products are obtained and released are implemented. They should ensure that only authorized entities can participate.

A procedure should exist describing how to act in case of non compliance of the transport conditions (*e.g.* temperature).

Personnel

Only trained personnel, receiving adequate initial and continued training, should participate in the distribution operations. Everybody should know their duties and responsibilities. Operators should wear adequate clothing for the activities they perform.

Premises

They should comply with GMP principles. Their design should be adequate to protect products from contamination. Operations should be organized as to diminish the risk of cross-contamination and mix-up.

Procedures should exist describing how to perform cleaning, prevent dust and control insects and pests.

Storage Conditions

The storage conditions of the products should be in compliance with the indications written on their labels (see chapter 1).

Procedures should specify how the thermal mapping of the storage areas should be realized, which the acceptance criteria are, how temperature will be controlled and which actions will be taken in case of non compliance. There should be preferably automatic continuous temperature monitoring, but when this is not possible temperatures should be frequently registered by independent personnel to provide faithful information on the evolution of temperature in the warehouse. Excursions from the established ranges should sound an alarm. See Table **2**.

Table 2. Storage conditions.

Topic	Requirement
Temperature mapping	Performed initially and then repeated periodically (2-3 years).
Temperature uniformity	There should not be significant differences within the premises.
Measure points	According to worst case (as shown by mapping).
Alarm	It should sound in case of excursions from the established temperature range (in the warehouse, in the cold chambers/refrigerators and in the freezers). Alarms should be periodically verified (at least yearly).

Table 2: contd...

Thermometers and hygrometers	Calibrated yearly.
Data	Registered, checked (at least monthly by independent personnel) and filed.

Vehicles and Equipment/Transportation

Vehicles should offer to the products the same conditions than storage areas in terms of temperature control, identification and safety. These topics should be validated and monitored (Table **3**).

Table 3. Validation/Monitoring of transportation.

Topic	Requirement
Temperature control	▪ Maintenance of the required conditions within the specified range during transport. ▪ There should be monitoring instrumentation. At least a high and low temperature thermometer strategically located. Thermometers should possess a battery system for 48 hours in case of electricity failure. Instrumentation should be calibrated. ▪ Establish loading patterns in order to ensure temperature uniformity. Include temperature probes within the load.
Temperature alarm	▪ Refrigerators and freezers provided with alarms. ▪ Temperature alarm displayed in the driver's cabin. ▪ Qualification of the disaster conditions (recovery time).
Vehicles	▪ Approved procedures for cleaning and controlling vermin. ▪ It is preferably to use dedicated vehicles, but if this is not possible it is necessary to ensure adequate cleaning. ▪ They should be qualified like small warehouses.
Transportation practices	▪ They should be periodically assessed. ▪ There should be a procedure describing the loading revision on arrival (checklist). ▪ Quick storage of products after reception. ▪ Delivery schedules and transport logistics should be planned for ensuring that products will be at any time under adequate conditions.
Safety	▪ Use of batch tracking systems during distribution. ▪ Restrict the need for intervention on equipment.

Their design and use should minimize the risk of contamination, mix-up and deterioration of the products. They should be clean and free of vermin at all times. It is preferable to use dedicated vehicles, but when this is not feasible there should be adequate procedures describing how to ensure that they are not going to put products at risk. Procedures should explain how to perform cleaning, prevent dust and control insects and pests.

As indicated by GMP, defective vehicles and equipment should be labeled as such and removed from service.

During transportation storage conditions should be monitored, adequate product segregation should be maintained and unauthorized access prevented. Any relevant deviation or incident should be communicated.

The storage and transport of dependence-producing products should be safe. Procedures should describe how to ensure the monitoring of temperature, taking into account the seasonal variations. Changes in packing should be documented.

There should be procedures describing how to act in case of damaged/broken containers.

Stock Management and Inventory

There should be procedures indicating how to manage product stocks (usually by means of computerized systems).

A system should be in place to ensure that the pharmaceutical products due to expire first are sold and/or distributed first (FEFO). Exceptions may be permitted as appropriate, provided that adequate controls are in place to prevent the distribution of expired products.

FEFO (first expiry/first out) is defined as a distribution procedure that ensures that the stock with the earliest expiry date is distributed and/or used before an identical stock item with a later expiry date is distributed and/or used.

The "expiry date" is the date given on the individual container (usually on the label) of a pharmaceutical product up to and including the date on which the product is expected to remain within specifications, if stored correctly. It is established for each batch by adding the shelf-life to the date of manufacture [4].

Shipment/Dispatch

Containers used for transportation of pharmaceuticals should keep them adequately protected and should bear labels with information on the product and on the handling and storage conditions. The aim is providing unequivocal product identification and information on how it has to be stored and if particular handling precautions are necessary. The name and the address of the manufacturer should also appear on the label if the container is transferred to another entity outside from the manufacturer's quality system.

When using dry ice to keep products refrigerated it should not come into contact with them. Products should only be supplied to authorized persons or entities (supplier should posses written proof that they are duly authorized), which possess adequate storage and transport conditions. There should be adequate procedures describing how products should be dispatched.

Records for the dispatch of pharmaceutical products should be prepared and should include at least the following information:

- *date of dispatch;*
- *complete business name and address (no acronyms), type of entity responsible for the transportation, telephone number and names of contact persons;*
- *complete business name, address (no acronyms), and status of the addressee (e.g. retail pharmacy, hospital or community clinic);*
- *a description of the products including, e.g. name, dosage form and strength (if applicable);*
- *quantity of the products, i.e. number of containers and quantity per container (if applicable);*
- *applicable transport and storage conditions;*
- *a unique number to allow identification of the delivery order;*

  and
- *assigned batch number and expiry date (where not possible at dispatch, this information should at least be kept at receipt to facilitate traceability) [5].*

There should be enough information for ensuring that in case of need the recall of a batch would be effectively performed.

Products should neither be supplied nor received when they are outdated or the expiry date is so near that patients will not be able to use it within its shelf life.

Procedures should specify which packaging will be used.

Repackaging/Relabeling

This activity is equivalent to the operations related to secondary packaging during manufacturing and as such it has to meet GMP and be authorized by the relevant authorities.

Complaints/Recalls/Rejected and Returned Products

All this cases have to be handled as described by GMP. There should be a procedure describing how to act in case of complaint. Transportation of recalled, rejected and returned products has to ensure that they are kept identified and segregated as such at all times.

Counterfeiting/Theft

Any counterfeit product or suspected of being such has to be immediately identified and segregated. Authorities should be informed.

A counterfeit pharmaceutical product is a *pharmaceutical product which is deliberately and fraudulently mislabeled with respect to identity and/or source. Counterfeiting can apply to both branded and generic products, and counterfeit pharmaceutical products may include products with the correct ingredients, with the wrong ingredients, without active ingredients, with an incorrect quantity of active ingredient or with fake packaging* [6].

Although the risk of theft of products exists at all times, even in the manufacturing laboratories, it increases during their distribution and this is why control on transportation is critical.

Contract Activities

A written contract should specify how these activities will be performed (see chapter 1). This contract should ensure the following points:

- Quality assurance terms.
- Supply terms.
- Documentation for the different parts (manufacturer, transporter, distributor, importer, *etc.*) establishing the mutual responsibilities, the registers and the filling terms.

- Conditions required for outsourcing.

Self-Inspection

As storage, distribution and transportation can affect the quality of a product all the elements described in GDPs should also be included in the self-inspection programs.

Spoiled Products

Products that are damaged or broken should be withdrawn and stored independently while it is decided how they are going to be handled.

GOOD LABORATORY PRACTICE

Good Laboratory Practice can be defined *as a quality system concerned with the organizational process and the conditions under which non-clinical health and environmental safety studies are planned, performed, monitored, recorded, archived and reported* [7].

Pharmacological studies on toxicology and safety are required to comply with GLP. Studies on pharmacokinetics and bioavailability can also be included in this requirement [8].

As it was discussed in chapter 11, the development of a new product involves periods, which are not covered by GMP requirements (they are however within the PQS of the company):

Stage 1 (Discovery): For the moment being there is not a regulatory standard dealing with the discovery of potential new drugs.

Stage 2 (Non-clinical): Good laboratory practice (GLP) is specifically devoted to this second stage, when studies are not performed in humans and their main purpose is safety testing (Fig. **1**).

Stage 3 (Clinical): Safety studies are followed by clinical studies in humans. Here, "Good Clinical Practice" (GCP) is the basis for quality standards, ethical conduct and regulatory compliance [9-11]. All clinical trials of phase I (for showing tolerance of the test drug and for determining human pharmacokinetics), phase II (for confirming the dose-effect relationship) and phase III (for showing clinical efficacy; they are carried out on hundreds of patients and often in several centers) should meet GCP.

Stage 4 (Post-approval): In this last stage the pharmaceutical product has already been registered and is available on the market. The use of the drug after marketing is monitored through formalized pharmacovigilance procedures. Any additional clinical trial (Phase IV) should also comply with GCP.

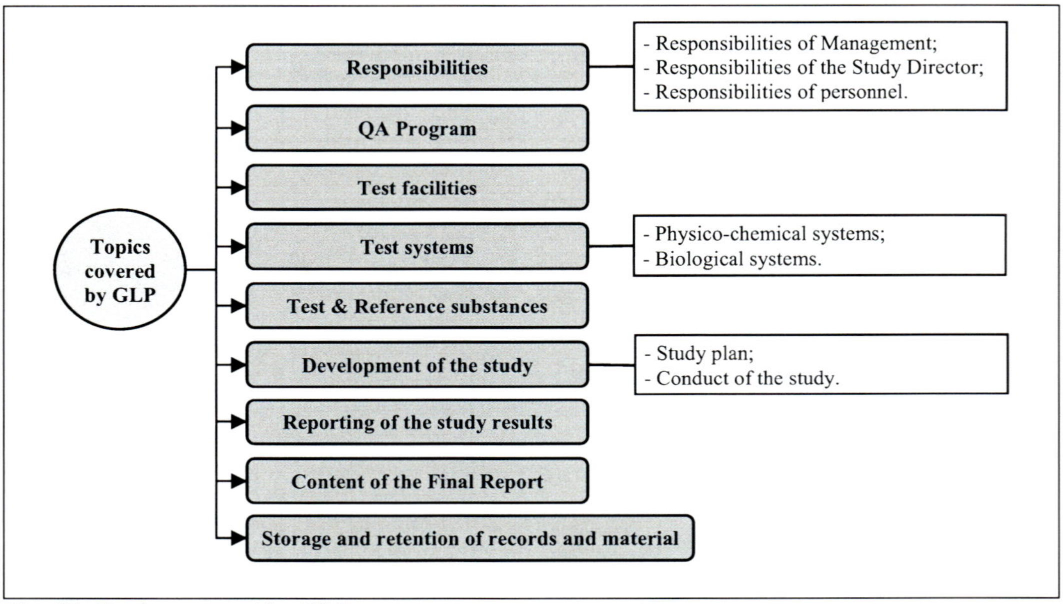

Fig. (1). Topics covered by GLP.

Responsibilities

Responsibilities of Management

They correspond basically to those described in GMP.

Management should ensure the availability of :

- Adequate and sufficient facilities, equipment, material and qualified personnel;
- Updated professional CVs showing qualification, experience and training of personnel;
- Job descriptions;

- A HSE (health, security and environment) program;
- A quality assurance program with the appropriate procedures (SOPs);
- Written study plans;
- A documented study director for each of program.

Management should ensure that:

- Personnel understand their functions and responsibilities;
- Procedures (SOPs) are understood and applied;
- Changes to procedures (SOPs) and study plans are made within a change management system;
- Study plans are approved by the sponsor and appropriately filed;
- Procedures (SOPs) and study plans are filed to keep historical traceability;
- There is a responsible of archiving documentation.

Responsibilities of the Study Director

She/he signs and dates the final study report and ensures that:

- The study plan and the procedures (SOPs) are followed;
- All data are recorded;
- All data and documentation are kept in the archive.

Responsibilities of Personnel

Personnel should perform safe working practice and protection (HSE).

Quality Assurance

Studies should be performed in compliance with GLP principles (Fig. **2**) and within the frame of the Quality System.

- Personnel in charge of QA should not be involved with the studies. They should report any finding in writing to management and to the study director;
- Study plan and SOPs should be accessible to personnel conducting the study;
- Periodic auditing to ensure compliance (with recording) should be realized;
- Final reports should be reviewed to confirm that they explain truly what has been done;
- Final reports should comprise an account of the dates of inspections and state that any finding was reported to the study director and to management.

Test Facilities

In order to ensure the validity of the study the location, construction and size of the facilities should be appropriate. It should also provide appropriate separation of the different activities and studies, taking into account the presence of known or suspected biohazardous substances.

Test Systems

It should be ensured that they will not be deteriorated by diseases.

There should be separated adequate storage areas for equipment and supplies (including refrigeration), separated from the test system areas, and protected from infestation and contamination.

Hazardous substances should be safely stored.

The areas for reception, storage and mixing of the test substances with a vehicle should be separated in order to prevent test and reference substances from mix-up and contamination.

Sufficient space should be available for the storage and safe retrieval of samples, specimens, raw data and reports.

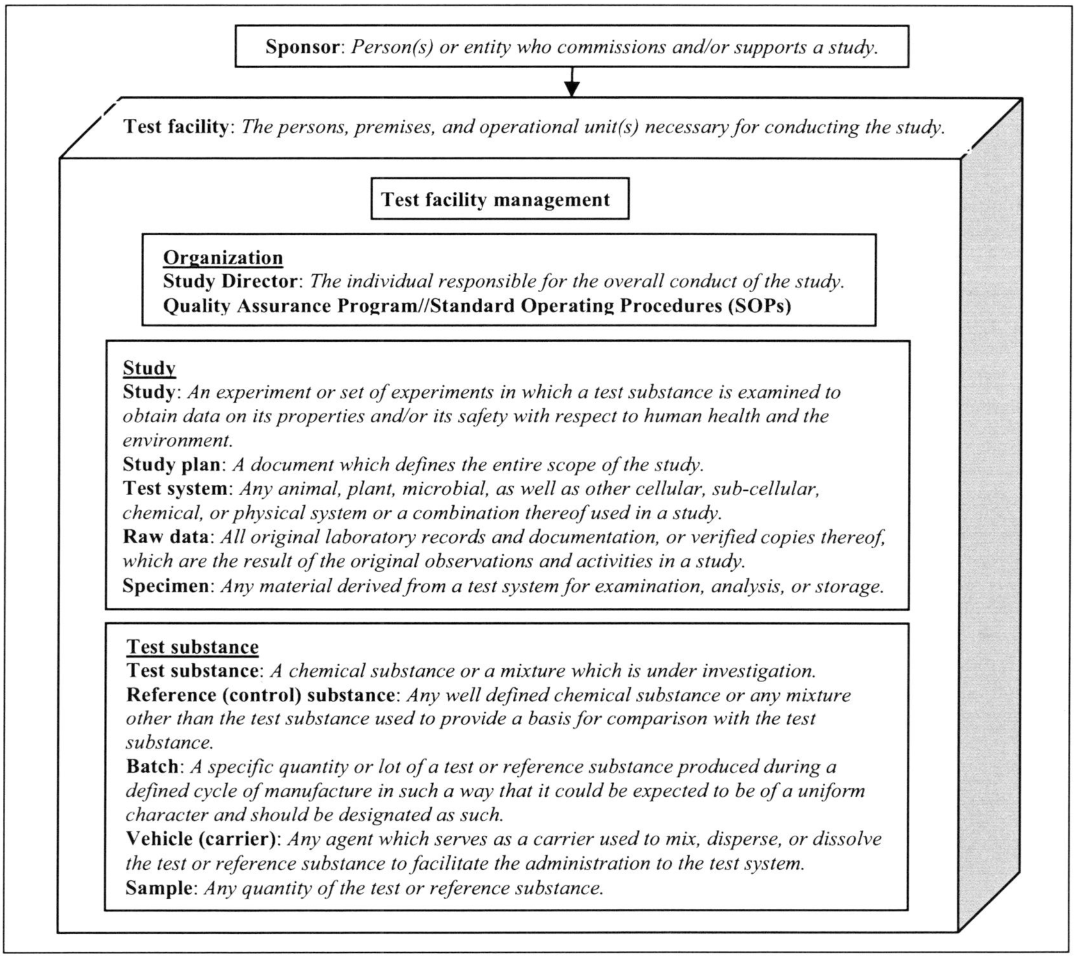

Fig. (2). GLP terms.

The safety of the studies should not be jeopardized by waste materials. These should be adequately handled and disposed of in accordance with regulatory requirements. Consequently there should be procedures and facilities for the gathering, storage, decontamination, transportation and disposal of waste materials. These activities should be recorded and records should be filed.

Physical/Chemical

Equipment should be adequately designed, placed and possess the appropriate capacity.

There should be SOPs describing how equipment has to be used, maintained and calibrated. These activities should be recorded in log-books.

Neither equipment nor materials should prevent the tests systems from working effectively. Reagents should be provided with labels containing adequate information (*i.e.* source, identity, concentration, stability, preparation date, responsible technician, expiration and specific storage instructions). The integrity of the physical/chemical test systems can be supported by using reference substances [12].

Biological

The quality of the data should be ensured by establishing and maintaining adequate conditions for the animals, plants and systems (microorganisms, cellular and sub-cellular) regarding housing, handling and care. These systems should meet applicable regulatory requirements regarding importation, collection, care and use.

Animal and plant systems upon arrival should be isolated to assess their health status. In case of abnormal morbidity or mortality, the lot should not be used in the studies and, if necessary, it should be humanely destroyed.

There should be kept records regarding the source, date of reception and condition of arrival. Before performing any study, the systems (either animal, plant, microbial or cellular) should be acclimatized during an adequate period of time to the test environment.

The housing or container of every system should be adequately identified with all necessary information. If during the study the system was diagnosed and treated of any disease this information should be recorded [13].

Test and Reference Substances

Each test and reference substance should be appropriately identified. For example: code, chemical abstract (CAS) number and name.

Records should be kept of both test and reference substances indicating:

- Substance characterization;
- Date of receipt;
- Quantity received;
- Quantity used in studies.

In order to ensure as much as possible the homogeneity and stability of these substances and to prevent mix-up and contamination there should be written procedures (SOPs) regarding their handling, sampling and storage (Fig. **3** and Table **4**).

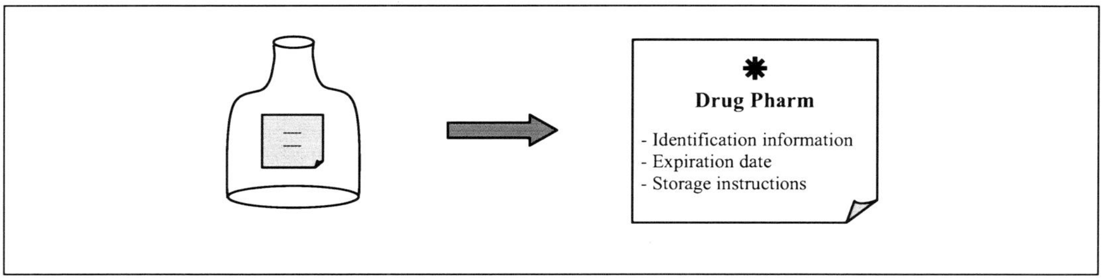

Fig. (3). Labeling on storage containers.

- Each batch of the test or reference substance used in the study should be known and identified (*i.e.* batch number, purity, composition, concentration, *etc.*).
- The stability of test and reference substances under conditions of storage should be known for all studies.
- It should also be known the stability of the test and reference substances under the test conditions.
- When a substance is administered in a vehicle there should be a procedure (SOP) describing how to test the homogeneity and stability of the substance in the vehicle.
- A sample of each batch of test substance should be retained to repeat testing, if necessary, when the substance is tested longer than four weeks during the study.

In each separated laboratory current written procedures (SOPs) should be available to personnel. Procedures may be complemented with books and articles.

Table 4. Topics that should be handled in procedures (SOPs).

Topic	Contents
Test & reference substances	Reception, identification, labeling, handling, sampling, and storage.
Equipment	Use, maintenance, cleaning, calibration of measuring instruments and environmental control equipment

Table 4: contd...

Reagents	Directions for the preparation of reagents
Record keeping, Reporting, Storage, and Retrieval	Coding of studies, data collection, preparation of reports, indexing systems, handling of data, including the use of computerized data systems.
Test system	Room preparation and environmental room conditions for the test system.
	Procedures for reception, transfer, arrangement, characterization, identification, and handling of the test system.
	Preparation, handling and examination of the test system, before, during and at termination of the study.
	Handling of test system individuals found moribund or dead during the study.
	Collection, identification and handling of specimens including necropsy and histopathology.
Quality assurance	Information on how QA personnel should perform and report audits, inspections and reviews of the final reports
Health and Safety Precautions	As required by national and/or international legislation or guidelines

Development of the Study

Study Plan

Before starting a study it is necessary to write a plan. This study plan should be considered as raw data and filed as such. Any change, modification or revision of the study plan should be documented and approved by the Study Director (*i.e.* description, justification, date and signature) and filed as previously mentioned.

The study plan should contain, at least, the information which is summarized in Table **5**.

Table 5. Content of the study plan.

	Topic	Contents
1	Identification of the study, the test and reference Substances	▪ A descriptive title; ▪ A declaration which shows the nature and reason of the study; ▪ Identification of the test substance by code or name (IUPAC; CAS number, *etc.*); ▪ Identification of the reference substance to be used.
2	Information concerning the Sponsor and the Test Facility	▪ Name and address of the Sponsor; ▪ Name and address of the Test Facility; ▪ Name and address of the Study Director.
3	Dates	▪ The date and signature of the Study Director (and when adequate, those of the sponsor and/or the test facility management) making evident the approval of the study plan; ▪ The proposed starting and conclusion dates.

Table 5: contd...

4	Test methods	▪ Reference to OECD Guideline or other test guidelines to be used.
5	Issues (where applicable)	▪ Rationale for the selection of the test system; ▪ Description of the test system (*i.e.* species, strain, sub-strain, source of supply, number, body weight range, sex, age, and other relevant information); ▪ Rationale for the selection of the method of administration; ▪ Information on the dose levels and/or concentration(s), frequency and duration of administration; ▪ Comprehensive information on the experimental design (*e.g.* description of the chronogram of the study; account of the methods and materials to be employed and of the conditions of use; explanation of the type and frequency of observation, testing, measurement and examination to be realized).
6	Records	▪ A list of the records to be retained.

Conduct of the Study

Every study should carry an identification being only one of its kind and all the items related to it should bear this identification.

The study should accurately follow the study plan.

All data generated during the study should be recorded as described by GMP (*i.e.* directly on the notebook or computer as soon as they are obtained; accurately and legibly; dated and signed by the person entering the data).

Changes in the raw data should also follow GMP requirements (*i.e.* dated and signed; the previous entry should not be obscured by the new one; if necessary the person entering the data should indicate the reason for the change).

GMP requirements should be met when entering data to a computer too (*i.e.* personal identification, data and time, reason for the change, traceability in the modifications).

Reporting of the Study Results

Once the study is finished a final report should be written. It is recommended to use the International System of Units (SI) in it.

This final report is dated and signed by the Study Director (and also by principal scientists of complementary scientific areas if they have contributed to the report with specialized information).

If it is necessary to correct or add information to the final report this should be made in the form of an amendment which should detail the reasons for the corrections or additions. The amendment should be dated and signed by the Study Director and by the principal scientists involved by the changes.

Content of the Final Report

The final report should contain, at least, the information which is summarized in Table **6**.

Table 6. Contents of the final report.

	Topic	Contents
1	Identification of the study, the test and reference substance	▪ A descriptive title; ▪ Identification of the test substance by code or name (IUPAC, CAS number, *etc.*); ▪ Identification of the reference substance by chemical name; ▪ Characterization of the test substance including purity, stability and homogeneity.
2	Information concerning the Test Facility	▪ Name and address; ▪ Name of the Study Director; ▪ Name of other principal personnel having contributed with specific parts to the final report.
3	Dates	▪ Dates on which the study was initiated and completed.
4	Statement	▪ A statement by QA certifying at which dates of the inspections were performed and at which dates any findings were reported to the Study Director and to management.
5	Description of materials and test methods	▪ Description of methods and materials used; ▪ Reference to OECD guidelines or to other test guidelines taken into account in the study
6	Results	▪ A summary of results; ▪ All information and data required in the study plan; ▪ A presentation of the results, including calculations and statistical methods; ▪ An evaluation and discussion of the results and conclusions (if appropriate).
7	Storage	▪ The location where all samples, specimens, raw data, and the final report are stored.

Storage and Retention of Records and Material

Archives should provide the safe maintenance and retrieval of all the data and samples related to the studies. See Table **7**.

Table 7. Storage and retention of records and material.

Topic		Contents
Storage and retrieval	1	Archives should provide an adequate and secure storage of: ▪ The study plans; ▪ The raw data; ▪ The final reports; ▪ The reports of laboratory inspections and study audits performed according to the Quality Assurance Program; ▪ Samples and specimens.
	2	Material retained in the archives should be indexed so as to facilitate orderly storage and rapid retrieval.
	3	Only personnel authorized by management should have access to the archives. Movement of material in and out of the archives should be appropriately recorded.
Retention	1	The following should be retained for the period specified by the appropriate authorities: ▪ The study plan, raw data, samples, specimens, and the final report of each study; ▪ Records of all inspections and audits performed by the Quality Assurance Program; ▪ Summary of qualifications, training, experience and job descriptions of personnel; ▪ Records and reports of the maintenance and calibration of equipment; ▪ The historical file of Standard Operating Procedures.
	2	Samples and specimens should be retained only as long as the quality of the preparation permits evaluation.
	3	If a test facility or an archive contracting facility goes out of business and has no legal successor, the archive should be transferred to the archives of the Sponsor(s) of the study(s).

PHARMACOVIGILANCE

Medicinal products are submitted to clinical studies for testing short-term safety and efficacy before being granted marketing permission. However, these studies are realized on a limited quantity of individuals, ranging from a few hundreds to a few thousands. Thus, after approval it is necessary to corroborate efficacy and specific safety issues in the varied real-life conditions. This monitoring process performed on approved pharmaceutical products is known as "pharmacovigilance". The aim of pharmacovigilance is to watch the behavior of pharmaceutical products on varied population groups, the efficacy and safety of their chronic use and their interactions with other medicines or foods.

Pharmacovigilance (PV) can be defined as *the science and activities relating to the detection, assessment, understanding and prevention of adverse effects or any other possible drug-related problems* [14].

In order to put pharmacovigilance into practice, and following the path of GMP, it is spoken of "Good Pharmacovigilance Practices" (GVP) that are defined *as the measures drawn up to facilitate the performance of pharmacovigilance and apply both to holders of a marketing authorization and to medicines regulatory authorities. The aim of GVP is the identification, quantification, evaluation and prevention of the risks associated to the use of pharmaceutical products after registration* [15].

Problems Posed by Medicinal Products

The problems posed by drug products can be practically summarized as follows:

- Adverse drug reaction (ADR): Any inconvenient and unplanned response to a medicinal product.

- Serious adverse drug reaction (SADR): Any harmful medical occurrence that at any dose results in death, is life-threatening, requires patient hospitalization or results in prolongation of existing hospitalization, results in persistent or significant disability/incapacity, is a congenital anomaly/birth defect, is a medically important event or reaction. Any suspicion will be considered as such and the transmission of an infective agent through a pharmaceutical too.

- Unexpected ADR: Any ADR whose nature, severity, specificity, or result is not consistent with the term or description used in the product labeling.

- Medication error: Any unintentional error in the prescription, dispensing or administration of a drug product. When it results in patient's harm it will be considered SADR, excepting if the error is the consequence of treatment omission.

- Suspected counterfeit/substandard drug: Any pharmaceutical product which is suspected of being an imitation with intent of deceiving or of being below the requested standard.

Organization of Pharmacovigilance

Information on commercialized pharmaceutical products can be very varied and come from different sources. National systems of pharmacovigilance are in charge of collecting and handling this information. They are further coordinated by international organizations (*e.g.* WHO).

A "pharmacovigilance system" can be defined as *a system used by an organization to fulfill its legal tasks and responsibilities in relation to pharmacovigilance and designed to monitor the safety of authorized medicinal products and detect any change to their risk-benefit balance* [16].

A pharmacovigilance system should have the following elements (Fig. **4**):

- A clear communication strategy, both for routine and emergency contact;
- A national database or system for collating and handling information (reports);
- A national advisory committee providing support on technical matters (evaluation of causality, risk assessment and management, case investigation and, if necessary, crisis management and communication).
- A national spontaneous reporting system with a national ADR reporting form.
- The functions of a National Pharmacovigilance Center can be summarized as follows:
- Provides support in follow-up programs;
- Identifies signals of medicine safety (*i.e.* unknown or poorly characterized adverse events in relation to a medicine or a combination of medicines and/or its use);
- Takes the responsibility of risk assessment and management;
- Identifies if there are quality problems in drug products leading to ADRs (*i.e.* supports the identification of medicine quality issues).
- Provides effective communication on aspects related to medicine safety, including removal of unfounded rumors on toxicity attributed to medicinal products and/or vaccines.
- Applies the information derived from pharmacovigilance to public health programs, to individual patients and to national policies regarding medicinal products and treatment guidelines;
- Manages information in respect of the use of drug products;

- Recognizes problems derived from unregulated prescribing and dispensing of medicinal products.

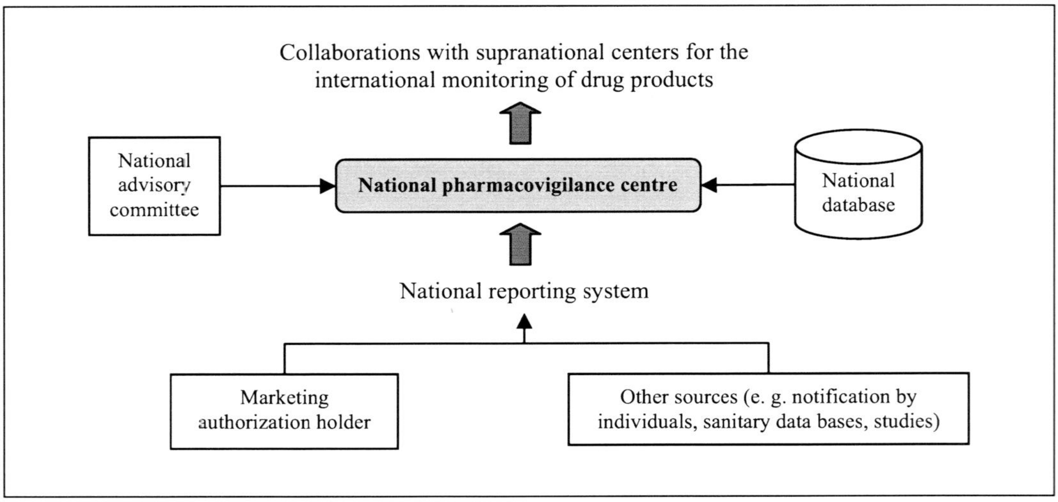

Fig. (4). National system of pharmacovigilance.

Duties of the Marketing Authorization Holders Regarding Pharmacovigilance

A marketing authorization holder (MAH) should provide safety data for the continued evaluation of the risk associated to the use of authorized medicinal products (Table **8**). This is why the MAHs have the responsibility of fulfilling all the legal requirements established for pharmacovigilance and consequently they have to establish a pharmacovigilance system for their authorized pharmaceutical products and they have to appoint in the company a responsible for pharmacovigilance. This latter person should be fully empowered in pharmacovigilance matters and keep in contact with the regulatory authorities.

Table 8. Activities of pharmacovigilance.

▪ Risks associated to the use of a medicinal: Any risk for the public health or the health of a patient regarding the quality, security or efficacy of the drug, including undesired effects on the environment.
▪ Periodical safety report: The holder gathers information on drug, including scientific evaluation of the benefit/risk balance.
▪ Post-authorization study: Clinical study or observational of a drug post-authorization.
▪ Post-authorization safety study: Study with the aim of identifying any risk, safety profile or evaluate risk management measures.
▪ Benefit-risk evaluation: Evaluation of the favorable therapeutic effects with use risks.

Table 8: contd…

▪ Risk management plan: Ensemble of activities of pharmacovigilance to determine, characterize, prevent or minimize the risks related to a pharmaceutical, including the evaluation of the effectiveness of these activities. For each identified risk it should be indicated which measures will be taken to improve the characterization of the risk and increase the level of information. It can be limited to pharmacovigilance activities or it can include other activities such as the realization of studies.   ▪ Signal (or alert): Conveyed information regarding a possible causal relation between an adverse reaction and a pharmaceutical product, when this relation was previously unknown or it was incompletely documented. Usually it is required more than a single notification to generate a signal, although it depends on the seriousness of the event and on the quality of the information.

The responsible of pharmacovigilance (RPV) fulfills the following tasks:

- Organizes the pharmacovigilance system;
- Monitors continuously pharmacovigilance data by gathering, collating and analyzing all the adverse drug reactions (ADRs) known to the company;
- Examines options for the minimization and prevention of risk,
- Reviews bibliography in search of citations of ADRs;
- For each pharmaceutical product it is kept a risk management plan;
- Provides the authorities with periodic safety update reports (PSURs), delivered within the established time-limits. She/he verifies the quality, integrity and comprehensiveness of the information regarding the risks of drug products. She/he applies processes to avoid duplicate submissions and to validate signals;
- Reviews post-authorization clinical studies regarding products for which the company holds marketing authorization;
- Commissions, when this is required, post-authorization studies on safety and/or efficacy for the products for which the company holds marketing authorization;
- Communicates with competent regulatory authorities in matters regarding pharmacovigilance (*e.g.* notifies relevant safety information, new or changed risks, risk management, risk minimization, corrective and preventive actions);
- Updates product information in the light of scientific knowledge;

- Keeps updated the pharmacovigilance system master file (PVSMF), including its human resource management;
- Performs continual benefit-risk evaluation for the products for which the company holds marketing authorization;
- Performs periodical and independent audits to verify the performance of the pharmacovigilance system.

Organization of the Pharmacovigilance System

The pharmacovigilance system should follow in its organization the same principles previously described (see chapter 5) for the pharmaceutical quality system (*i.e.* management responsibilities, provision of adequate resources, adequate training of personnel, definition of job profiles and their organizational chart, documentation, safe information archival and retrieval, *etc.*). See Table **9**.

Table 9. Summary of topics that should be dealt with by the documents of the Pharmacovigilance system.

- Activities of RPV and of her/his substitute/s. Communication o the regulatory authorities of their names.
- An organizational chart defining the hierarchical relationships of supervisory and managerial staff;
- Job descriptions which define the duties of the supervisory and managerial staff (*i.e.* assignments of tasks, responsibilities and hierarchies to the personnel directly involved in pharmacovigilance tasks);
- Compilation, coding, register, evaluation, follow-up, detection of duplicate cases and communication of adverse reactions (ADRs);
- Notification to the authorities of serious cases;
- Writing, approval and submission of periodic safety update reports (PSUR);
- Instructions on critical processes in the pharmacovigilance system master file (PVSMF);
- Management of information request to the authorities;
- Continual evaluation of the benefit-risk safety profile of the products of the company and communication of changes;
- Preparation, application and follow-up of plans of pharmacovigilance and of risk management;
- Action and follow-up for safety and modifications;
- Diffusion of technical files of authorized drugs;
- Coordination in case of safety issues;
- Pharmacovigilance data base management;
- Post-authorization studies;
- Training;
- Audits;
- Archive.

CONCLUDING REMARKS

The development and application of a Pharmaceutical Quality System ensures GMP-compliance. Thus, it is possible to manufacture quality products which were developed to possess quality by design. GDPs complete GMP for securing that the quality of the drug products is not lost during the period of time comprised between the dispatch of the laboratory warehouse and the reception by the patient. The intent of GLP is making sure the equivalence of studies realized in different laboratories. And, finally, pharmacovigilance keeps updated the information on adverse reactions after a pharmaceutical product has been marketed in order to know at any time its benefit-risk balance.

CONFLICT OF INTEREST

The author confirms that this chapter contents have no conflict of interest.

ACKNOWLEDGEMENT

Declared None.

REFERENCES

[1] WHO (World Health Organisation). WHO good distribution practices for pharmaceutical products. In: WHO Expert Committee on Specifications for Pharmaceutical Preparations. Forty-fourth report (WHO Technical Report Series, No. 957). WHO, Geneva, Switzerland, 2010. Annex 5. Glossary.

[2] European Commission. Guidelines of 5 November 2013 on Good Distribution Practice of medicinal products for human use. Information from European Union Institutions, Bodies, Offices and Agencies. Official Journal of the European Union, C 343/1, 23.11.2013.

[3] PDA (Parenteral Drug Association). Last Mile: Guidance for good distribution practices for pharmaceutical products to the end user. Technical Report No. 46. PDA, Bethesda, MD, USA, 2009

[4] WHO (World Health Organisation). WHO good distribution practices for pharmaceutical products. In: WHO Expert Committee on Specifications for Pharmaceutical Preparations. Forty-fourth report (WHO Technical Report Series, No. 957). WHO, Geneva, Switzerland, 2010. Annex 5. 3. Glossary.

[5] Ibid. 12.5.

[6] WHO (World Health Organisation). WHO good distribution practices for pharmaceutical products. In: WHO Expert Committee on Specifications for Pharmaceutical Preparations. Forty-fourth report (WHO Technical Report Series, No. 957). WHO, Geneva, Switzerland, 2010. Annex 5. 3. Glossary.

[7] OECD (Organisation for Economic Co-operation and Development). Environment Directorate. Chemicals Group and Management Committee. OECD Principles on Good Laboratory Practice (as revised in 1997). OECD series on principles of Good Laboratory Practice and compliance monitoring. No. 1. ENV/MC/CHEM(98)17. OECD, Paris, France, 1998.

[8] UNDP (United Nations Development Program)/World Bank/WHO (World Health Organisation). Handbook: Good Laboratory Practice (GLP). Quality practices for regulated non-clinical research and development. Special Programme for Research and Training in Tropical Diseases. TDR/WHO, Geneva, Switzerland, 2000.

[9] ICH (International Conference on Harmonisation of Technical Requirements for registration of Pharmaceuticals for Human Use). Guideline for Good Clinical Practice. Harmonised Tripartite Guideline. E6(R1). ICH, Geneva, Switzerland, 1996.

[10] Commission of the European Communities. Directive 2005/28/EC of 8 April 2005 laying down principles and detailed guidelines for good clinical practice as regards investigational medicinal products for human use, as well as the requirements for authorisation of the manufacturing or importation of such products. Official Journal of the European Union. L 91/13, 9.4.2005.

[11] WHO (World Health Organisation). Handbook for Good Clinical Research Practice (GCP). Guidance for implementation. WHO, Geneva, Switzerland, 2002.

[12] WHO (World Health Organisation). WHO good practices for pharmaceutical quality control laboratories. In: WHO Expert Committee on Specifications for Pharmaceutical Preparations. Forty-fourth report (WHO Technical Report Series, No. 957). WHO, Geneva, Switzerland, 2010. Annex 1.

[13] WHO (World Health Organisation). WHO good practices for pharmaceutical microbiology laboratories. In: WHO Expert Committee on Specifications for Pharmaceutical Preparations. Forty-fifth report (WHO Technical Report Series, No. 961). WHO, Geneva, Switzerland, 2011. Annex 2.

[14] WHO (World Health Organisation). Pharmacovigilance: ensuring the safe use of medicines. WHO, Geneva, Switzerland, 2004.

[15] EMA (European Medicines Agency). Guidelines on good pharmacovigilance practices (GVP). EMA/475236/2014. EMA, London, 2014.

[16] HMA (Heads of Medicine Agencies). EMA (European Medicines Agency). Guideline on good pharmacovigilance practices (GVP). Definitions. EMA/876333/2011. Revision 3. EMA, London, UK, 2011. Annex I.

Bibliography

PUBLICATIONS

[1] ANVISA (Agência Nacional de Vigilância Sanitária). Guia de qualidade para sistemas de purificação de água para uso farmacêutico. ANVISA, Brasília, Brazil, 2013.

[2] Avery R E, Keith Raney R. Rouging in stainless steel equipment for hygienic services. EJPPS, 13 (1), 2008, 21-24

[3] CEN (European Committee for Standardization). High efficiency air filters (EPA, HEPA and ULPA). Part 1: Classification, testing, marking. Standard EN 1822-1: 2009. CEN, Brussels, Belgium, 2009.

[4] CEN (European Committee for Standardization). High efficiency air filters (EPA, HEPA and ULPA). Part 2: Aerosol production, measuring equipment, particle counting statistics. Standard EN 1822-2: 2009. CEN, Brussels, Belgium, 2009.

[5] CEN (European Committee for Standardization). High efficiency air filters (EPA, HEPA and ULPA). Part 3: Testing flat sheet filter media. Standard EN 1822-3: 2009. CEN, Brussels, Belgium, 2009.

[6] CEN (European Committee for Standardization). High efficiency air filters (EPA, HEPA and ULPA). Part 4: Determining leakage of filter element (scan method). Standard EN 1822-4: 2009. CEN, Brussels, Belgium, 2009.

[7] CEN (European Committee for Standardization). High efficiency air filters (EPA, HEPA and ULPA). Part 5: Determining the efficiency of filter elements. Standard EN 1822-5: 2009. CEN, Brussels, Belgium, 2009.

[8] Clontz L, Wagner C. (editors). Biofilm control in drug manufacturing. PDA, Bethesda, MD, USA, 2012,

[9] Commission of the European Communities. Directive 2005/28/EC of 8 April 2005 laying down principles and detailed guidelines for good clinical practice as regards investigational medicinal products for human use, as well as the requirements for authorisation of the manufacturing or importation of such products. Official Journal of the European Union, L 91/13, 9.4.2005.

[10] Commission of the European Communities. Guidelines on Pharmacovigilance for Medicinal Products for veterinary Use. The Rules Governing Medicinal Products in the European Union. Volume 9B.

[11] Deeks T, Ginsbury K, Schniepp S. Pharmaceutical outsourcing: quality management and project delivery. PDA Bethesda, MD, USA 2013.

[12] Department of Health and Human Services. U.S Food and Drug Administration. Pharmaceutical cGMPs for the 21st Century: A Risk-Based Approach. Final Report. FDA, Rockville, MD, USA, 2004.

[13] Department of Health and Human Services. U.S. Food and Drug Risk-Based Method for Prioritizing CGMP Inspections of Pharmaceutical Manufacturing Sites – A Pilot Risk Ranking Model. FDA, Rockville, MD, USA, 2004.

[14] EMA (European Medicines Agency). CHMP (Committee for Medicinal Products for Human Use), CVMP (Committee for Medicinal Products for Veterinary Use). Guideline on setting health based exposure limits for use in risk identification in the manufacture of different medicinal products in shared facilities. EMA/CHMP/ CVMP/ SWP/169430/2012. EMA, London, 2014.

[15] EMA (European Medicines Agency). Guidelines on good pharmacovigilance practices (GVP). EMA/475236/2014. EMA, London, 2014.

[16] EMA (European Medicines Agency). CPMP (Committee for Proprietary Medicinal Products). CVMP (Committee for Veterinary Medicinal Products). Note for guidance on quality of water for pharmaceutical use. CPMP/QWP/158/01 Revision. EMEA/CVMP/115/01 Revision. EMA, London, UK, 2002.

[17] European Commission. Directorate General for Health and Food Safety. Qualification and Validation. In: EudraLex. The Rules Governing Medicinal Products in the European Union. Volume 4. EU Guidelines to Good Manufacturing Practice for Medicinal Products for Human and Veterinary Use. European Commission, Brussels, Belgium, 2015. Annex 15.

Jordi Botet

[18] European Commission. Health and Consumers Directorate General. Certification by a Qualified Person and Batch Release. In: EudraLex. The Rules Governing Medicinal Products in the European Union. Volume 4. Good Manufacturing Practice. Medicinal Products for Human and Veterinary Use. European Commission. Brussels, Belgium, 2015. Annex 16.
[19] European Commission. Guidelines of 5 November 2013 on Good Distribution Practice of medicinal products for human use. Information from European Union Institutions, Bodies, Offices and Agencies. Official Journal of the European Union, C 343/1, 23.11.2013.
[20] European Commission. Health and Consumers Directorate General. Computerised Systems. In: EudraLex. The Rules Governing Medicinal Products in the European Union. Volume 4. Good Manufacturing Practice. Medicinal Products for Human and Veterinary Use. European Commission. Brussels, Belgium, 2010. Annex 11.
[21] European Commission. Enterprise and Industry Directorate-General. Investigational Medicinal Products. In: EudraLex. The Rules Governing Medicinal Products in the European Union. Volume 4. EU Guidelines to Good Manufacturing Practice. Medicinal Products for Human and Veterinary Use. European Commission, Brussels, Belgium, 2010. Annex 13.
[22] European Commission. Enterprise and Industry Directorate. Manufacture of Sterile Medicinal Products. In: EudraLex. The Rules Governing Medicinal Products in the European Union. Volume 4. EU Guidelines to Good Manufacturing Practice. Medicinal Products for Human and Veterinary Use. European Commission, Brussels, Belgium, 2008. Annex 1.
[23] European Commission. Enterprise and Industry Directorate. Reference and Retention samples. In: EudraLex. The Rules Governing Medicinal Products in the European Union. Volume 4. EU Guidelines to Good Manufacturing Practice. Medicinal Products for Human and Veterinary Use. European Commission, Brussels, Belgium, 2005. Annex 19.
[24] European Commission. Enterprise Directorate-General. Parametric Release. In: EudraLex. The Rules Governing Medicinal Products in the European Union. Volume 4. EU Guidelines to Good Manufacturing Practice. Medicinal Products for Human and Veterinary Use. European Commission, Brussels, Belgium, 2001. Annex 17.
[25] European Commission. Good manufacturing practices. Medicinal products for human and veterinary use. The rules governing medicinal products in the European Union. Volume 4. Brussels.
[26] European Directorate for the Quality of Medicines & HealthCare. Council of Europe. Qualification of equipment. Annex 8: Qualification of balances. OMCL Network of the Council of Europe. Quality Management Document. PA/PH/OMCL (12) 77 7R. Council of Europe, Strasbourg, France, 2013.
[27] Gough J, Nettleton D. Risk-based software validation. PDA Bethesda, MD, USA 2006.
[28] Hornback L. A. Combination products: Implementation of CGMP requirements. PDA Bethesda, MD, USA 2013
[29] HMA (Heads of Medicine Agencies). EMA (European Medicines Agency). Guideline on good pharmacovigilance practices (GVP). Definitions. EMA/876333/2011. Revision 3. EMA, London, UK, 2011. Annex I.
[30] ICH (International Conference on Harmonisation of Technical Requirements for registration of Pharmaceuticals for Human Use). Development and manufacture of drug substances (chemical entities and biotechnological/biological entities). Harmonised Tripartite Guideline Q11. ICH, Geneva, Switzerland, 2012.
[31] ICH (International Conference on Harmonisation of Technical Requirements for registration of Pharmaceuticals for Human Use). Pharmaceutical development. Harmonised Tripartite Guideline. Q8(R2). ICH, Geneva, Switzerland, 2009.
[32] ICH (International Conference on Harmonisation of Technical Requirements for registration of Pharmaceuticals for Human Use). Pharmaceutical Quality System. Harmonised Tripartite Guideline. Q10. ICH, Geneva, Switzerland, 2008.
[33] ICH (International Conference on Harmonisation of Technical Requirements for registration of Pharmaceuticals for Human Use). Validation of Analytical Procedures: Text and Methodology. Harmonised Tripartite Guideline. Q2(R1). ICH, Geneva, Switzerland, 2005.
[34] ICH (International Conference on Harmonisation of Technical Requirements for registration of Pharmaceuticals for Human Use). Quality Risk Management. Q9. ICH, Geneva, Switzerland, 2005.
[35] ICH (International Conference on Harmonisation of Technical Requirements for registration of Pharmaceuticals for Human Use). Stability testing of new drug substances and products. Harmonised Tripartite Guideline Q1A(R2). ICH, Geneva, Switzerland, 2003.

[36] ICH (International Conference on Harmonisation of Technical Requirements for registration of Pharmaceuticals for Human Use). Evaluation for stability data. Harmonised Tripartite Guideline Q1E. ICH, Geneva, Switzerland, 2003.

[37] ICH (International Conference on Harmonisation of Technical Requirements for registration of Pharmaceuticals for Human Use). Stability data package for registration applications in climatic zones III and IV. Harmonised Tripartite Guideline Q1F. ICH, Geneva, Switzerland, 2003.

[38] ICH (International Conference on Harmonisation of Technical Requirements for registration of Pharmaceuticals for Human Use). Bracketing and matrixing designs for stability testing of new drug substances and products. Harmonised Tripartite Guideline Q1D. ICH, Geneva, Switzerland, 2002.

[39] ICH (International Conference on Harmonisation of Technical Requirements for registration of Pharmaceuticals for Human Use). Active Pharmaceutical Ingredients. Harmonised Tripartite Guideline Q7. ICH, Geneva, Switzerland, 2000.

[40] ICH (International Conference on Harmonisation of Technical Requirements for registration of Pharmaceuticals for Human Use). Guideline for Good Clinical Practice. Harmonised Tripartite Guideline. E6(R1). ICH, Geneva, Switzerland, 1996.

[41] ICH (International Conference on Harmonisation of Technical Requirements for registration of Pharmaceuticals for Human Use). Stability testing for new dosage forms. Annex to the ICH Harmonised Tripartite Guideline on Stability Testing for New Drugs and Products. Harmonised Tripartite Guideline Q1C. ICH, Geneva, Switzerland, 1996.

[42] ICH (International Conference on Harmonisation of Technical Requirements for registration of Pharmaceuticals for Human Use). Stability testing: Photostability testing of new drug substances and products. Harmonised Tripartite Guideline Q1B. ICH, Geneva, Switzerland, 1996.

[43] IEC (International Electrotechnical Commission). Hazard and operability studies (HAZOP studies) – Application guide. Standard CEI/IEC 61882:2001. IEC, Geneva, Switzerland, 2001.

[44] IEC (International Electrotechnical Commission). Fault tree analysis (FTA). Standard CEI/IEC 1025:1990. IEC, Geneva, Switzerland, 1990.

[45] IEC (International Electrotechnical Commission). Analysis techniques for system reliability – Procedure for failure mode and effects analysis (FMEA). International Standard IEC 60812:2006(E). IEC, Geneva, Switzerland, 1985.

[46] IES (Institute of Environmental Sciences). U.S. General Services Administration. Federal Standard 209E. Airborne Particulate Cleanliness Classes in Cleanrooms and Clean Zones. IES, Mount Prospect, Illinois, USA, 1992.

[47] IPEC (The International Pharmaceutical Excipients Council). PQG (Pharmaceutical Quality Group). The Joint IPEC – PQG Good Manufacturing Practices Guide for Pharmaceutical Excipients. IPEQ, PQG, Arlington, VA, USA, 2006.

[48] IPEC (The International Pharmaceutical Excipients Council). The IPEC Good Distribution Practices Guide for Pharmaceutical Excipients. IPEC, Arlington, VA, USA, 2006.

[49] ISO (International Organization for Standardization). Control charts. Part 1: General guidelines. International Standard ISO 7870-1:2014(E). ISO, Geneva, Switzerland, 2014.

[50] ISO (International Organization for Standardization). Control charts. Part 5: Specialized control charts. International Standard ISO 7870-5:2014(E). ISO, Geneva, Switzerland, 2014.

[51] ISO (International Organization for Standardization). Control charts. Part 2: Shewhart control charts. International Standard ISO 7870-2:2013(E). ISO, Geneva, Switzerland, 2013.

[52] ISO (International Organization for Standardization). Cleanrooms and associated controlled environments. Part 8: Classification of air cleanliness by chemical concentration (ACC). International standard ISO 14644-8:2013(en). ISO, Geneva, Switzerland, 2013.

[53] ISO (International Organization for Standardization). Cleanrooms and associated controlled environments. Part 10: Classification of surface cleanliness by chemical concentration. International standard ISO 14644-10:2013(en). ISO, Geneva, Switzerland, 2013.

[54] ISO (International Organization for Standardization). Cleanrooms and associated controlled environments. Part 9: Classification of surface cleanliness by particle concentration. International standard ISO 14644-9:2012(en). ISO, Geneva, Switzerland, 2012.

[55] ISO (International Organization for Standardization). Control charts. Part 3: Acceptance control charts. International Standard ISO 7870-3:2012(E). ISO, Geneva, Switzerland, 2012.

[56] ISO (International Organization for Standardization). Control charts. Part 4: Cumulative sum charts. International Standard ISO 7870-4:2011(E). ISO, Geneva, Switzerland, 2011.
[57] ISO (International Organization for Standardization). Compressed air. Part 1: Contaminants and purity classes. International standard ISO 8573-1:2010(en). ISO, Geneva, Switzerland, 2010.
[58] ISO (International Organization for Standardization). Managing for the sustained success of an organization — A quality management approach. International Standard ISO 9004:2009. ISO, Geneva, Switzerland, 2009.
[59] ISO (International Organization for Standardization). Quality management systems – Requirements. International standard ISO 9001:2008(en). ISO, Geneva, Switzerland, 2008.
[60] ISO (International Organization for Standardization). Compressed air. Part 2: Test methods for oil aerosol content. International standard ISO 8573-2:2007(en). ISO, Geneva, Switzerland, 2007.
[61] ISO (International Organization for Standardization). Primary packaging materials for medicinal products. Particular requirements for the application of ISO 9001:2005 with reference to GMP. International standard ISO 15378:2006(en). ISO, Geneva, Switzerland, 2006.
[62] ISO (International Organization for Standardization). Quality management systems – Fundamentals and vocabulary. International standard ISO 9000:2005(en). ISO, Geneva, Switzerland, 2005.
[63] ISO (International Organization for Standardization). Cleanrooms and associated controlled environments. Part 3: Test methods. International standard ISO 14644-3:2005(en). ISO, Geneva, Switzerland, 2005.
[64] ISO (International Organization for Standardization). Cleanrooms and associated controlled environments. Part 5: Operations. International standard ISO 14644-5:2004(en). ISO, Geneva, Switzerland, 2004.
[65] ISO (International Organization for Standardization). Cleanrooms and associated controlled environments. Part 7: Separative devices (clean air hoods, gloveboxes, isolators and mini-environments). International standard ISO 14644-7:2004(en). ISO, Geneva, Switzerland, 2004.
[66] ISO (International Organization for Standardization). Environmental management systems – Requirements with guidance for use. International standard ISO 14001:2004(en). ISO, Geneva, Switzerland, 2004
[67] ISO (International Organization for Standardization). Compressed air. Part 6: Test methods for gaseous contaminant content. International standard ISO 8573-6:2003(en). ISO, Geneva, Switzerland, 2003.
[68] ISO (International Organization for Standardization). Compressed air. Part 7: Test method for viable microbiological contaminant content. International standard ISO 8573-7:2003(en). ISO, Geneva, Switzerland, 2003.
[69] ISO (International Organization for Standardization). Guidelines for quality and/or environmental management systems auditing. International standard ISO 19011:2002(en). ISO, Geneva, Switzerland, 2002.
[70] ISO (International Organization for Standardization). Guidelines for quality and/or environmental management systems auditing. International standard ISO 19011:2002(en). ISO, Geneva, Switzerland, 2002.
[71] ISO (International Organization for Standardization). Cleanrooms and associated controlled environments. Part 4: Design, construction and start-up. International standard ISO 14644-4:2001(en). ISO, Geneva, Switzerland, 2001.
[72] ISO (International Organization for Standardization). Compressed air. Part 4: Test methods for solid particle content. International standard ISO 8573-4:2001(en). ISO, Geneva, Switzerland, 2001.
[73] ISO (International Organization for Standardization). Compressed air. Part 5: Test methods for oil vapour and organic solvent content. International standard ISO 8573-5:2001(en). ISO, Geneva, Switzerland, 2001.
[74] ISO (International Organization for Standardization). Cleanrooms and associated controlled environments. Part 2: Specifications for testing and monitoring continued compliance with ISO 14644-1. International standard ISO 14644-2:2000(en). ISO, Geneva, Switzerland, 2000.
[75] ISO (International Organization for Standardization). Cleanrooms and associated controlled environments. Part 6: Vocabulary. International standard ISO 14644-6:2007(en). ISO, Geneva, Switzerland, 2000.

[76] ISO (International Organization for Standardization). Cleanrooms and associated controlled environments. Part 1: Classification of air cleanliness. International standard ISO 14644-1:1999(en). ISO, Geneva, Switzerland, 1999.

[77] ISO (International Organization for Standardization). Compressed air. Part 3: Test methods for measurement of humidity. International standard ISO 8573-3:1999(en). ISO, Geneva, Switzerland, 1999.

[78] ISPE (International Society of Pharmaceutical Engineering). Technology transfer. Second edition. Good practice guide. ISPE, Tampa, Florida, USA, 2014.

[79] ISPE (International Society of Pharmaceutical Engineering). Biopharmaceutical Manufacturing Facilities. Baseline Pharmaceutical engineering guides. 2nd edition. ISPE, Tampa, Florida, USA 2013.

[80] ISPE (International Society of Pharmaceutical Engineering). Quality laboratory facilities. Good practice guide. ISPE, Tampa, Florida, USA, 2012.

[81] ISPE (International Society of Pharmaceutical Engineering). GAMP: A risk-based approach to GXP process control systems. Second edition. ISPE, Tampa, Florida, USA 2011.

[82] ISPE (International Society of Pharmaceutical Engineering). Sterile manufacturing facilities. Baseline pharmaceutical engineering guides. Second edition. ISPE, Tampa, Florida, USA, 2011.

[83] ISPE (International Society of Pharmaceutical Engineering). Process gases. ISPE Good Practice Guide, Tampa, Florida, USA, 2011.

[84] ISPE (International Society of Pharmaceutical Engineering). Cold chain management. Good practice guide. ISPE, Tampa, Florida, USA, 2011.

[85] ISPE (International Society of Pharmaceutical Engineering). Water and steam systems. ISPE Baseline Pharmaceutical Engineering Guides. 2nd edition. ISPE, Tampa, Florida, USA, 2011.

[86] ISPE (International Society of Pharmaceutical Engineering). Risk-based manufacture of Pharmaceutical Products. Baseline pharmaceutical engineering guides. ISPE, Tampa, Florida, USA, 2010.

[87] ISPE (International Society of Pharmaceutical Engineering). A risk-based approach to calibration management. GAMP guidance document. Second edition. ISPE, Tampa, Florida, USA, 2010.

[88] ISPE (International Society of Pharmaceutical Engineering). Oral solid dosage forms. Baseline pharmaceutical engineering guides Tampa, Florida, USA, 2009.

[89] ISPE (International Society of Pharmaceutical Engineering). Heating, Ventilation, and Air Conditioning (HVAC). Good practice guide. ISPE, Tampa, Florida, USA, 2009.

[90] ISPE (International Society of Pharmaceutical Engineering). Maintenance. Good practice guide. ISPE, Tampa, Florida, USA, 2009.

[91] ISPE (International Society of Pharmaceutical Engineering). Good Engineering Practice. ISPE Good Practice Guide. ISPE, Tampa, Florida, USA, 2008.

[92] ISPE (International Society of Pharmaceutical Engineering). GAMP: Electronic Data archiving. ISPE, Tampa, Florida, USA, 2007.

[93] ISPE (International Society of Pharmaceutical Engineering). Active Pharmaceutical Ingredients. Baseline Pharmaceutical engineering guides. ISPE, Tampa, Florida, USA 2007.

[94] ISPE (International Society of Pharmaceutical Engineering). GAMP: A risk-based approach to compliant electronic records and signatures. ISPE, Tampa, Florida, USA, 2005.

[95] ISPE (International Society of Pharmaceutical Engineering). Commissioning and qualification. ISPE Baseline Pharmaceutical Engineering Guides. ISPE, Tampa, Florida, USA, 2001.

[96] Kirkpatrick DL, Kirkpatrick JD. Evaluating training programs: The four levels. Berrett-Koehler Publishers. San Francisco, CA, USA, 2006.

[97] Le Hir A, Chaumeil JC, Brossard D. Pharmacie galénique. Bonnes pratiques de fabrication des médicaments. 9th Edition. Elsevier Masson, Issy-les-Moulineaux, France, 2009.

[98] Lysfjord J. Practical aseptic processing: Fill and finish. Volume I and II. PDA Bethesda, MD, USA 2009

[99] OECD (Organisation for Economic Co-operation and Development). Environment Directorate. Chemicals Group and Management Committee. OECD Principles on Good Laboratory Practice (as revised in 1997). OECD series on principles of Good Laboratory Practice and compliance monitoring. No. 1. ENV/MC/CHEM(98)17. OECD, Paris, France, 1998.

[100] PDA (Parenteral Drug Association). Fundamentals of an environmental monitoring program. Technical Report No. 13. Revised. PDA, Bethesda, MD, USA, 2014.

[101] PDA (Parenteral Drug Association). Application of single-use systems in pharmaceutical manufacturing. Technical Report No. 66. PDA, Bethesda, MD, USA, 2014.
[102] PDA (Parenteral Drug Association). Risk-based approach for prevention and management of drug shortages. Technical Report No. 68. PDA, Bethesda, MD, USA, 2014.
[103] PDA (Parenteral Drug Association). Exclusion of objectionable microorganisms from nonsterile pharmaceuticals, medical devices, and cosmetics. Technical Report No. 67. PDA, Bethesda, MD, USA, 2014.
[104] PDA (Parenteral Drug Association). Technology transfer. Technical Report No. 65. PDA, Bethesda, MD, USA, 2014.
[105] PDA (Parenteral Drug Association). Recommended practices for manual aseptic processes. Technical Report No. 62. PDA, Bethesda, MD, USA, 2013.
[106] PDA (Parenteral Drug Association). Biological indicators for gas and vapor-phase decontamination processes: specification, manufacture, control and use. Technical Report No. 51. PDA, Bethesda, MD, USA, 2010.
[107] PDA (Parenteral Drug Association). Moist Heat Sterilizer Systems: Design, Commissioning, Operation, Qualification and Maintenance. Technical Report No. 48. PDA, Bethesda, MD, USA, 2010.
[108] PDA (Parenteral Drug Association). Last Mile: Guidance for good distribution practices for pharmaceutical products to the end user. Technical Report No. 46. PDA, Bethesda, MD, USA, 2009
[109] PIC/S (Pharmaceutical Inspection Convention. Pharmaceutical Inspection Co-Operation Scheme). Good Distribution Practice for medicinal Products. Guide PE 011-1. PIC/S, Geneva, Switzerland, 2014.
[110] PIC/S (Pharmaceutical Inspection Convention. Pharmaceutical Inspection Co-Operation Scheme). Good Manufacturing Practice for Medicinal Products. Guide PE 009-11. PIC/S, Geneva, Switzerland, 2014.
[111] PIC/S (Pharmaceutical Inspection Convention / Pharmaceutical Inspection Co-Operation Scheme). A recommended model for risk-based inspection planning in the GMP environment. Recommendation PI 037-1. PIC/S, Geneva, Switzerland, 2012.
[112] PIC/S (Pharmaceutical Inspection Convention / Pharmaceutical Inspection Co-Operation Scheme). Assessment of quality risk management implementation. Aide-Memoire PI 038-1. PIC/S, Geneva, Switzerland, 2012.
[113] PIC/S (Pharmaceutical Inspection Convention / Pharmaceutical Inspection Co-Operation Scheme). Explanatory notes for pharmaceutical manufacturers on the preparation of a Site Master File. PE 008-4. PIC/S, Geneva, Switzerland, 2011.
[114] PIC/S (Pharmaceutical Inspection Convention / Pharmaceutical Inspection Co-Operation Scheme). Validation of Aseptic Processes. Recommendation PI 007-6. PIC/S, Geneva, Switzerland, 2011.
[115] PIC/S (Pharmaceutical Inspection Convention / Pharmaceutical Inspection Co-Operation Scheme). Recommendation on GMP Annex 1 Revision 2008, Interpretation of most important changes for the manufacture of sterile medicinal products. PI 032-2. PIC/S, Geneva, Switzerland, 2010.
[116] PIC/S (Pharmaceutical Inspection Convention / Pharmaceutical Inspection Co-Operation Scheme). Aide-memoire on GMP Inspection related to Packaging. PI 028-1. PIC/S, Geneva, Switzerland, 2009.
[117] PIC/S (Pharmaceutical Inspection Convention / Pharmaceutical Inspection Co-Operation Scheme). Inspection of Active Pharmaceutical Ingredients. Aide-Memoire PI 030-1. PIC/S, Geneva, Switzerland, 2009.
[118] PIC/S (Pharmaceutical Inspection Convention. Pharmaceutical Inspection Co-Operation Scheme). Good Practices for Computerised systems in regulated "GXP" environments. Guidance PI 011-3. PIC/S, Geneva, Switzerland, 2007.
[119] PIC/S (Pharmaceutical Inspection Convention / Pharmaceutical Inspection Co-Operation Scheme). Inspection of Medicinal Gases. Aide-Memoire PI 025-2. PIC/S, Geneva, Switzerland, 2007.
[120] PIC/S (Pharmaceutical Inspection Convention. Pharmaceutical Inspection Co-Operation Scheme). Recommendation on Isolators used for aseptic processing and sterility testing. PE 014-3. PIC/S, Geneva, Switzerland, 2007.
[121] PIC/S (Pharmaceutical Inspection Convention. Pharmaceutical Inspection Co-Operation Scheme). Inspection of utilities. Aide-memoire PI 009-3. PIC/S, Geneva, Switzerland, 2007.

[122] PIC/S (Pharmaceutical Inspection Convention. Pharmaceutical Inspection Co-Operation Scheme). Sterility testing. Recommendation PI 012-3. PIC/S, Geneva, Switzerland, 2007.
[123] PIC/S (Pharmaceutical Inspection Convention / Pharmaceutical Inspection Co-Operation Scheme). Inspection of Biotechnology Manufacturers. Aide-memoires PI 024-2. PIC/S, Geneva, Switzerland, 2007.
[124] PIC/S (Pharmaceutical Inspection Convention / Pharmaceutical Inspection Co-Operation Scheme). Validation Master Plan, Installation and Operational Qualification, Non-sterile Process Validation, Cleaning Validation. Recommendations PI 006-3. PIC/S, Geneva, Switzerland, 2007.
[125] PIC/S (Pharmaceutical Inspection Convention / Pharmaceutical Inspection Co-Operation Scheme). Guidance on Parametric Release. Recommendation PI 005-3. PIC/S, Geneva, Switzerland, 2007.
[126] PIC/S (Pharmaceutical Inspection Convention / Pharmaceutical Inspection Co-Operation Scheme). Inspection of Pharmaceutical Quality Control Laboratories. Aide-memoire PI 023-2. PIC/S, Geneva, Switzerland, 2007.
[127] Rosetto Y (editor). φ41. Pharmacotechnie industrielle. I.M.T. Editions, Tours, France, 1998.
[128] Sandle T. Sterility testing of pharmaceutical products, PDA Bethesda, MD, USA 2013.
[129] Schmitt S. Quality by design: Putting theory into practice. PDA Bethesda, MD, USA, 2011.
[130] The Commission of the European Communities. Commission directive 2003/94/EC of 8 October 2003 laying down the principles and guidelines of good manufacturing practice in respect of medicinal products for human use and investigational medicinal products for human use. Official Journal of the European Union L 262/22 of 14.10.2003.
[131] The European Parliament and the Council of the European Union. Directive 2003/10/EC of 6 February 2003 on the minimum health and safety requirements regarding the exposure of workers to the risks arising from physical agents (noise). Official Journal of the European Union L 42/38 of 15.02.2003.
[132] The Commission of the European Communities. Commission directive 91/412/EEC of 23 July 1991 laying down the principles and guidelines of good manufacturing practice for veterinary medicinal products. Official Journal of the European Union L 228 of 17.8.1991.
[133] TIMET (Titanium Metals Corporation). Titanium design and fabrication handbook for industrial applications. HQ-10/97-BG104-4M. TIMET, Denver, Colorado, USA, 1997.
[134] Tuthill A H. Fabrication and post-fabrication cleanup of stainless steels. Chemical Engineering, September 1986, 1-5.
[135] UNDP (United Nations Development Program)/World Bank/WHO (World Health Organisation). Handbook: Good Laboratory Practice (GLP). Quality practices for regulated non-clinical research and development. Special Programme for Research and Training in Tropical Diseases. TDR/WHO, Geneva, Switzerland, 2000.
[136] U.S. Department of Health and Human Services. Food and Drug Administration. Center for Drug Evaluation and Research (CDER). Non-Penicillin Beta-Lactam Drugs: A CGMP Framework for Preventing Cross-Contamination. Guidance for Industry. Current Good Manufacturing Practices (CGMPs). FDA, Rockville, MD, USA, 2013.
[137] U.S. Department of Health and Human Services. Food and Drug Administration (FDA). Center for Drug Evaluation and Research (CDER). Center for Biologics Evaluation and Research (CBER). Center for Veterinary Medicine (CVM). Process Validation: General Principles and Practices. Guidance for industry. Current Good Manufacturing Practices (CGMP). Revision 1. FDA, Rockville, MD, USA. 2011.
[138] US Department of Health and Human Services. Public health Service Centers for Disease Control and Prevention. National Institutes of Health. Biosafety in Microbiology and Biomedical Laboratories. HHS Publication No. (CDC) 21-1112. 5th edition revised. CDC, Atlanta, Georgia, USA, 2009.
[139] U.S. Department of Health and Human Services Food and Drug Administration Center for Drug Evaluation and Research (CDER) Center for Biologics Evaluation and Research (CBER) Office of Regulatory Affairs (ORA). CGMP for Phase 1 Investigational Drugs. Guidance for Industry. CGMP. FDA, Rockville, MD, USA, 2008.
[140] U.S. Department of Health and Human Services. Food and Drug Administration. Center for Drug Evaluation and Research (CDER). Center for Biologics Evaluation and Research (CBER). Center for Veterinary Medicine (CVM). Office of Regulatory Affairs (ORA). Quality systems approach to

pharmaceutical CGMP regulations. Guidance for industry, Pharmaceutical CGMPs. Rockville, MD, USA, 2006

[141] U.S. Department of Health and Human Services. Food and Drug Administration. Center for Drug Evaluation and Research (CDER). Investigating Out-of-Specification (OOS) Test Results for Pharmaceutical Production. Guidance for industry. Pharmaceutical CGMPs. FDA, Rockville, MD, USA, 2006

[142] U.S. Department of Health and Human Services. Food and Drug Administration. Center for Drug Evaluation and Research (CDER). Center for Biologics Evaluation and Research (CBER). Good Pharmacovigilance Practices and Pharmacoepidemiologic Assessment. Guidance for industry. FDA, Rockville, MD, USA, 2005.

[143] U.S. Department of Health and Human Services. Food and Drug Administration. Center for Drug Evaluation and Research (CDER). Center for Biologics Evaluation and Research (CBER). Office of Regulatory Affairs (ORA). Sterile drug products produced by aseptic processing – Current Good Manufacturing Practice. Guidance for Industry. FDA, Rockville, MD, USA, 2004.

[144] U.S. Department of Health and Human Services. Food and Drug Administration. Center for Drug Evaluation and Research (CDER). Center for Veterinary Medicine (CVM). Office of Regulatory Affairs (ORA). PAT – A Framework for Innovative Pharmaceutical Development, Manufacturing, and Quality Assurance. Guidance for industry, FDA, Rockville, MD, USA, 2004.

[145] U.S. Department of Health and Human Services. Food and Drug Administration. Center for Drug Evaluation and Research (CDER). Center for Biologics Evaluation and Research (CBER). Center for Devices and Radiological Health (CDRH). Center for Food Safety and Applied Nutrition (CFSAN). Center for Veterinary Medicine (CVM). Office of Regulatory Affairs (ORA). Part 11, Electronic Records; Electronic Signatures — Scope and Application. Guidance for Industry. Pharmaceutical CGMPs. FDA, Rockville, MD, USA, 2003.

[146] U.S. FDA (U.S. Food and Drug Administration). Guide to inspections of high purity water systems. FDA, Inspection Technical Guides, 7/93. FDA, Rockville, MD, USA, 1993.

[147] US National Archives & Records Administration. Federal Register. Code of Federal Regulations (CFR). Title 21 (Food & drugs). Parts 210 through 226.

[148] Vesper J. Risk assessment and risk management in the pharmaceutical industry: clear and simple. PDA Bethesda, MD, USA 2006.

[149] WHO (World Health Organization). WHO Good manufacturing practices for pharmaceutical products: main principles. In: WHO Expert Committee on Specifications for Pharmaceutical Preparations. Forty-eighth report (WHO Technical Report Series, No. 986). WHO, Geneva, Switzerland, 2014. Annex 2.

[150] WHO (World Health Organisation). WHO guidelines on quality risk management. In: WHO Expert Committee on Specifications for Pharmaceutical Preparations. Forty-seventh report (WHO Technical Report Series, No. 981). WHO, Geneva, Switzerland, 2013. Annex 2.

[151] WHO (World Health Organisation). Development of pediatric medicines: points to consider in formulation. In: WHO Expert Committee on Specifications for Pharmaceutical Preparations. Forty-sixth report (WHO Technical Report Series, No. 970). WHO, Geneva, Switzerland, 2012. Annex 5.

[152] WHO (World Health Organization). WHO Good manufacturing practices. Water for pharmaceutical use. In: WHO Expert Committee on Specifications for Pharmaceutical Preparations. Forty-sixth report (WHO Technical Report Series, No. 970). WHO, Geneva, Switzerland, 2012. Annex 2.

[153] WHO (World Health Organisation). WHO good practices for pharmaceutical microbiology laboratories. In: WHO Expert Committee on Specifications for Pharmaceutical Preparations. Forty-fifth report (WHO Technical Report Series, No. 961). WHO, Geneva, Switzerland, 2011. Annex 2.

[154] WHO (World Health Organisation). Model guidance for the storage and transport of time- and temperature-sensitive pharmaceutical products (jointly with the Expert Committee on Biological Standardization). In: WHO Expert Committee on Specifications for Pharmaceutical Preparations. Forty-fifth report (WHO Technical Report Series, No. 961). WHO, Geneva, Switzerland, 2011. Annex 9.

[155] WHO (World Health Organisation). WHO guidelines on good manufacturing practices for heating, ventilation and air-conditioning systems for non-sterile pharmaceutical dosage forms. In: WHO Expert Committee on Specifications for Pharmaceutical Preparations. Forty-fiftieth report (WHO Technical Report Series, No. 961). WHO, Geneva, Switzerland, 2011. Annex 5.

[156] WHO (World Health Organization). WHO guidelines for preparing a laboratory information file. In: WHO Expert Committee on Specifications for Pharmaceutical Preparations. Forty-fifth report (WHO Technical Report Series, No. 961). WHO, Geneva, Switzerland, 2011. Annex 13.

[157] WHO (World Health Organisation). Good manufacturing practices for sterile pharmaceutical products. In: WHO Expert Committee on Specifications for Pharmaceutical Preparations. Forty-fifth report (WHO Technical Report Series, No. 961). WHO, Geneva, Switzerland, 2011. Annex 6.

[158] WHO (World Health Organization). WHO guidelines for drafting a site master file. In: WHO Expert Committee on Specifications for Pharmaceutical Preparations. Forty-fifth report (WHO Technical Report Series, No. 961). WHO, Geneva, Switzerland, 2011. Annex 14.

[159] WHO (World Health Organisation). WHO good manufacturing practices for active pharmaceutical ingredients. In: WHO Expert Committee on Specifications for Pharmaceutical Preparations. Forty-fourth report (WHO Technical Report Series, No. 957). WHO, Geneva, Switzerland, 2010. Annex 2.

[160] WHO (World Health Organisation). WHO good distribution practices for pharmaceutical products. In: WHO Expert Committee on Specifications for Pharmaceutical Preparations. Forty-fourth report (WHO Technical Report Series, No. 957). WHO, Geneva, Switzerland, 2010. Annex 5.

[161] WHO (World Health Organisation). WHO good practices for pharmaceutical quality control laboratories. In: WHO Expert Committee on Specifications for Pharmaceutical Preparations. Forty-fourth report (WHO Technical Report Series, No. 957). WHO, Geneva, Switzerland, 2010. Annex 1.

[162] WHO (World Health Organisation). WHO good manufacturing practices for pharmaceutical products containing hazardous substances. In: WHO Expert Committee on Specifications for Pharmaceutical Preparations. Forty-fourth report (WHO Technical Report Series, No. 957). WHO, Geneva, Switzerland, 2010, Annex 3.

[163] WHO (World Health Organization). Stability testing of active pharmaceutical ingredients and finished pharmaceutical products. In: WHO Expert Committee on Specifications for Pharmaceutical Preparations. Forty-third report (WHO Technical Report Series, No. 953). WHO, Geneva, Switzerland, 2009. Annex 2.

[164] WHO (World Health Organisation). Supplementary guidelines on good manufacturing practices for the manufacture of herbal medicines. In: WHO Expert Committee on Specifications for Pharmaceutical Preparations. Fortieth report (WHO Technical Report Series, No. 937). WHO, Geneva, Switzerland, 2006. Annex 3.

[165] WHO (World Health Organisation). Supplementary guidelines on good manufacturing practices: validation. In: WHO Expert Committee on Specifications for Pharmaceutical Preparations. Fortieth report (WHO Technical Report Series, No. 937). WHO, Geneva, Switzerland, 2006. Annex 4 (Appendix 1: Validation of heating, ventilation and air-conditioning systems. Appendix 2: Validation of water systems for pharmaceutical use. Appendix 3: Cleaning validation. Appendix 4: Analytical method validation. Appendix 5: Validation of computerized systems. Appendix 6: Qualification of systems and equipment. Appendix 7: Non-sterile process validation).

[166] WHO (World Health Organisation). Good manufacturing practices: requirement for the sampling of starting materials (amendment). In: WHO Expert Committee on Specifications for Pharmaceutical Preparations. Thirty-ninth report (WHO Technical Report Series, No. 929). WHO, Geneva, Switzerland, 2005. Annex 2.

[167] WHO (World Health Organisation). WHO guidelines for sampling of pharmaceutical products and related materials. In: WHO Expert Committee on Specifications for Pharmaceutical Preparations. Thirty-ninth report (WHO Technical Report Series, No. 929). WHO, Geneva, Switzerland, 2005. Annex 4.

[168] WHO (World Health Organization). Laboratory biosafety manual. 3rd edition. WHO, Geneva, Switzerland, 2004.

[169] WHO (World Health Organisation). Good trade and distribution practices for pharmaceutical starting materials. In: WHO Expert Committee on Specifications for Pharmaceutical Preparations. Thirty-eighth report (WHO Technical Report Series, No. 917). WHO, Geneva, Switzerland, 2003. Annex 2.

[170] WHO (World Health Organisation). WHO guide to good storage practices for pharmaceuticals. In: WHO Expert Committee on Specifications for Pharmaceutical Preparations. Thirty-seventh report (WHO Technical Report Series, No. 908). WHO, Geneva, Switzerland, 2003, Annex 9.

[171] WHO (World Health Organisation). Guidelines on Good Manufacturing Practices for radiopharmaceutical products. In: WHO Expert Committee on Specifications for Pharmaceutical

Preparations. Thirty-seven report (WHO Technical Report Series, No. 908). WHO, Geneva, Switzerland, 2003, Annex 3.
[172] WHO (World Health Organisation). Application of Hazard Analysis and Critical Control Point (HACCP) method to pharmaceuticals. In: WHO Expert Committee on Specifications for Pharmaceutical Preparations. Thirty-seventh report (WHO Technical Report Series, No. 908). WHO, Geneva, Switzerland, 2003. Annex 7.
[173] WHO (World Health Organisation). Handbook for Good Clinical Research Practice (GCP). Guidance for implementation. WHO, Geneva, Switzerland, 2002.
[174] WHO (World Health Organisation). Good Manufacturing Practices: Supplementary guidelines for the manufacture of Pharmaceutical Excipients. In: WHO Expert Committee on Specifications for Pharmaceutical Preparations. Thirty-fifth report (WHO Technical Report Series, No. 885). WHO, Geneva, Switzerland, 1999. Annex 5.
[175] WHO (World Health Organisation). Good Manufacturing Practices: Authorized person – role, functions and training. In: WHO Expert Committee on Specifications for Pharmaceutical Preparations. Thirty-fifth report (WHO Technical Report Series, No. 885). WHO, Geneva, Switzerland, 1999. Annex 4.
[176] WHO (World Health Organisation). Good Manufacturing Practices: Supplementary guidelines for the manufacture of investigational pharmaceutical products for clinical trials in humans. In: WHO Expert Committee on Specifications for Pharmaceutical Preparations. Thirty-fourth report (WHO Technical Report Series, No. 863). WHO, Geneva, Switzerland, 1996. Annex 7.
[177] WHO (World Health Organisation). WHO Good manufacturing practices for biological products. In: WHO Expert Committee on Specifications for Pharmaceutical Preparations. Thirty-third report (WHO Technical Report Series, No. 834). WHO, Geneva, Switzerland, 1993. Annex 3.
[178] WHO (World Health Organisation). Sampling procedure for industrially manufactured pharmaceuticals. In: WHO Expert Committee on Specifications for Pharmaceutical Preparations. Thirty-first report (WHO Technical Report Series, No. 790). WHO, Geneva, Switzerland, 1990. Annex 2.
[179] WHO (World Health Organisation). Quality requirements for pharmaceutical aids. In: WHO Expert Committee on Specifications for Pharmaceutical Preparations. Twenty-ninth report (WHO Technical Report Series, No. 704). WHO, Geneva, Switzerland, 1984. Annex 2.
[180] WHO (World Health Organisation). Tests for solid oral dosage forms. In: WHO Expert Committee on Specifications for Pharmaceutical Preparations. Twenty-seventh report (WHO Technical Report Series, No. 645). WHO, Geneva, Switzerland, 1980, Annex 2.
[181] WHO (World Health Organisation). Good practices in the manufacture and quality control of drugs. In: WHO Expert Committee on Specifications for Pharmaceutical Preparations. Twenty-second report (WHO Technical Report Series, No. 418). WHO, Geneva, Switzerland, 1969. Annex 2.
[182] WHO (World Health Organisation). Principles of pharmaceutical quality control. In: WHO Expert Committee on Specifications for Pharmaceutical Preparations. Twenty-second report (WHO Technical Report Series, No. 418). WHO, Geneva, Switzerland, 1969. Annex 1.

WEBS

01 ANVISA: http://www.anvisa.gov.br
02 CEN: http://www.cen.eu
03 EMA: http://www.ema.europa.eu
04 European Commission: http://ec.europa.eu
05 IEC: http:// www.iec.ch
06 ICH: http://www.ich.org
07 IPEC: http://www.ipec.org
08 ISO: http://www.iso.org
09 ISPE: http://www.ispe.org
10 OECD: http://www.oecd.org

11 PDA: http://www.pda.org
12 PIC/S: http://www.picscheme.org
13 TIMET: http://www.timet.org
14 U.S. FDA: http://www.fda.gov
15 WHO: http://www.who.int

SUBJECT INDEX

Subject Index

A

B

C

D

E

J

K

L

M

N

O

P

Q

R

S

T

Made in United States
North Haven, CT
05 November 2026

21764582R60283